SITE-SPECIFIC CANCER SERIES

Lung Cancer

Edited by
Nancy G. Houlihan, RN, MA, AOCN®

Oncology Nursing Society
Pittsburgh, Pennsylvania

ONS Publishing Division
Publisher: Leonard Mafrica, MBA, CAE
Director, Commercial Publishing/Technical Editor: Barbara Sigler, RN, MNEd
Production Managers: Lisa M. George, BA, Anne H. Snively, BS
Staff Editor: Lori Wilson, BA
Graphic Designer: Dany Sjoen

Site-Specific Cancer Series: Lung Cancer

First printing June 2004
Second printing January 2005

Library of Congress Control Number: 2004107737

ISBN 1-890504-48-3

Publisher's Note

This book is published by the Oncology Nursing Society (ONS). ONS neither represents nor guarantees that the practices described herein will, if followed, ensure safe and effective patient care. The recommendations contained in this book reflect ONS's judgment regarding the state of general knowledge and practice in the field as of the date of publication. The recommendations may not be appropriate for use in all circumstances. Those who use this book should make their own determinations regarding specific safe and appropriate patient-care practices, taking into account the personnel, equipment, and practices available at the hospital or other facility at which they are located. The editor and publisher cannot be held responsible for any liability incurred as a consequence from the use or application of any of the contents of this book. Figures and tables are used as examples only. They are not meant to be all-inclusive, nor do they represent endorsement of any particular institution by ONS. Mention of specific products and opinions related to those products do not indicate or imply endorsement by ONS.

ONS publications are originally published in English. Permission has been granted by the ONS Board of Directors has granted permission for foreign translation. (Individual tables and figures that are reprinted or adapted require additional permission from the original source.) However, because translations from English may not always be accurate and precise, ONS disclaims any responsibility for inaccuracies in words or meaning that may occur as a result of the translation. Readers relying on precise information should check the original English version.

Printed in the United States of America

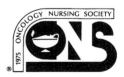

Oncology Nursing Society
Integrity • Innovation • Stewardship • Advocacy • Excellence • Inclusiveness

Contributors

Editor

Nancy G. Houlihan, RN, MA, AOCN®
Nurse Leader
Division of Nursing, Ambulatory Thoracic Oncology Service
Memorial Sloan-Kettering Cancer Center
New York, New York

Authors

Marianne Davies, RN, MSN, ACNP, OCN®
Oncology Nurse Practitioner, Coordinator
Yale University Section of Medical Oncology
New Haven, Connecticut

Nancy G. Houlihan, RN, MA, AOCN®
Nurse Leader
Division of Nursing, Ambulatory Thoracic
   Oncology Service
Memorial Sloan-Kettering Cancer Center
New York, New York

Dana Inzeo, RN, MA, AOCN®
Clinical Nurse Specialist, Thoracic Oncology Service
Memorial Sloan-Kettering Cancer Center
New York, New York

Margaret Joyce, MSN, RN, AOCN®
Advanced Practice Nurse
The Cancer Institute of New Jersey
New Brunswick, New Jersey

Leslie B. Tyson, MS, ANP-C, OCN®
Nurse Practitioner, Thoracic Oncology Service
Memorial Sloan-Kettering Cancer Center
New York, New York

Contents

Preface

The inspiration for this book came first from the many people with lung cancer for whom we have cared. We share in the triumph of the survivors; for those living with the disease, and for the many more who have died, we share hope for the future. Never before has there been so much evidence that new treatments hold the chance for cure. Yet, we face a future with more than 50 million current and former smokers with the potential to create another generation of people with lung cancer. Although we are hopeful about treatment, we are equally hopeful that the movement to curtail the use of tobacco will grow in strength. Second, we recognize our fellow thoracic oncology colleagues who have done so much to further the care of people with lung cancer. Current advances in science, technology, screening, treatment, and symptom management have produced a change in the lung cancer paradigm, and we share an excitement that has never before existed in the thoracic oncology specialty.

CHAPTER 1

Overview

Nancy G. Houlihan, RN, MA, AOCN®

Introduction

Lung cancer represents one of the most challenging health threats in the United States and around the world. Despite progress over the last decade in the control or cure of many cancers, lung cancer continues to occur at high rates and kill most of its victims. This is true for many reasons, including ineffective prevention programs, lack of a good population-based screening test, and controversy over the most effective treatment strategies. In addition, research funding for lung cancer has lagged behind that appropriated for other diseases, possibly because of its association with tobacco products and the related political and financial implications (Kennedy, Miller, & Prindiville, 2000). Despite the persistent poor statistics, the 1990s marked the beginning of a shift in the lung cancer paradigm. Technological advances with low-dose computed tomography (CT) scans offer hope for earlier diagnosis and treatment. Clinical research has identified more effective treatments with improved survival and quality of life for patients at every stage of disease. Greater understanding of the genetic alterations in lung cancer has led to investigations into novel approaches and advances in early diagnostic and treatment strategies. In addition, national legislation, education on prevention, and availability of effective smoking cessation interventions have led to changes in the tobacco usage trends in the United States. Although lung cancer persists as the most deadly cancer, there is hope that the future will bring improvements in outcomes.

Nursing care of those with lung cancer also has advanced during this time as a result of the development of more effective, research-based interventions for managing symptoms. Care of patients with lung cancer incorporates all aspects of oncology nursing, including direct care delivery, patient education and counseling, treatment side effect management, and palliation. This book will review the current knowledge related to the disease and its properties, including prevention, screening, diagnosis, clinical manifestations, treatment and research, and nursing management.

Lung Cancer Overview

Lung cancer is the third most commonly occurring cancer in the United States, with an estimated 173,770 new cases developing in 2004. Cancers of the breast and prostate occur more frequently, with estimates of 217,440 and 230,110 cases, respectively. However, lung cancer also is associated with the highest cancer-related mortality, with an estimated 160,440 deaths occurring in 2004. This far outweighs deaths from breast (40,580) and prostate cancers (29,900) (Jemal et al., 2004).

Overall five-year survival from lung cancer is approximately 14%. Treatment of early-stage disease can produce cures, with five-year survival from treated stage I lung cancers as high as 70%. Unfortunately, less than 15% of lung cancers are localized at the time of diagnosis. Most lung cancers are diagnosed in advanced stages, and five-year survival in patients with locally advanced and metastatic disease is less than 10% (Jemal et al., 2004). Late diagnosis is attributed to multiple factors. First, there is no proven tool or recommendation for screening or early detection in high-risk individuals. Although most patients present with symptoms, symptoms such as cough and exertional dyspnea often can be subtle and attributed to chronic symptoms of smoking. These topics will be explored further in this publication.

According to data gathered by the National Cancer Institute Surveillance, Epidemiology, and End Results Program (n.d.), the age-adjusted rate for lung cancer for all race and sex groups combined has risen sharply since 1950. From 1969 to 1991, the overall incidence almost doubled, with rates diminishing over the last decade. Lung cancer rates for African American and White men peaked and began to decrease around 1984. Although incidence for women of both races continues to rise, the rate at which it occurs is diminishing, as well (Travis, Linder, & Mackay, 2000).

Lung cancer was thought to be a disease of elderly men until the last half of the 20th century, when incidence in women rose sharply. Women now represent almost half of all new cases, with 2004 estimates of 93,110 for men versus 80,660 for women (Jemal et al., 2004). In addition, lung cancer surpassed breast cancer in 1987 as the leading cause of cancer-related deaths in women and currently accounts for more deaths than breast and all gynecologic cancers (i.e., ovarian, vulvar, vaginal, uterine) combined and breast and colorectal cancer, the other leading causes of death, combined. Lung cancer is expected to account for 25% of all female cancer deaths in 2003 (Jemal et al.) (see Table 1-1).

Most lung cancers are attributed to tobacco exposure. At least 79% of lung cancer cases in women are related to smoking. Although smoking rates have declined since the 1960s, the current prevalence of smoking among U.S. women is still high—estimated at 26%—and smoking rates are highest among teenage girls (Baldini & Strauss, 1997). Whether the association between smoking and lung cancer is stronger for women than men is unclear. Many epidemiologic studies have provided evidence that women are more susceptible than men to the adverse effects of tobacco smoke, whereas other studies suggest that estrogen plays a role in lung carcinogenesis. The presence of estrogen receptors on lung cancer cells has been documented, with evidence that estrogen induces cell proliferation and stimulates growth factors in the lung (Stabile et al., 2002).

The magnitude of the effect of smoking on lung cancer risk may not differ across the genders, but smoking appears to have an impact on the type of lung cancer that develops in each gender. Women smokers have a greater risk of developing small cell lung cancer (SCLC) than men smokers. Also, women are more likely to develop adenocarcinoma than men, and evidence suggests that this may be related to the role of estrogen (Baldini & Strauss, 1997). The inclusion of women in lung cancer screening and treatment trials has not been adequate in the past. Active recruitment of women for trials with specific reference to gender is needed to investigate this phenomenon further (Baldini & Strauss).

Male African Americans experience higher lung cancer incidence and mortality rates than all other male racial groupings, including Whites, Asian/Pacific Islanders, American Indians/Alaska Natives, and Latinos. This is not true for women, who demonstrate similar incidence and death rates among Whites and African Americans. Incidence and mortality in the other female ethnic groups is half of that for Whites and African Americans (Jemal et al., 2004).

Histologic Classification

The World Health Organization classification of lung cancer includes four major histologic types: squamous cell carcinoma, adenocarcinoma, small cell lung carcinoma, and large cell carcinoma. These classes are further subdivided more specifically, and there are other, less common, lung tumors, such as carcinoid. For clinical purposes, the histologic classes are grouped into two main categories of lung cancer: SCLC and non-small cell lung cancer (NSCLC). SCLC includes a category called combined small cell carcinoma. NSCLC includes squamous cell carcinoma (SCC), large cell carcinoma, and adenocarcinoma (Travis et al., 2000) (see Table 1-2).

Non-Small Cell Lung Cancer

Approximately 75%–80% of all lung cancers in the United States are NSCLC. Although the subtypes may differ in incidence according to sex, race, and age, they are grouped because of similarities in course and response to treatment. SCC arises most frequently in the proximal segmental bronchi and is associated with squamous metaplasia. Tumors are composed of sheets of epithelial cells, which may be poorly or well differentiated. At one time, SCC was the most frequently occurring lung cancer in North America, but its incidence is decreasing and has been surpassed by adenocarcinoma for reasons that are thought to be related to changes in tobacco use (Ginsberg, Vokes, & Rosenzwieg, 2001). SCC can be detected by cytologic examination of exfoliated cells in its earliest form, carcinoma in situ, where stratified squamous epithelium is replaced with malignant squamous cells. Unchecked, the tumor eventually invades and obstructs the bronchial lumen. SCC tends to be slow growing and can take three to four years to develop from a carcinoma in situ to a clinically evident tumor (Ginsberg et al.).

Adenocarcinoma is the most common form of lung cancer in North America, accounting for almost 40% of all lung cancers. It presents as a peripheral tumor, arising from the alveolar surface epithelium or the bronchial mucosal glands. Tumors also can arise from areas of previous infections or scars. Adenocarcinoma tumors are mucin-producing and form glands. Other than very early stage tumors, adenocarcinoma appears to have a worse prognosis than SCC. Bronchoalveolar carcinoma (BAC) is a subclassification of adenocarcinoma that appears to have distinct clinical and pathologic properties (Ginsberg et al., 2001).

Table 1-1. Estimated Leading Cancer Incidence and Mortality by Sex, 2004			
Sex	Cancer Type	Incidence	Mortality
Male	Prostate	33%	10%
	Lung	13%	32%
	Colorectal	11%	10%
Female	Breast	32%	15%
	Lung	12%	25%
	Colorectal	11%	11%
Note. Based on information from Jemal et al., 2004.			

Table 1-2. Histologic Groups of Lung Cancers	
Category	**Lung Cancer Diagnoses**
Non-small cell lung cancer	Squamous cell carcinoma Adenocarcinoma Large cell carcinoma
Small cell lung cancer	Combined small cell carcinoma

Large cell lung carcinoma (LCLC) is the least common of all NSCLC tumors, representing about 15% of all lung tumors. As diagnostic techniques have improved, tumors originally thought to be LCLC have been more appropriately diagnosed as poorly differentiated adenocarcinoma or SCC (Ginsberg et al., 2001). The prognosis of LCLC appears to be the same as for adenocarcinoma except for those with neuroendocrine features. These tumors appear to have a worse prognosis, and their relation to SCLC is still undefined (Ginsberg et al.).

Small Cell Lung Cancer

SCLC is less common than NSCLC, representing fewer than 20% of all lung cancers or approximately 30,000 cases per year in the United States. The latest World Health Organization classification of SCLC includes a variant known as combined small cell carcinoma, which is defined as a small cell carcinoma with a component of any histologic subtype of NSCLC (Travis et al., 2000). SCLC is a neuroendocrine tumor that routinely occurs in the central airways. Among the subtypes of lung cancer, the highest association between the extent of tobacco exposure and risk occurs in SCLC and SCC. SCLC also has a higher incidence in women than men (Murren, Glatstein, & Pass, 2000).

Although SCLC officially is staged according to the International System for Staging Lung Cancer, a more common clinical staging introduced by the Veterans Administration Lung Study Group generally is used. SCLC is staged as either limited or extensive disease. Nearly one-third of patients present with limited-stage disease, which is defined as disease that is confined to one hemithorax, without pericardial or pleural effusion, and encompassable by a single radiotherapy port (Kristjansen & Hansen, 1990). Extensive is the term applied to all other presentations of the disease. SCLC is an aggressive disease, in which limited stage is more curable than extensive-stage disease. Prior to the use of chemotherapy, patients diagnosed with limited-stage disease survived about three months. Median survival with chemotherapy is 10–14 months, with a five-year survival of 2%–8% (Murren et al., 2000). SCLC exhibits a high degree of neuroendocrine differentiation with expression of a wide variety of neuropeptides and neuropeptide receptors. Several of these neuropeptides have mitogenetic potential and have been shown to be mediators of SCLC proliferation.

Staging of Lung Cancer

Staging is a major indicator of prognosis and treatment for lung cancer. The International System for Staging Lung Cancer was adopted by the American Joint Committee on Cancer and the International Union Against Cancer in 1986 as a means of unifying variations in definitions and providing consistent meaning and interpretation among clinicians and scientists throughout the world. The system was revised in 1996 to improve the rules for TNM subsets and incorporate a new schema for regional lymph node mapping (Mountain, 1997).

The primary tumor is subdivided into four categories (T1–T4) and reflects size, site, and local involvement. Lymph node spread is subdivided into bronchopulmonary (N1), ipsilateral mediastinal (N2), and contralateral or supraclavicular disease (N3). Metastatic spread is either absent (M0) or present (M1) (Ginsberg et al., 2001). The purpose of clinical stage classification is to facilitate the accurate, concise description of the extent of disease in a way that can be communicated and replicated (the TNM classification) and to facilitate comparison of differing therapeutic approaches by combining patients with certain common attributes (TNM subsets) into groups or stages with generally similar prognoses and treatment options (Mountain, 2000). Four stages of lung cancer have been identified depending on the presentation at diagnosis, and treatment is prescribed accordingly. The accuracy of the system in predicting survival has been confirmed by many investigators (Ginsberg et al.).

The International System for Staging Lung Cancer is relevant for classifying the major types of lung cancer. Even though SCLC stages commonly are designated as either "limited" or "extensive" diseases, the TNM system can be useful and often is required for participation in multimodality programs or clinical trials (Mountain, 1997).

Prognostic Factors

Clinical stage is the most important prognostic indicator for lung cancer survival. The size and location of the tumor at the time of diagnosis is tied directly to the ability to achieve cure. Other factors have been known to affect survival. Male gender and age greater than 60 years have been found to adversely affect survival. Numerous studies have shown that women generally survive longer than men (Baldini & Strauss, 1997). Tumor expression of mucin, seen in adenocarcinoma, has been identified as an adverse factor in early-stage disease because mucin may facilitate formation of metastases. In those with advanced stages at diagnosis, performance status, weight loss, and elevated serum lactate dehydrogenase have been associated with poor outcomes, whereas histologic subtype is of no prognostic importance (Ginsberg et al., 2001).

The significance of specific metastatic sites is unclear, although presence of liver and bone metastases is reported to be associated with shorter survival. Total number of metastatic sites or degree of tumor burden does seem to be associated with survival. This is most clearly evident in the longer duration of survival associated with a single site of metastasis (Ginsberg et al., 2001).

Advances in molecular testing have produced a variety of novel potentially useful prognostic factors. The connection between activated oncogenes and loss of tumor suppressor gene function offers targets for determining prognostic outcomes. These targets include the significance of the presence of epidermal growth factor receptors on lung cancer cells, neuroendocrine markers, blood group antigen, and genetic markers such as K-*ras* mutations, *p53* mutations, *bcl-2* expression, *Fas* expression, and angiogenic indicators, to name a few (Ginsberg et al., 2001).

Histogenesis

More than 90% of primary lung cancers begin with an epithelial stem cell in the bronchial epithelium (Elpern, 1993) (see Figure 1-1). This stem cell normally differentiates to those cells found in the tracheobronchial tree, including pseudostratified reserved cells, ciliated goblet columnar cells, neuroendocrine cells, and pneumocytes lining the alveoli (Ginsberg et al., 2001). The columnar epithelial cells line the area from the trachea to the terminal bronchioles resting on a basement membrane. Some of these cells are ciliated, and some are mucin producing (goblet cells). Between the colum-

nar cells and the bronchial lumen are the smaller, shorter basal cells, some of which differentiate to become columnar cells. Others contain secretory granules and are thought to have a neurosecretory or endocrine function (Elpern).

Normal bronchial epithelial cells function as a lining and offer protection to the tracheobronchial tree. As a protective layer, the bronchial epithelium is continually damaged, shed, and replaced. Cellular abnormalities occur as the epithelium is chronically exposed to irritating inhaled substances, as most commonly is seen with tobacco smoke (see Figure 1-2). Exposure of the cell results in various combined genetic muta-

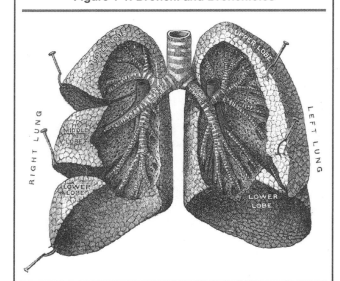

Figure 1-1. Bronchi and Bronchioles

Note. From *Anatomy of the Human Body,* by H. Gray, 1918, Philadelphia: Lea and Febiger. Retrieved June, 27, 2003, from www.bartleby.com/107/. Copyright 2000 by Bartleby.com, Inc. Reprinted with permission.

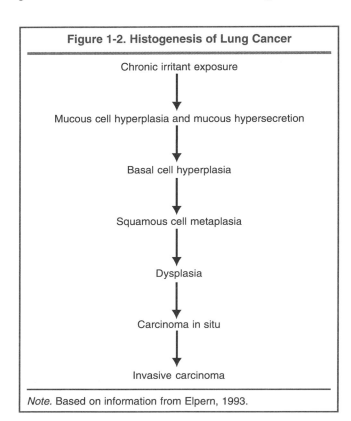

Figure 1-2. Histogenesis of Lung Cancer

Chronic irritant exposure

↓

Mucous cell hyperplasia and mucous hypersecretion

↓

Basal cell hyperplasia

↓

Squamous cell metaplasia

↓

Dysplasia

↓

Carcinoma in situ

↓

Invasive carcinoma

Note. Based on information from Elpern, 1993.

tions that contribute to malignant transformation, taking a normal cell through the morphologic evolution of hyperplasia; metaplasia; mild, moderate, and severe dysplasia; carcinoma in situ; and invasive carcinoma (Ginsberg et al., 2001).

Short-term exposure to irritants changes ciliary structure and function and leads to mucous cell hyperplasia and hypersecretion of mucus. With continued exposure, ciliated cells are repeatedly damaged and shed from the basement membrane, leading to basal cell hyperplasia. Repeated insult causes the rapidly proliferating basal cells to become less able to differentiate, leading to squamous cell metaplasia. The protective ciliated and mucus-producing cells are replaced by these dysplastic cells, allowing even greater exposure to irritants and carcinogens. Even at the point of squamous metaplasia, injury is reversible if the cause is removed. With continued exposure, atypia of the cell progresses, leading to intraepithelial carcinomas in both bronchi that do not invade the basement membrane (carcinoma in situ). Although not all of these cells progress to become invasive tumors, over time, many invade through the basement membrane with downgrowth of the tumor. Continued replication of mutant cells results in progression through carcinogenesis with further proliferation, angiogenesis, metastasis, and resistance (Sekido, Fong, & Minna, 2001).

Transformation of the bronchial epithelium occurs over extended periods of time, usually several decades, and depends on the duration and degree of exposure to lung irritants and carcinogens (Elpern, 1993). However, only 5%–10% of heavy smokers develop lung cancer, implying a genetic susceptibility (Deveraux, Taylor, & Barrett, 1996). Genetic susceptibility may involve individual variability in genes that encode proteins that are responsible for activation and detoxification of environmental carcinogens. An inherited variability also may exist in the tumor suppressor genes and oncogenes, which also influence a person's susceptibility to developing lung cancer (Deveraux et al.). Chapter 2 will further discuss the genetic development of lung cancer.

References

Baldini, E., & Strauss, G. (1997). Women and lung cancer: Waiting to exhale. *Chest, 112*(Suppl. 4), 229S–239S.

Deveraux, T., Taylor, J., & Barrett, J. (1996). Molecular mechanisms of lung cancer: Interaction of environmental and genetic factors: Giles F. Filley lecture. *Chest, 109*(Suppl. 3), 14S–19S.

Elpern, E.H. (1993). Lung cancer. In S.L. Groenwald, M.H. Frogge, M. Goodman, & C.H. Yarbro (Eds.), *Cancer nursing: Principles and practice* (3rd ed., pp. 1174–1199). Sudbury, MA: Jones and Bartlett.

Ginsberg, R., Vokes, E., & Rosenzweig, K. (2001). Non-small cell lung cancer. In V.T. DeVita, S. Hellman, & S.A. Rosenberg (Eds.), *Cancer: Principles and practice of oncology* (6th ed., pp. 925–975). Philadelphia: Lippincott Williams & Wilkins.

Jemal, A., Tiwari, R.C., Murray, T., Ghafoor, A., Samuels, A., Ward, E., et al. (2004). Cancer statistics, 2004. *CA: A Cancer Journal for Clinicians, 54,* 8–29.

Kennedy, T.C., Miller, Y., & Prindiville, S. (2000). Screening for lung cancer revisited and the role of sputum cytology and fluorescence bronchoscopy in a high risk group. *Chest, 117*(Suppl. 1), 72S–79S.

Kristjansen, P., & Hansen, H. (1990). Management of small cell lung cancer: A summary of the Third International Association for the Study of Lung Cancer Workshop on Small Cell Lung Cancer. *Journal of the National Cancer Institute, 82,* 263–266.

Mountain, C. (1997). Revisions in the international staging system for lung cancer. *Chest, 111,* 1710–1717.

Mountain, C. (2000). International staging system for lung cancer. In H. Pass, J. Mitchell, D. Johnson, A. Turrisi, & J. Minna (Eds.), *Lung cancer: Principles and practice* (2nd ed., pp. 591–601). Philadelphia: Lippincott Williams & Wilkins.

Murren, J.R., Glatstein, I., & Pass, H. (2000). Small cell lung cancer. In H. Pass, J. Mitchell, D. Johnson, A. Turrisi, & J. Minna (Eds.), *Lung cancer: Principles and practice* (2nd ed., pp. 983–1018). Philadelphia: Lippincott Williams & Wilkins.

National Cancer Institute Surveillance, Epidemiology and End Results (SEER) Program. (n.d.). *Incidence: Lung and bronchus cancer.* Retrieved February 12, 2003, from http://seer.cancer.gov/faststats/html/inc_lungb.html

Sekido, Y., Fong, K.M., & Minna, J.D. (2001). Molecular biology of lung cancer. In V.T. DeVita, S. Hellman, & S.A. Rosenberg (Eds.), *Cancer: Principles and practice of oncology* (6th ed., pp. 917–924). Philadelphia: Lippincott Williams & Wilkins.

Stabile, L.P., Gaither-Davis, A.L., Gubish, C.T., Hopkins, T.M., Luketich, J.D., Cristie, N., et al. (2002). Human non-small cell lung tumors and cells derived from normal lung express both estrogen receptor alpha and beta and show biological responses to estrogen. *Cancer Research, 62,* 2141–2150.

Travis, W.D., Linder, J., & Mackay, B. (2000). Classification, histology, cytology and electron microscopy. In H. Pass, J. Mitchell, D. Johnson, A. Turrisi, & J. Minna (Eds.), *Lung cancer: Principles and practice* (2nd ed., pp. 453–495). Philadelphia: Lippincott Williams & Wilkins.

CHAPTER 2

Biology of Lung Cancer and Therapeutic Implications

Nancy G. Houlihan, RN, MA, AOCN®

Introduction

Lung cancer occurs as a result of the deregulation of normal gene expression (Mulligan-Kehoe & Russo, 2000). Molecular biology provides a framework for explaining and extending the phenomena of gene regulation and expression as they relate to lung cancer. Advances in the understanding of the molecular biology of lung cancer are guiding the development of strategies for prevention, early detection, prediction of prognosis, and treatment (Gazdar, 1993). This chapter will review the specific molecular alterations and carcinogenesis of lung cancer with an introduction to related therapeutics.

Lung Cancer Carcinogenesis

Lung cancer begins as a single genetic mutation of a bronchial epithelial cell in response to exposure to a carcinogen. The single mutant cell has the potential to further develop through clonal expansion (Aberle & McLeskey, 2003). A complex interaction exists between the molecular changes and the activation of key pathways for the regulation and control of cells. The loss of cellular control results in further proliferation of the mutant cells (Sekido, Fong, & Minna, 2001). Tumor development occurs as a result of a concept known as field cancerization, whereby the gradual accrual of sequential genetic and morphologic changes results in the formation of an invasive tumor (Mulligan-Kehoe & Russo, 2000; Valle, Chavany, Zhokov, & Jendoubi, 2003).

Carcinogenesis is a multistep process occurring over time. The stages of carcinogenesis include initiation, promotion, and progression. Initiation refers to the irreversible, nonlethal genetic damage to a cell. Cigarette smoke, the number-one cause of lung cancer, contains more than 4,000 chemicals and 55 known carcinogens. Components of cigarette smoke, such as polyaromatic hydrocarbons and the nitrosamine metabolite of nicotine, specifically react with DNA-forming adducts,

causing genetic point mutations, translocations, and amplification (Valle et al., 2003; Works & Gallucci, 1996). If cellular damage is not repaired, the daughter cells inherit the abnormal DNA sequences and become what are called initiated cells. In tumor promotion, clonal expansion of an initiated cell together with accumulation of genetic alterations causes excessive proliferation of the initiated cells and malignant tumor growth. The final step, tumor progression, refers to invasion and metastases (Bale & Brown, 2001; Valle et al.).

Normal Cellular Behavior

Normally, all of the body's cells are held under rigid growth control. Cell division is carefully regulated by two opposing sets of genes, one promoting growth and the other inhibiting growth. The number of times a cell is allowed to replicate is controlled by an internal mechanism. Genetic damage that occurs during the growth process is carefully repaired by enzymes coded by DNA repair genes. When damage is unable to be repaired, the cell is destroyed (Yarbro, 2000).

Cellular development involves a chain of activities that include the cell life cycle and its regulatory mechanisms. The cell cycle consists of stages: DNA synthesis; two development stages, G1 and G2; and mitosis, or cell division. G0 is a quiescent or nondividing phase in which the cell remains metabolically active but is not progressing through the cell cycle toward division. G1 is the gap prior to replication where the cell prepares for DNA replication and division by accumulating the molecules necessary for cell cycle transit, and some cellular differentiation begins. Growth factors stimulate cells in G0 or G1 to divide in response to an extracellular signal. During the S phase, DNA synthesis occurs with replication of the entire cellular DNA content and associated structure. G2 is the gap phase following replication when, prior to cell division, any necessary repair of DNA synthesis occurs. If unable to be repaired, cell death, or apoptosis, is induced

(Gupta, Harris, Bernhard, Muschel, & McKenna, 2000; Works & Gallucci, 1996) (see Table 2-1).

The proliferation of normal cells is controlled by a series of chemical signals. The transmission of these signals follows a pathway that involves growth factors, their receptors, transmitting proteins in the cytoplasm, and regulatory proteins in the nucleus. The process requires release of a growth factor, which travels to its respective receptor on the cell membrane or in the cytoplasm. The growth factor, also known as the ligand, binds to its receptor, activating the signal transduction proteins, which carry the message to the nucleus. Most signal transduction pathways activate tyrosine kinase enzymes (Carpenter & Cantley, 2001). Activated tyrosine kinases signal adjacent molecules, *Ras* and *Rho*, which affect delivery, or transduction, of the signal through the cytoplasm to the nucleus. *Ras* and *Rho* are proteins attached to the inner aspect of the plasma membrane by a farnesyl group and are regulated by an enzyme called farnesyl transferase (Aberle & McLeskey, 2003). Once the signal reaches the nucleus, the nuclear regulatory proteins oversee cell division. Growth pathways also are involved in the transmission of signals that can interfere with apoptotic, or cell death, signals (Kalemkerian, 2000). Activation of growth signaling pathways results in cellular proliferation and decreased apoptosis, or programmed cell death (see Figure 2-1).

The growth factors, growth factor receptors, signal-transducing proteins, and nuclear regulatory proteins are called proto-oncogenes (Ross, 2003). Proto-oncogenes that are damaged by exposure to carcinogens, radiation, or viruses and contain proteins that are genetically altered or overexpressed are called **oncogenes** (Gupta et al., 2000). Genetically mutated or overexpressed oncogenes cause continuous cell growth and proliferation.

Normal cell division is regulated not only by proto-oncogenes but also by inhibitory genes called **tumor suppressor genes** (TSGs). TSGs are negative growth regulators functioning to turn off cellular proliferation. In normal tissue, there is a counterbalance between cell proliferation and programmed cell death, or apoptosis. In addition to controlling normal cellular proliferation, TSGs are involved in suppression of cellular malignant transformation and proliferation by repairing DNA or initiating apoptosis.

Apoptosis is a genetically regulated form of cell death that normally is involved in organogenesis, tissue homeostasis, and the regulation of the immune system to remove autoreactive clones (Gupta et al., 2000). Apoptosis is the cell's suicidal functionality that induces cell destruction rather than replicating genetic mutations. Apoptosis is linked to cellular proliferation and can be triggered by the loss of cell cycle controls associated with the activation of oncogenes and cellular transformation. In addition, apoptosis can be triggered in response to external stimuli, including hormonal or growth factor manipulation, and in response to toxic agents, such as chemotherapy and x-rays (Aberle & McLeskey, 2003).

Inactivation of TSG function, through genetic mutation or overexpression, results in uncontrolled growth. A characteristic feature of many tumors, including lung cancer, is the loss of the specific TSG regulators of cell proliferation. If tumor cells are to continue to proliferate and increase in number, they must lose the apoptotic response as well as undergo growth stimulation. The activation of oncogenes causes persistent cell growth, whereas inactivation of TSGs causes loss of growth inhibition (Gupta et al., 2000; Sekido et al., 2001).

Chromosomal Abnormalities in Lung Cancer

The genetic damage causing lung tumor development occurs in the form of point mutations, chromosomal translocations, and gene amplification (Phillips & Nuwayhid, 1993; Sekido et al., 2001). In point mutations, the most common type of mutation, a single amino acid in the gene's protein product is altered. Chromosomal translocation refers to the transfer of a gene from its usual chromosome to a new position on another chromosome. In both cases, the genes behave abnormally as a result of the change. Amplification refers to the repeated duplication of the gene. Both translocation and amplification result in overexpression, or overproduction, of the gene product (Works & Gallucci, 1996). The specific chromosomal abnormalities found in lung cancer cell lines include DNA nuclear changes and chromosomal abnormalities (allele losses and gains or amplification); microsatellite instability (mismatching in short DNA sequences); and aberrant DNA methylation (Sekido et al.; Valle et al., 2003). These alterations are significant in view of their potential use as markers for early diagnosis or prognosis of the disease.

Deletion of the short arm of chromosome 3 is the most frequent genetic event, occurring in more than 90% of small cell lung cancers (SCLCs) and 50% of non-small cell lung

Table 2-1. Stages of the Cell Cycle	
Stage	**Activity**
G0	Resting phase; nondividing; metabolically active but not progressing.
G1	Gap prior to DNA replication; cell prepares by accumulating molecules necessary for transit; some differentiation occurs.
S	DNA synthesis occurs with replication of the entire DNA content and associated structure.
G2	Gap following replication where any required DNA repair occurs.
M	Mitosis, or cell division, occurs.

Note. Based on information from Gupta et al., 2000.

Figure 2-1. Growth Factor Signaling Pathway

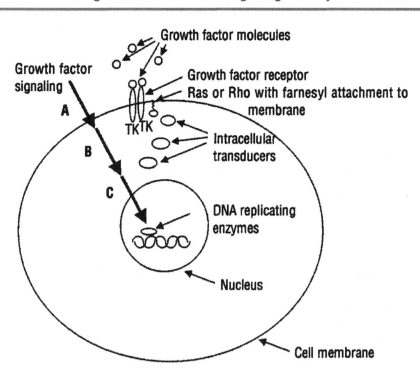

Growth factor signaling begins outside of the cell **(A)** where molecules of growth factors are present. The signal is transmitted to the inside of the cell when growth factor molecules (e.g., epidermal growth factor) bind to growth factor receptors (e.g., epidermal growth factor receptor). The growth factor receptors are tyrosine kinase enzymes that are activated when growth factor is bound to them. The tyrosine kinase activity is a signal that activates adjacent small molecules called Ras or Rho. These molecules, in turn, activate cytosolic signaling molecules (transducers) that transmit the growth factor signal to the nucleus **(B)**. In the nucleus, the receipt of the growth factor signal **(C)** causes a series of events including duplication of the chromosomes by DNA replicating enzymes and culminating in mitosis, the splitting of the parent cell into two daughter cells.

Note. From "Biology of Lung Cancer With Implications for New Therapies," by M.F. Aberle and S.W. McLeskey, 2003, *Oncology Nursing Forum, 30,* p. 275. Copyright 2003 by the Oncology Nursing Society. Reprinted with permission.

cancers (NSCLCs), and often includes the fragile histidine triad (FIHT) gene (Valle et al., 2003). This deletion is considered to be a critical early event in lung cancer pathogenesis, as alterations in 3p are identified in the bronchial epithelium of current and former smokers (Witsuba, Lam, & Behrens, 1997). Other predominant chromosomal losses for SCLC include 5q, 15q, and 17p. In NSCLC, deletions of 9p and 17p together with +7, i(5),(p10), and i(8)(q10) often are seen (Sekido et al., 2001).

Lung cancer frequently exhibits microsatellite instability, which occurs as a result of a mutation known as the replication error repair phenotype. Overall, about 35% of SCLCs and 22% of NSCLCs demonstrate this alteration, which is associated with younger age at diagnosis, reduced survival, and advanced tumor stage. The possibility of using microsatellite alteration phenotype for early diagnosis is being tested in sputum, bronchial washings, and blood (Sekido et al., 2001).

Another acquired tumor abnormality is the alteration of genomic imprinting, or DNA methylation. Aberrantly methylated DNA sequences, which can be sensitively detected among a background of normal DNA, can be used for early molecular detection. Hypermethylation of the $p16^{INK4A}$ gene in a subset of NSCLC results in its downregulation and may be an early event in lung cancer pathogenesis. Other sites of hypermethylation, including 3p, 4q34, 10q26, and 17p13, have been implicated in lung cancer pathogenesis, although the precise gene targets are uncertain. Loss of methylation also occurs in lung cancer as seen in the insulin-like growth factor-2 (*IGF-2*) gene and the *H19* gene (associated with hypomethylation of its promoter region) (Sekido et al., 2001).

Other molecular alterations demonstrated in lung cancer include upregulation or activation of oncogenes—*ras, myc, bcl-2,* and *c-erb-2*—and downregulation or loss of tumor suppressor genes—*p53, RB,* and *p16*[INK4A] (Gupta et al., 2000). These specific genes will be discussed further in the following sections.

Growth Factors

Various growth factors and receptors have been implicated in the pathogenesis and progression of both SCLC and NSCLC (Kalemkerian, 2000). The dysregulation of the expression or function of growth factors, receptors, or signal transduction mediators can result in cellular proliferation and malignant transformation (see Figure 2-1).

In keeping with the neuroendocrine properties of SCLC, a wide variety of neuropeptides and neuropeptide receptors are expressed by SCLC cell lines and tumors, of which many are mitogenic and shown to be mediators of SCLC proliferation. These include the following peptides and receptors: bombesin-like peptides, including gastrin-releasing peptide (GRP) and neuromedin B (NMB); vasopressin; bradykinin; gastrin and cholecystokinin peptides; vasoactive intestinal peptide (VIP); and neurotensin (Kalemkerian, 2000). Specific factors will be further discussed in Chapter 7.

Distinct growth factors and receptors are involved in the regulation of NSCLC. Epidermal growth factor receptor (EGFR) can be activated by several growth factors or ligands, including epidermal growth factor (EGF), transforming growth factor-alpha (TGFα), and amphiregulin. EGF is a major growth factor for NSCLC and will be discussed further in the section on *ErbB* family of oncogenes. Other stimulatory growth factors/receptors include platelet-derived growth factor (PDGF) receptor, IGF receptor, parathyroid hormone-related peptide (PTHrP), VIP receptor, transferrin, and p185HER2 (*HER2/neu*). Inhibitory factors/receptors include transforming growth factor-beta (TGFß) receptor, interleukin-6 (IL-6) receptor; and tumor necrosis factor-alpha (TNFα) receptor (Kalemkerian, 2000).

Oncogenes

As described earlier, genetic mutation or overexpression of oncogenes results in uncontrolled cellular proliferation and loss of apoptosis. Multiple oncogene aberrations have been found to be associated with lung cancer (see Table 2-2).

Ras

Ras is a guanine binding protein that acts as a switch to transduce signals from the ligand-stimulated receptor on the extracellular membrane to the nucleus. An example of *ras* signal transduction is the EGFR and *erbB2* heterodimer receptor. When the effector ligand, TGFα, binds to this receptor complex, the *Ras* protein is activated, inducing nuclear transcription factors that enhance cellular proliferation. In the process, the receptor is phosphorylated and the associated tyrosine kinase is transported across the nuclear membrane.

Mutations that occur as a result of carcinogens can cause activation of *Ras* with a resulting exaggeration of the downstream effects, especially cell division (Lechner & Fugaro, 2000).

Three members of the Ras family of genes are differentiated by their homology to different sarcoma oncogenes: H-*ras,* K-*ras,* and N-*ras.* H-*ras* is homologous to the Harvey murine sarcoma virus oncogene; K-*ras* is homologous to the Kirsten murine sarcoma virus; and N-*ras* initially was isolated from a neuroblastoma cell line (Lechner & Fugaro, 2000). Activating mutations of *Ras* can be seen in up to 30% of all human tumors. In the absence of mutation, there is also overexpression of *Ras.* Although mutational activation of H-*ras* and N-*ras* is rare in lung cancer, K-*ras* has been shown to be mutated or overexpressed in 30% of adenocarcinomas, 30% of carcinoid tumors, 13% of large cell tumors, and none of the squamous cell tumors (Lechner & Fugaro; Sekido et al., 2001).

The *Ras* protein has a historical role in molecular oncology, as it provided the first direct link of genetics to malignancy. It has been studied in lung cancer for its usefulness as a biomarker for early detection, as a predictor of prognosis, and as a target for antitumor therapy (Lechner & Fugaro, 2000). Studies to identify individuals at high risk for lung cancer have evaluated bronchial cells for K-*ras* mutations. These studies show that

Table 2-2. Genetic Mutations or Overexpressions in Lung Cancer

Oncogenes	NSCLC	SCLC
ras	30% adenocarcinoma 13% LCC	Rare
myc	5%–10%	15%–30%
bcl-2	25% SCC 12% adenocarcinoma	75%–80%
erbB2	25%–60% in all NSCLC (highest in adenocarcinoma)	Rare

Tumor Suppressor Genes	NSCLC	SCLC
p53	50% in all NSCLC • 50% SCC • 53% LCC • 38% adenocarcinoma	90%
p16[INK4A] (CDKN2)	0%–10%	30%–70%
RB	15%–30%	90%

LCC—large cell carcinoma; NSCLC—non-small cell lung cancer; SCC—squamous cell carcinoma; SCLC—small cell lung cancer

Note. Based on information from Gupta et al., 2000; Sekido et al., 2001.

although mutations can predict the presence of carcinogen-damaged epithelium, they do not necessarily predict malignancy (Yakubovskaya et al., 1995). Therefore, a positive *ras* assay may correlate to DNA damage without necessarily predicting malignant potential (Lechner & Fugaro).

Studies suggest that K-*ras* mutations predict a poor clinical prognosis for patients with advanced lung cancer because of therapeutic resistance, whereas other studies have shown that K-*ras* mutations have no correlation with late-stage cancer survival or chemosensitivity (Rosell et al., 1993; Slebos et al., 1991). The survival advantage of patients without K-*ras* mutations is seemingly limited to early stages of lung cancer (Sugio et al., 1992.)

Understanding the biochemistry of *Ras* protein (p21) has prompted many studies targeting inhibition of protein activity as an antitumor therapy. Many pharmacologic approaches are aimed at blocking expression, interfering in membrane localization and signal transduction, and activating proteins that deactivate *Ras* (Lechner & Fugaro, 2000). However, *Ras* is only one of many proteins that are responsible for signal transduction and cell fate determination. Mutation and overexpression of *Ras* is not sufficient alone to transform normal epithelial cells, requiring further clarification of its mechanism and utility as a focus of treatment (Hahn et al., 1999).

Ras and *Rho* protein, a gene similar to *Ras*, are attached to the inner aspect of the plasma membrane of the intracellular domain of the cell by a farnesyl protein called farnesyl transferase. Inhibition of farnesyl transferase prevents the activation of *Ras* and *Rho,* interfering with the signal transduction pathway. Farnesyl transferase inhibitors currently are under clinical investigation for the treatment of lung cancer (Aberle & McLeskey, 2003; Bunn, Soriano, Johnson, & Heasley, 2000; Sekido et al., 2001).

Myc

Myc proteins are transcription factors involved in both cell proliferation and apoptosis (Janne & Johnson, 2000). Three forms of *Myc* have been described: C-*myc* is cellular, N-*myc* was isolated from a neuroblastoma cell, and L-*myc* was isolated from an SCLC cell. *Myc* genes usually are not mutated in carcinogenesis but are activated by overexpression by either upregulation or gene amplification. *Myc* oncogene is an "early response" gene with involvement in the cell cycle at G0–1 and early S phase, but *Myc* expression also is sustained throughout the cell cycle. In addition to its proliferative function, *Myc* also can induce apoptosis in G0 and G1. The regulation of the *Myc* protein expression is crucial for normal cellular proliferation (Lechner & Fugaro, 2000).

In lung cancer, *Myc* amplification most commonly is found in SCLC and is predominantly L-*myc* and N-*myc*. In NSCLC, *Myc* amplification is rare (adenocarcinoma, 5%–10%). *Myc* amplification in SCLC is associated with variant morphology and occurs in approximately 15%–30%, depending on cell morphology.

In preclinical models, *Myc* can be inhibited by antisense oligonucleotides and by transfection of mutant *Myc* genes. The difficulties associated with systemic gene delivery limit the clinical evaluation of *Myc* as a treatment approach (Bunn et al., 2000). *Myc* overexpression is associated with poor survival (Lechner & Fugaro, 2000).

Bcl-2

Bcl-2 is expressed in tissues that are renewed from stem cells, have proliferative ability, or that are long-lived. In the past, the function of *bcl-2* was viewed like that of many other oncogenes, as promoting proliferation. More recently, expression has been shown to delay or even prevent apoptosis (Gupta et al., 2000). Expression of *bcl-2* in SCLC is as high as 80%. In NSCLC, it is found in 25% of squamous cell carcinomas (SCCs) and 12% of adenocarcinomas. It is unclear if it plays a role in prognosis, but studies demonstrate a trend toward longer survival in patients whose tumors express *bcl-2* (Kaiser et al., 1996; Pezzella et al., 1993).

ErbB

Ligand binding is the characteristic used to describe the members of the *ErbB* gene family of cell membrane receptor tyrosine kinases: EGFR (HER1 or *erbB1*), *erbB2* (HER2), *erbB3* (HER3), and *erbB4* (HER4). These receptors are transmembrane glycoproteins that consist of an extracellular ligand-binding domain, a transmembrane domain, and an intracellular domain with tyrosine kinase activity for signal transduction. As described previously, when growth factors bind with a receptor, a strong, constant growth signal results.

EGFR (erbB1)

Activation of EGFR occurs when a specific ligand, EGF, TGFα, or amphiregulin, binds to the extracellular domain. Receptors exist as inactive single units or monomers that, on activation by ligand binding, pair to form an active dimer. The receptor dimerizes with either another EGFR monomer (homodimer) or another member of the *ErbB* family (heterodimer) to form a pair. These events lead to activation of a cascade of biochemical and physiologic responses that are involved in the mitogenic signal transduction of cancer cells. Following pairing, or dimerization, a signal is sent across the membrane into the intracellular domain activating tyrosine kinase and leading to mitogenic signaling and other cellular activities regulating apoptosis, gene expression, and cellular proliferation (Baselga, 2002) (see Figure 2-2). There is now a body of evidence to show that the EGFR-mediated drive is increased in a wide variety of epithelial solid tumors, including NSCLC, and cancers of the prostate, breast, stomach, and head and neck (Salomon, Brandt, Ciardello, & Normanno, 1995). In these cancers, where growth factors and growth factor receptors are overexpressed, inappropriate, constant signaling occurs leading to uncontrolled cellular growth. Activation of EGFR in lung cancer results in

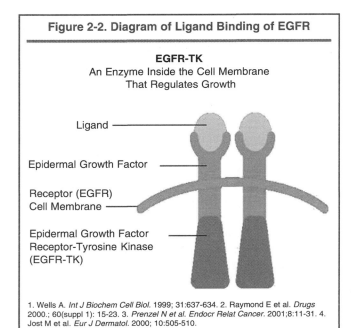

Figure 2-2. Diagram of Ligand Binding of EGFR

EGFR-TK
An Enzyme Inside the Cell Membrane
That Regulates Growth

Ligand

Epidermal Growth Factor

Receptor (EGFR)
Cell Membrane

Epidermal Growth Factor
Receptor-Tyrosine Kinase
(EGFR-TK)

1. Wells A. *Int J Biochem Cell Biol.* 1999; 31:637-634. 2. Raymond E et al. *Drugs* 2000.; 60(suppl 1): 15-23. 3. Prenzel N et al. *Endocr Relat Cancer.* 2001;8:11-31. 4. Jost M et al. *Eur J Dermatol.* 2000; 10:505-510.

Note. From *Inside Cancer* [slide kit], by the Alliance for Scientific Affairs and Publications, Inc. Copyright 2003 by the Alliance for Scientific Affairs and Publications, Inc. Reprinted with permission.

tumor growth and progression, including promotion of proliferation, angiogenesis, invasion and metastases, and inhibition of apoptosis.

EGFR is not expressed at high levels, if at all, in SCLC. Consequently, EGFR has little effect on tumor cell growth and progression (Nakagawa, 2001). EGFR overexpression is pronounced in NSCLC (13%–80%) including virtually all SCCs and 65% of large cell and adenocarcinomas (Franklin, Veve, Hirsch, Helfrich, & Bunn, 2002). Furthermore, some clinical data suggest that overexpression of these receptors is known to correlate with advanced disease, development with a metastatic phenotype, and poor disease prognosis (Nakagawa; Salomon et al., 1995).

The clear potential for EGFR-targeted therapies in the treatment of lung cancer has prompted the development of a variety of agents targeted to the extracellular ligand-binding domain, to the intracellular tyrosine kinase domain, to the ligand, or to the synthesis of EGFR. Two therapeutic approaches have been shown to be most promising: monoclonal antibodies and small molecule inhibitors of the EGFR to block ligand binding and receptor activation. These agents are being investigated as monotherapy and in combination with conventional therapies (Baselga, 2000).

erbB2

The second gene, *erbB2*, or *HER2/neu,* more often is expressed in breast cancer but also is overexpressed in approxi-

mately 25%–60% of all NSCLCs, with highest expression levels found in adenocarcinomas (Bunn et al., 2000; Gupta et al., 2000). Gene amplification or overexpression is rare in SCLC. *ErbB2* overexpression has been shown to correlate with decreased survival and chemoresistance (Aberle & McLeskey, 2003).

The use of monoclonal antibodies (MoAbs) against the *ErbB* family of receptors has been validated with trastuzumab (Herceptin®, Genentech, San Francisco, CA), a humanized MoAb targeting the extracellular domain of *erbB2;* trastuzumab is approved by the U.S. Food and Drug Administration (FDA) for treatment of metastatic breast cancer. Trastuzumab also is used in clinical trials for NSCLC in combination with conventional chemotherapy (Baselga, 2002). The MoAb C-225, or cetuximab (Erbitux™, ImClone, New York, NY), is directed against the extracellular ligand-binding domain of the EGFR *(erbB1).* Preclinical data show inhibition of the growth of NSCLC xenografts in monotherapy. Clinical trial data demonstrate that therapy was well tolerated and antitumor activity was noted in some patients with NSCLC (Nakagawa, 2001). Other MoAbs targeting EGFR are under development.

Several agents recently have completed phase III clinical trials or procured approval by the FDA. Small-molecule, orally active, intracellular tyrosine kinase inhibitors (TKI) are now available. These compounds directly inhibit tyrosine kinase phosphorylation, blocking EGFR drive and inhibiting tumor cell proliferation (Baselga, 2002; Nakagawa, 2001). Gefitinib (Iressa®, AstraZeneca, Wilmington, DE) and erlotinib (Tarceva™, Genentech) are examples of EGFR-TKI that have the ability to cross the cell membrane into the cytoplasm and turn off the signal at the source. Phase I and II trials demonstrated disease response or stabilization, improved survival, and improved symptom control in people with advanced NSCLC (Baselga, 2002; Bunn et al., 2000; Kris et al., 2002). In addition, side effects were reported as mild and included reversible rash and diarrhea (Baselga; Kris et al.). Phase III trials of gefitinib showed no survival benefit when added to chemotherapy (Giaccone et al., 2002; Johnson et al., 2002). Daily oral dose of erlotinib is 150 mg, and gefitinib is 250 mg. These new agents increase the options in extending survival with fewer side effects while improving symptoms and quality of life for patients with advanced lung cancer. Gefitinib received FDA approval in 2003.

Tumor Suppressor Genes and Growth Suppression

p53

p53 is a TSG that is activated in cells that have undergone stress, such as exposure to genotoxic agents or oncogene activation. Once active, *p53* initiates cell cycle arrest or apoptosis. Mutation of *p53* allows for continued malignant cell growth (Szak, Pietenpol, & Carbone, 2000).

p53 levels in normal cells are very low. When cells suffer DNA damage, the level and activity of *p53* increases and causes cell cycle arrest at the G1 or 2 phases. This arrest permits repair to take place and prevents accumulation of mutant sequences. If DNA damage is extensive, *p53* is thought to stimulate apoptosis. Otherwise, *p53* mediates cell cycle arrest, allowing for repair before the cell resumes cycling. If *p53* is absent or mutant in a cell, it is unable to mediate cell cycle arrest or apoptosis, and any mutations from DNA damage are perpetuated (Liotta & Liu, 2001; Szak et al., 2000).

p53 is the most frequently altered TSG in human malignancies, with mutations affecting 80% of SCLCs and 50% of NSCLCs (Gupta et al., 2000). In NSCLC, *p53* alterations occur most frequently in SCC (51.2%), large cell carcinoma (53.7%), and adenocarcinoma (38.8%) (Szak et al., 2000). Mutations of *p53* in lung cancer are of all types: missense, nonsense, splicing, and large deletions. *p53* mutations are correlated closely with chronic exposure to cigarette smoke (Sekido et al., 2001).

The usefulness of *p53* in lung cancer therapeutics is under study as a clinical marker for early diagnosis and as a prognostic and treatment response predictor. Preneoplastic lung tissue from cigarette smokers shows allele loss, gene mutation, and other abnormalities of *p53*. Sputum analysis in presymptomatic populations could be used to detect occult *p53* genetic damage leading to lung cancer (Szak et al., 2000). Studies show that response of clinical lung cancers to radiation and chemotherapy appears to be worse in the presence of the *p53* mutation (Szak et al.). If larger prospective studies confirm this data, *p53* status could be used to select subsets of patients for more aggressive treatments and allow those with a smaller potential benefit to avoid the toxicities of treatment. Lastly, the presence of antibodies to *p53* has been detected in 13% of patients with lung cancer with missense mutations of *p53* and may precede the development of a clinical cancer. The significance of these antibodies and association with outcome currently is under investigation (Szak et al.).

Discovery of *p53* mutations in lung cancer has led to the hypothesis that replacement of the defective gene protein or decreasing the expression of the overexpressed ones may lead to a potential treatment. Laboratory studies of delivering *p53* through the airways of mice with *p53* deletions showed inhibition of lung tumor formation. Administration of adenoviral *p53* vector to NSCLC patients demonstrated increased sensitivity to chemotherapy with little toxicity. Investigations of *p53* as a treatment are dependent on development of more effective means of delivering the gene to affected tissues (Gupta et al., 2000; Sekido et al., 2001).

p16^INK4A^-Cyclin D1-Cyclin-Dependent Kinase-4-Retinoblastoma Protein Pathway

The *p16*[INK4A]-cyclin D1-cyclin-dependent kinase-4 retinoblastoma protein pathway is composed of three genes. The retinoblastoma (RB) gene encodes a growth-suppressive nuclear phosphoprotein. When active, RB binds and inactivates proteins essential for G1/S phase transition of the cell cycle. RB mutations have been demonstrated in lung cancers. The RB protein is mutated or absent in more than 80% of SCLCs and 40% of NSCLCs. In addition, disruptions of the RB pathway can be seen in 90% of NSCLCs. Thus, the RB pathway plays an important role in tumorigenesis in lung cancer. Although no correlation has been found in RB presence and clinical outcome, it has been shown to be correlated to the multidrug resistance gene and may be a marker for the assessment of sensitivity to some chemotherapeutic drugs (Claudio & Giordano, 2000).

The *p16*[INK4A] (also called CDKN2) is the inhibitor of cycline dependent kinases (CDK), especially CDK4 or CDK6, which phosphorylate and keep RB in an inactive state. Its normal role is to positively regulate RB's growth-controlling function by keeping RB unphosphorylated. If *p16*[INK4A] is inactivated by mutation, RB remains chronically phosphorylated and cannot function to regulate growth (Gupta et al., 2000). Aberrant methylation of *p16*[INK4A] has been found to be an early event in lung cancer, with its frequency increasing with disease progression from basal cell hyperplasia (17%) to squamous metaplasia (24%) to carcinoma in situ (50%). Application of this data is under study for early detection of lung cancer (Gupta et al.).

The *p16*[INK4A] gene locus often is abnormal in human malignancies. In lung cancer, its abnormalities frequently are found in NSCLC (50%) and not reported in SCLC (Gupta et al., 2000). RB is mutated in the majority of SCLCs. Thus, the two major histologic lung cancer types have this pathway inactivated by mutation of one gene or the other (Sekido et al., 2001).

Metastases and Angiogenesis

Blood vessels are integral to the growth and metastases of solid tumors. Angiogenesis is the phenomenon of the development of new blood vessels from preexisting vessels, which is called neovascularization. Tumor angiogenesis is necessary for a mass to grow beyond a few millimeters in size. Development of metastases involves a sequential cascade of events beginning with angiogenesis and growth of tumor cells at the primary site, followed by invasion, intravasation, transport, arrest, attachment, and extravasation. This cascade of events repeats itself at the metastatic site. Multiple factors inherent to lung tumors predispose them to early growth and metastases and explain why many lung cancers advance so rapidly. This has generated research into angiogenesis as a potential prognostic indicator and a target for therapeutic interventions against tumor growth and metastases (Ohta & Watanabe, 2000).

Angiogenesis currently is thought to be regulated by the balance of inducers and inhibitors that are released by tumor cells and host cells. Vascular endothelial growth factor (VEGF) and basic fibroblastic growth factor are two major angiogenesis inducers produced by human lung tumors, with VEGF being the most powerful endothelial cell-specific mitogen associated with tumor neovascularization (Ohta & Watanabe, 2000; Sekido et al., 2001). EGFR activation is linked to the production of VEGF and promotes the ability of tumor cells to invade neighboring tissues, especially the vascular endothelium, thus giving access to the circulation (Salomon et al., 1995). Mutations in *p53, Ras,* and other oncogenes appear to have a connection with VEGF expression in tumor angiogenesis (Ohta & Watanabe). Strong VEGF expression in tumors seems to predict a poor outcome in patients with lung cancer. Mutations in *p53* also lead to decreased expression of thrombospondin, a negative regulator of angiogenesis. Folkman, considered the father of angiogenesis research, also discovered that many tumors themselves secrete antiangiogenic factors (Folkman, 1995). Overall, it is thought that lung tumors produce factors that stimulate angiogenesis and stop producing others that would inhibit this process (Ohta & Watanabe).

Tumor angiogenesis is of particular interest as a promising prognostic indicator and as a target for innovative therapeutic interventions against tumor growth and metastases. Clinical trials with humanized recombinant anti-VEGF MoAb combined with chemotherapy in NSCLC are under way, as are studies of other agents that inhibit the tyrosine kinase activity of the VEGF receptors (Conti, 2002; Sekido et al., 2001). The antiangiogenic factors endostatin and angiostatin are under study in phase I clinical trials. Although not well studied in lung cancer, thalidomide also is considered to have potential use for its interference in angiogenesis activity. The matrix metalloproteinases (MMPs) are enzymes used by tumor cells to invade and destroy the basement membrane of normal cells, promoting metastases. Lung tumors both produce MMPs and induce other, neighboring cells to secrete MMPs. MMP inhibitors such as marimastat (British Biotech, Larden, United Kingdom), Ag 33340 (Agouron Pharmaceuticals, LaJolla, CA), and Bay 12-9566 (Bayer Corporation, West Haven, CT) are in clinical trials for SCLC and NSCLC (Bunn et al., 2000).

Tumor Markers

Identification of specific molecular characteristics of lung cancer has led to the investigation of possible prognostic and diagnostic markers in serum and sputum, but none have achieved a significantly clinical value. As mentioned previously, studies are under way examining the predictive nature

of chromosomal abnormalities and mutation or overexpression of oncogenes and TSGs (Valle et al., 2003). hnRNP A2/B1, an immunoreactive protein identified by the National Cancer Institute, has shown promise as a marker for early lung cancer detection, as its expression has been detected in resected lung tumors and in sputum cells shed from premalignant bronchial epithelium. Studies show that the protein is two- to threefold more sensitive for detection of lung cancer than chest x-ray or conventional sputum cytology. hnRNP A2/B1 currently is being tested in clinical trials for sensitivity and specificity (Tockman, 2000; Valle et al.).

Future Directions

The failure to significantly improve the course of lung cancer in the last few decades has led to a search for innovations. Development of the scientific knowledge of the pathogenesis of lung cancer has provided new directions for research. Application of this knowledge already is being applied in clinical settings for prevention, early detection, prognostic forecasting, and therapeutic treatments. Advances in science and technology, combined with successful efforts at tobacco control, will direct the future for the next generation of actual and potential patients with lung cancer.

References

Aberle, M.F., & McLeskey, S.W. (2003). Biology of lung cancer with implications for new therapies. *Oncology Nursing Forum, 30,* 273–278.

Bale, A., & Brown S. (2001). Etiology of cancer: Cancer genetics. In V.T. DeVita, S. Hellman, & S.A. Rosenberg (Eds.), *Cancer: Principles and practice of oncology* (6th ed., pp. 207–218). Philadelphia: Lippincott Williams & Wilkins.

Baselga, J. (2000). New therapeutic agents targeting the epidermal growth factor receptor. *Journal of Clinical Oncology, 18*(Suppl. 21), 54S–59S.

Baselga, J. (2002). Why the epidermal growth factor receptor? Rationale for cancer therapy. *Oncologist, 7*(Suppl. 4) 2–8.

Bunn, P., Soriano, A., Johnson, G., & Heasley, L. (2000). New therapeutic strategies for lung cancer: Biology and molecular biology come of age. *Chest, 117*(Suppl. 4), 163S–168S.

Carpenter, C.L., & Cantley, L.C. (2001). Essentials of signal transduction. In V.T. DeVita, S. Hellman, & S.A. Rosenberg (Eds.), *Cancer: Principles and practice of oncology* (6th ed., pp. 31–42). Philadelphia: Lippincott Williams & Wilkins.

Claudio, P.P., & Giordano, A. (2000). RB1 and RB2. In H. Pass, J. Mitchell, D. Johnson, A. Turrisi, & J. Minna (Eds.), *Lung cancer: Principles and practice* (2nd ed., pp. 133–155). Philadelphia: Lippincott Williams & Wilkins.

Conti, C.J. (2002). Vascular endothelial growth factor: Regulation in the mouse skin carcinogenesis model and use in angiogenesis cancer therapy. *Oncologist, 7*(Suppl. 3), 4–11.

Folkman, J. (1995). Clinical application of research on angiogenesis. *New England Journal of Medicine, 333,* 1757–1763.

Franklin, W.A., Veve, R., Hirsch, F.R., Helfrich, B.A., & Bunn, P.A. (2002). Epidermal growth factor receptor family in lung cancer and premalignancy. *Seminars in Oncology, 29*(Suppl. 4), 3–14.

Gazdar, A.F. (1993). Pathology's impact on lung cancer therapy. *Contemporary Oncology, 3*, 22–31.

Giaccone, G., Johnson, D.H., Manegold, C., Scagliotti, G.V., Rosell, R., Wolf, M., et al. (2002). A phase III clinical trial of ZD 1829 (Iressa®) in combination with gemcitabine and cisplatin in chemotherapy naïve patients with advanced non-small cell lung cancer (INTACT 1) [Abstract 4]. *Annals of Oncology, 13*(Suppl. 5), 2–3.

Gupta, A.K., Harris, E.R., Bernhard, E.J., Muschel, R.J., & McKenna, W.G. (2000). Overview of cell cycle and apoptosis. In H. Pass, J. Mitchell, D. Johnson, A. Turrisi, & J. Minna (Eds.), *Lung cancer: Principles and practice* (2nd ed., pp. 67–81). Philadelphia: Lippincott Williams & Wilkins.

Hahn, W.C., Counter, C.M., Lundberg, A.S., Beijersbergen, R.L., Brooks, M.W., & Weinberg, R.A. (1999). Creation of human tumour cells with defined genetic elements. *Nature, 400,* 464–468.

Janne, P.A., & Johnson, B.E. (2000). The role of MYC, JUN, and FOS oncogenes. In H. Pass, J. Mitchell, D. Johnson, A. Turrisi, & J. Minna (Eds.), *Lung cancer: Principles and practice* (2nd ed., pp. 98–119). Philadelphia: Lippincott Williams & Wilkins.

Johnson, D.H., Herbst, R., Giaccone, G., Schiller, J., Natale, R.B., Miller, V., et al. (2002). ZD 1839 (Iressa®) in combination with paclitaxel and carboplatin in chemotherapy-naïve patients with advanced non-small cell lung cancer (NSCLC): Results from a phase III clinical trial (INTACT 2) [Abstract 468]. *Annals of Oncology, 13*(Suppl. 5), 127–128,

Kaiser, U., Schilli, M., Haag, U., Neumann, K., Kreipe, H., Kogan, E., et al. (1996). Expression of bcl-2 protein in small cell lung cancer. *Lung Cancer, 15*(1), 31–40.

Kalemkerian, G.P. (2000). Growth factors. In H. Pass, J. Mitchell, D. Johnson, A. Turrisi, & J. Minna (Eds.), *Lung cancer: Principles and practice* (2nd ed., pp. 181–198). Philadelphia: Lippincott Williams & Wilkins.

Kris, M.G., Natale, R.B., Herbst, R.S., Lunch, T.J., Prager, D., Belani, C.P., et al. (2002). A phase II trial of ZD1839 (Iressa®) in advanced non-small cell lung cancer (NSCLC) patients who had failed platinum and docetaxel based regimens (IDEAL II) [Abstract]. *Proceedings of the American Society of Clinical Oncology, 12,* 292.

Lechner, J.F., & Fugaro, J.M. (2000). RAS and erbB2. In H. Pass, J. Mitchell, D. Johnson, A. Turrisi, & J. Minna (Eds.), *Lung cancer: Principles and practice* (2nd ed., pp. 89–97). Philadelphia: Lippincott Williams & Wilkins.

Liotta, L., & Liu, E. (2001). Essentials of molecular biology In V.T. DeVita, S. Hellman, & S.A. Rosenberg (Eds.), *Cancer: Principles and practice of oncology* (6th ed., pp. 3–17). Philadelphia: Lippincott Williams & Wilkins.

Mulligan-Kehoe, M.J., & Russo, A. (2000). General concepts of molecular biology related to lung cancer. In H. Pass, J. Mitchell, D. Johnson, A. Turrisi, & J. Minna (Eds.), *Lung cancer: Principles and practice* (2nd ed., pp. 5–66). Philadelphia: Lippincott Williams & Wilkins.

Nakagawa, K. (2001). Targeting the epidermal growth factor receptor in lung cancer: 9th World Lung Cancer Conference. *Signal, 2*(1), 17–20.

Ohta, Y., & Watanabe, Y. (2000). Current concepts of angiogenesis related to primary lung cancer. In H. Pass, J. Mitchell, D. Johnson, A. Turrisi, & J. Minna (Eds.), *Lung cancer: Principles and practice* (2nd ed., pp. 199–212). Philadelphia: Lippincott Williams & Wilkins.

Pezzella, F., Turley, H., Kuzu, I., Tungekar, M.F., Dunnill, M.S., Pierce, C.B., et al. (1993). bcl-2 protein in NSCLC. *New England Journal of Medicine, 329,* 690–694.

Phillips, C.A., & Nuwayhid, N.F. (1993). The malignant state: The molecular, cytogenetic and immunologic basis of cancer. In G.R. Weiss (Ed.), *Clinical oncology* (pp. 3–10). Norwalk, CT: Appleton and Lange.

Rosell, R., Li, S., Skacel, Z., Mate, J.L., Maestre, J., Canela, M., et al. (1993). Prognostic impact of mutated K-ras gene in surgically resected non-small cell lung cancer patients. *Oncogene, 8,* 2407–2412.

Ross, J. (2003). Biology of lung cancer. In M. Haas (Ed.), *Contemporary issues in lung cancer: A nursing perspective* (pp. 11–23). Sudbury, MA: Jones and Bartlett.

Salomon, D.S., Brandt, R., Ciardello, F., & Normanno, N. (1995). Epidermal growth factor-related peptides and their receptors in human malignancies. *Critical Reviews in Oncology/Hematology, 19,* 183–232.

Sekido, Y., Fong, K.M., & Minna, J.D. (2001). Molecular biology of lung cancer. In V.T. DeVita, S. Hellman, & S.A. Rosenberg (Eds.), *Cancer: Principles and practice of oncology* (6th ed., pp. 917–924). Philadelphia: Lippincott Williams & Wilkins.

Slebos, R.J., Kibbelaar, R.E., Dalesio, O., Kooistra, A., Stam, J., Meijer, C.J., et al. (1991). K-ras oncogene activation as a prognostic marker in adenocarcinoma of the lung. *New England Journal of Medicine, 323,* 561–565.

Sugio, K., Ishida, T., Yokoyama, H., Inoue, T., Sugimachi, K., & Sasazuki, T. (1992). Ras gene mutations as a prognostic marker in adenocarcinoma of the human lung without lymph node metastasis. *Cancer Research, 52,* 2903–2906.

Szak, S.T., Pietenpol, J., & Carbone, D.P. (2000). p53. In H. Pass, J. Mitchell, D. Johnson, A. Turrisi, & J. Minna (Eds.), *Lung cancer: Principles and practice* (2nd ed., pp. 120–132). Philadelphia: Lippincott Williams & Wilkins.

Tockman, M.S. (2000). Advances in sputum analysis for screening and early detection of lung cancer. *Cancer Control: Journal of the Moffitt Cancer Center, 7*(1), 19–24.

Valle, R., Chavany, C., Zhokov, T.A., & Jendoubi, M. (2003). New approaches for biomarker discovery in lung cancer. *Expert Review of Molecular Diagnostics, 3*(1), 55–67.

Witsuba, I., Lam, S., & Behrens, C. (1997). Molecular damages in the bronchial epithelium of current and former smokers. *Journal of the National Cancer Institute, 89,* 1966–1973.

Works, C., & Gallucci, B. (1996). Biology of lung cancer. *Seminars in Oncology Nursing, 12,* 276–284.

Yakubovskaya, M., Spiegelman, V., Luo, F., Malaev, S., Salnev, A., Zborovskaya, I., et al. (1995). High frequency of K-ras mutations in normal appearing lung tissues and sputum of patients with lung cancer. *International Journal of Cancer, 63,* 810–814.

Yarbro, J. (2000). Carcinogenesis. In C.H. Yarbro, M.H. Frogge, M. Goodman, & S.L. Groenwald (Eds.), *Cancer nursing: Principles and practice* (5th ed., pp. 48–54). Sudbury, MA: Jones and Bartlett.

CHAPTER 3

Lung Cancer Control

Marianne Davies, RN, MSN, ACNP, OCN®, Nancy G. Houlihan, RN, MA, AOCN®, and Margaret Joyce, MSN, RN, AOCN®

Introduction

Lung cancer is one of the leading causes of preventable death among men and women in the United States (Alberg & Samet, 2003) and has reached epidemic proportions since the middle of the 20th century. Although some progress is being made in treatment, efforts to control lung cancer have been modest compared with other major health threats. A reduction in smoking rates has led to decreased lung cancer incidence and mortality in men, but this trend is not expected to continue unless smoking is eliminated (Alberg & Samet). In addition to prevention efforts, an effective screening method is necessary so that early detection and intervention can alter the outcomes for those at high risk for developing lung cancer.

Lung cancer control entails multiple initiatives. This chapter will review the epidemiologic evidence for the disease; primary, secondary, and tertiary prevention strategies; tobacco control efforts; smoking cessation recommendations; and screening and early detection approaches.

Risk Factors in Lung Cancer

Smoking

Since the 1950s, smoking has been well established as the single most important risk factor for development of lung cancer (Doll & Hill, 1952; Levin & Gerhardt, 1950). Tobacco smoking is responsible for 80%–90% of lung cancers (Schottenfeld, 1995), and smokers are 20–40 times more likely to develop lung cancer than nonsmokers (Peto et al., 2000; Simonato et al., 2001).

The risk of lung cancer varies widely among smokers (Bach, Kattan, et al., 2003). A dose-exposure relationship exists between the development of lung cancer and (a) the number of cigarettes smoked per day, (b) duration of smoking, (c) degree of inhalation, (d) smoking of unfiltered cigarettes, and (e) age at which smoking is initiated (Bach, Kattan,

et al.; Gilliland & Samet, 1994; Hart et al., 2001; Kreuzer, Gerkin, Kreienbrock, Wellmann, & Wichmann, 2001; Kreuzer et al., 2002; Mao, 2001; Wynder & Kabat, 1988). Evidence to support age at initiation of smoking as an independent risk factor for lung cancer is conflicting (Benhamou & Benhamou, 1994; Hegmann et al., 1993). The risk may be attributable to increased length of smoking history (Samet, 1993).

The type of cigarette smoked also may have an impact on cancer risk. Those who smoke filtered cigarettes have a lower lifetime risk than those who smoke nonfiltered cigarettes (Lubin, 1984). One would postulate that those who smoke lower tar-content cigarettes would have a lower risk of lung cancer. However, often when smokers choose low-tar cigarettes, they smoke more and take deeper inspirations that negate the potential benefit of low tar content (Benhamou, Benhamou, Auquier, & Flamant, 1994; Zang & Wynder, 1992).

Smoking cessation reduces the risk of lung cancer development. Early studies indicate that the risk of lung cancer decreases in proportion to the number of years after smoking cessation and may reach 50% (Burns, 2000; Ebbert et al., 2003; Samet, 1992). Risk reduction after cessation also depends on the number of cigarettes smoked per day and how deeply the smoker inhales (Halpern, Gillespie, & Warner, 1993). The risk decline varies between heavier and lighter smokers and tumor type (Speizer, Colditz, Hunter, Rosner, & Hennekens, 1999). Significant benefits are not seen until five years after smoking cessation. Former smokers have an elevated risk of lung cancer for up to 30 years after smoking cessation (Ebbert et al.). This is consistent with recent evidence of cancer-associated genetic alterations in former smokers (Fearon, 1997; Mao et al., 1997).

Smoking of cigars, cigarillos, and pipe tobacco also increases lung cancer risk. A dose-response relationship is evident for the duration of use, cumulative consumption, and depth of inhalation (Baker et al., 2000; Boffetta et al., 1999; Iribarren, Tekawa, Sidney, & Friedman, 1999). Evidence indicates that age at the start of smoking is strongly related to risk, with smokers who start before the age of 20 having a fivefold increased risk compared with those who start after age 26 (Benhamou & Benhamou, 1994). In addition, the risk is higher among cigar smokers who were previously cigarette smokers.

Environmental Exposures

Passive exposure to environmental tobacco smoke is associated with increased risk of lung cancer in nonsmoking populations (Hu, Mao, Dryer, & White, 2002). Environmental tobacco smoke contains various toxic compounds that often are measured in higher amounts than inhaled smoke products because they are unfiltered (Tredaniel, Boffetta, Saracci, & Hirsch, 1994). The risk for developing lung cancer may increase by as much as 30% for people exposed to secondhand smoke for 25 or more years (Hackshaw, Law, & Wald, 1997; Janerich et al., 1990; Trendaniel et al.). Cardenas et al. (1997), using data from the Cancer Protection Study II, showed that lung cancer death rates were 20% higher in women married to smokers than in women married to nonsmokers. The risk was higher for women whose husbands smoked more than two packs per day, supporting a dose-response relationship.

Another form of environmental exposure is radon gas. Radon is a colorless, odorless, inert, radioactive gas found in the earth's crust that can accumulate in homes. As radon decays, it emits particles that damage the respiratory epithelium. Indoor radon exposure accounts for approximately 50%–80% of the total radiation transferred to humans, on average, in the United States (Lubin & Boice, 1989). The amount of radon in a home depends on ventilation and distance from the source. At high concentrations, radon has been shown to cause lung cancer among uranium miners and has a synergistic relationship with smoking (Lubin et al., 1995; Samet, Kutvirt, Waxweiler, & Key, 1984). Studies exploring the impact of residential radon have been controversial (Axelson et al., 1988; Blot et al., 1990; Kreuzer et al., 2002). A meta-analysis of eight studies examining the impact of residential radon on lung cancer supported an increased risk with exposure (Lubin & Boice, 1997). More recently, Kreuzer et al. (2002) found no significant trend in lung cancer risk with increasing residential radon levels.

Several air pollutants have been identified as possible contributors to lung cancer risk in industrialized countries (Caputi, Esposito, Mancini, & Giordano, 2002). Although evidence supports an association between pollution and lung cancer, most studies do not adequately control for confounding factors, such as smoking and occupational exposures.

Occupational Exposures

Occupational exposures account for up to 20% of lung cancers (Samet et al., 1984). Lung cancer mortality is higher among manual workers than non–manual workers, an effect that is only partially explained by smoking patterns (Hart et al., 2001). The International Agency for Research on Cancer has classified occupations that are associated with exposure to substances known to cause lung cancer and occupations that are suspected to increase the risk of developing lung cancer. A strong positive association has been found between lung cancer and occupational exposure to asbestos, coal tar, soot, creosote, asphalt, ether, chromium, nickel, and vinyl chloride (Mao, 2001; Samet et al., 1984). Occupations that pose the highest risk to men include miners; shipyard, dockyard, and railroad manufacture workers exposed to diesel exhaust; workers in nonferrous metal business and coal plants; and carpenters, roofers, painters, bus and truck drivers, mechanics, and welders. Occupations suspected of causing lung cancer in women are laundry and dry cleaner workers and glass workers (Doll, 1976; Garshick et al., 1988; Hammond, Selikoff, Lawther, & Seidman, 1976; Pohlabeln et al., 2000). Exposure from many of these occupations acts synergistically with primary and secondary tobacco smoke to further increase the risk of lung cancer (Kreuzer et al., 2002).

Asbestos has been one of the most extensively reviewed occupational agents known to cause lung cancer (Koskinen, Pukkala, Martikainen, Reijula, & Karjalainen, 2002; Ulvestad et al., 2002). The risk depends on type of asbestos and nature of exposure, which may help to explain an increased risk in certain occupations (Lee, 2001). A synergistic increase in lung cancer exists in smokers exposed to asbestos (Hammond et al., 1976; Lee).

Social Class

Socioeconomic status has been considered an important contributing factor to the development of lung cancer. The incidence of lung cancer is higher in lower socioeconomic groups (Hein, Suadicani, & Gyntelberg, 1992; Mansson, Marklund, Bengtsson, & Oden, 1995; Mao, 2001; Pearce & Bethwaite, 1997; Vagero & Persson, 1986; van Loon, Goldbohm, & van den Brandt, 1995). Some studies have suggested that socioeconomic status is related to lifestyle behaviors, such as diet, smoking, and occupation, which contribute to the increased risk of lung cancer (Kabat, Ng, & Wynder, 1993; Thun, 1998; Ziegler, Mayne, & Swanson, 1996). In a large, population-based study in Canada, 3,280 newly diagnosed patients with lung cancer and 5,073 controls were studied over a four-year period. A strong inverse association was found among education, family income, and lung cancer, independent of other confounding risks (Mao). Long-term influence of poor social circumstances beginning early in life also contributed to increased lung cancer mortality (Hart et al., 2001; Smith, Hart, Blane, & Hole, 1998). This may be attributed to poor overall lung health (Hart et al.). Antismoking interventions targeted toward this population may reduce the risk of lung cancer.

Gender

Given the same level of lifelong exposure to cigarette smoke, women have a 150% higher relative risk of developing lung cancer than men (Dwyer, Blizzard, Shugg, Hill, & Ansari, 1994; McDuffie, 1991; Risch et al., 1993; Zang & Wynder, 1992). The estimated risk for women increases as the following increase: levels of lifelong exposure to cigarette smoke, a higher tar yield per amount smoked, age of smoking initiation, duration of smoking, and number of cigarettes smoked each day. The findings are unrelated to differences in body surface area. However, women with lung cancer are two to three times more likely to have never smoked than men, suggesting that women may have a greater susceptibility to the effects of lung carcinogens (Radzikowska & Roszkowski, 2002; Zang & Wynder, 1996).

Physiologic differences in drug metabolism between men and women may contribute to increased susceptibility. Metabolism of drugs and carcinogens by cytochrome P450 enzyme is decreased in women (Dresler et al., 2000; Kure et al., 1996). In addition, women with a mutant genotype for the detoxification enzyme CYP1A1 have a larger cancer risk than men. These factors contribute to prolonged exposure to carcinogens, increasing relative risks in women (Dresler et al.; Guengerich & Turvy, 1991).

Hormones also may play a role in the etiology of lung cancer in females. The impact of age, length of menstrual cycles, reproductive history, and age at menopause has been controversial (Adami, Persson, Hoover, Schairer, & Bergkvist, 1989; Kreuzer et al., 2002; Liao et al., 1996; Seow et al., 2002; Taioli & Wynder, 1994). Lung cancer risk has been reported to be higher in women receiving estrogen replacement therapy (Adami et al.; Taioli & Wynder). Estrogens are hypothesized to promote bronchial cell proliferation, influence metabolism of carcinogens, or precipitate development of lung disease, which predisposes women to lung cancer. The impact of smoking and estrogen is undergoing research. Some studies have reported an apparent synergism, with a 32-fold increased risk of developing lung cancer in women who smoke and take estrogens, compared to women who never smoked (Taioli & Wynder, 1994). In contrast, Kreuzer et al. (2002) reported a reduced risk of lung cancer in women who were longtime users of hormone replacement therapy. As a result, the risk of estrogen and smoking remains unclear.

Age

Lung cancer is predominantly a disease of the elderly. Since 1990, the proportion of lung cancer cases in the United States occurring among patients 70 and older increased from 35% to 43% (Stewart, Bland, McGinnis, Morrow, & Eyre, 2000). The change in smoking prevalence in the same period has been reflected in a decreased incidence of lung cancer in younger people. Because of the latency of the disease, however, the incidence of lung cancer has not begun to decline in older patients. Of concern is the apparent rise in adolescent smoking patterns. Unless this pattern changes, lung cancer incidence in younger people can be expected to peak again in 30–40 years.

Race

Racial discrepancies for lung cancer are well documented (King & Brunetta, 1999). The National Cancer Institute's (NCI's) Surveillance, Epidemiology, and End Results Program provides a comparison of risks among various racial and ethnic groups in the United States. The most radical difference in incidence is between African Americans and Whites (Miller, 1993). The incidence among African American men is 122 per 100,000, compared to 78 per 100,000 among White men. African American women and White women have similar discrepancies in incidence rates (Howe et al., 2001). Racial differences in lung cancer mortality rates are explained by differences in the incidence of disease, but also reflect differences in survival rates. African American patients with lung cancer have a lower five-year survival rate (12%) than White patients (16%) (King & Brunetta). Researchers theorize that two factors contribute to this disparity: differences in the use of surgical treatment for early-stage lung cancer among African Americans and Whites and later-stage disease at time of diagnosis among African Americans (Bach, Cramer, Warren, & Begg, 1999; Greenwald, Polissar, Borgatta, McCorkle, & Goodman, 1998; King & Brunetta). Differences in rates also are assumed to be partially explained by different lifetime patterns of cigarette smoking (Schottenfeld, 1996). Compared with Whites, a higher percentage of African Americans are current smokers, smoke cigarettes higher in tar and nicotine, and prefer to smoke mentholated cigarettes, which may promote deeper inhalation. Among current smokers, African American males tend to smoke fewer cigarettes per day but start smoking at an earlier age and smoke longer. Reports of higher serum cotinine levels (a nicotine metabolite and marker of tobacco smoke exposure) in African Americans suggest differences in metabolism and excretion rates of tobacco carcinogens in African American smokers (Bach et al., 1999).

Physical Activity

Physical activity appears to be inversely associated with lung cancer incidence (Lee, Sesso, & Paffenbarger, 1999). In a prospective cohort study of 13,905 men between 1977 and 1993, the benefit was seen particularly with moderate levels of recreational physical activity for at least 6–8 hours per week. This effect was not appreciated with occupational physical activity at the same level (Thune & Lund, 1997). Increased pulmonary function that occurs with higher levels of physical activity may result in a decreased opportunity for interaction between inhaled carcinogens and the airways (Thune & Lund). However, in long-term smokers, neither occupational nor recreational physical activity has been shown to have an impact on lung cancer risk (Colbert et al., 2002).

Genetic Factors

Fewer than 20% of heavy smokers develop lung cancer, supporting the notion that genetic factors contribute to the development of lung cancer. In addition, first-degree relatives of patients with lung cancer have a significantly increased risk for developing lung cancer compared with controls (Ooi, Elston, Chen, Bailey-Wilson, & Rothschild, 1986; Samet, Humble, & Pathak, 1986). Several studies have begun to explore the relationship between genetic alterations and the risk of developing lung cancer. Certain genetic alterations may reduce the risk of lung cancer given the exposure factors previously identified (Ratnasinghe et al., 2003).

Researchers have studied the enzymes that are responsible for carcinogen activation and degradation (Goodman & Watson, 2002). The role of insulin-like growth factor-1 (IGF-1) and IGF-binding proteins has been studied in regard to carcinogenesis. Cells need IGF-1 to progress through the cell cycle; it promotes growth and reduces apoptosis. IGF-binding proteins have opposing actions; they inhibit cell proliferation and induce apoptosis (programmed cell death). In recent epidemiologic studies, high levels of plasma IGF-1 and low levels of IGF-binding proteins have been independently associated with greater risk of several cancers (Giovannucci, 1999a). In a prospective, case-controlled study of 18,000 patients, those with higher levels of IGF-binding protein-3 had a reduced risk of developing lung cancer (London et al., 2002).

Genetic alterations in the P450 family of hepatic enzymes affect the risk of developing lung cancer (Goodman & Watson, 2002). Cytochrome P4502A6 (CYP2A6) plays a role in the activation of tobacco-related carcinogens. Patients with a defect in this gene are twice as likely to develop lung cancer. In contrast, specific genetic modifications may cause gene instability and alter apoptosis, leading to increased incidence of cancer (Caputi, Groeger, et al. 2002; Garte, 1998). Although much research is necessary to understand the full role of genetics, these studies may help us to identify high-risk patients for whom early or more diligent screenings would be beneficial.

Prior Lung Dysfunction

Chronic bronchitis, emphysema, and asthma are associated with increased risk of lung cancer (Alavanja et al., 2001; Boffetta, Ye, Boman, & Nyren, 2002; Brownson & Alavanja, 2000; Mayne, Buenconsejo, & Janerich, 1999). The likelihood of developing lung cancer is increased when forced expiratory volume in one second is less than 60% (Kishi et al., 2002). In a multicenter study of 4,395 male smokers, the presence

of airway obstruction was found to be a stronger indicator in the development of lung cancer than age or degree of smoking, and the risk was proportional to the level of obstruction (Tockman, Anthonisen, Wright, & Donithan, 1987). Pulmonary function also is inversely related to mortality from lung cancer (Nomura, Stemmermann, Chyou, Marcus, & Buist, 1991). After adjustment for smoking history, women are at increased risk for developing lung cancer if they have a prior diagnosis of pneumonia or tuberculosis (Kreuzer et al., 2002).

Prior radiotherapy for breast cancer significantly increases the risk of developing lung cancer (Kreuzer et al., 2002; Neugut, Weinberg, Ahsan & Rescigno, 1999; Rubino et al., 2002). The risk is seen 10 years following radiation and for at least another 20 years. The risk is most notable in the ipsilateral lung in postmastectomy patients, while excessive risk is not identified in patients treated with breast-sparing lumpectomy (Zablotska & Neugut, 2003). Patients treated with radiation therapy for Hodgkin's disease are at particularly higher risk for developing lung cancer, as doses of radiation usually exceed 30 Gy. The risk increases even more for patients receiving concurrent alkylating agents and who have a history of smoking (Gilbert et al., 2003).

Dietary

Research suggests that poor diet is responsible for approximately 30% of all cancers (Willett & Trichopoulos, 1996). Several studies have shown an association between dietary intake of fruits and vegetables and reduced risk of lung cancer (Alavanja et al., 2001; Axelsson, Liljeqvist, Andersson, Bergman, & Rylander, 1996; Le Marchand, Yoshizawa, Kolonel, Hankin, & Goodman, 1989; Ziegler et al., 1986). The associated risk reduction may be as high as 30% with regular intake of fruits and vegetables. Risk reduction is greater when fruits and vegetables are consumed raw rather than cooked (Cooper, Eldridge, & Peters, 1999; Mayne, Handelman, & Beecher, 1996). Risk reduction also is related to the frequency and amount of consumption. Higher consumption is associated with lower risk (Feskanich et al., 2000). Although total intake of all fruits and vegetables is beneficial, the most protection appears to come from cruciferous vegetables, citrus fruits, and foods high in total carotenoids (DeStefani, Brennan, Boffetta, et al., 2002; DeStefani, Brennan, Ronco, et al., 2002; Feskanich et al.; Holick et al., 2002; Koo, 1988; Mao, 2001; Seow et al., 2002; Steinmetz & Potter, 1991; Steinmetz, Potter, & Folsom, 1993). This may be because of the anticarcinogenic, antioxidant action of carotenoids, such as lycopene; alpha carotene; beta carotene; lutein; vitamins A, C, and E; selenium; and flavonoids (Buring & Hennekens, 1995; DeStefani, Brennan, Boffetta, et al.; Le Marchand et al.; Michaud et al., 2000; Steinmetz & Potter; Ziegler et al., 1996). Smoking causes oxidative damage in the lungs. Antioxidants prevent this damage and later cancer development by neutralizing free radicals (Byers & Perry, 1992). The benefits of retinoids are seen specifically with natural dietary intake, whereas supplementation substantially increases lung cancer risk. Diets rich in alpha carotene and beta carotene are more predictive of reduced lung cancer risk; low intake of alpha carotene is associated with increased risk whereas low intake of beta carotene is not (Ziegler et al., 1996). Lycopene, the second most common carotenoid, is found predominantly in tomatoes. Dietary intake is inversely associated with lung cancer risk, independent of food preparation methods (Clinton et al., 1996; Giovannucci, 1999b). Flavonoids, found in apples and onions, have been associated with reduced risk. However, the bioavailability varies by part of food consumed and method of preparation (Knekt et al., 1997). A trend in reduction of lung cancer risk has been found with selenium supplementation in subjects with lower baseline levels; no impact has been identified in the general population (Reid et al., 2002).

Other areas of dietary analysis have included red meats, fish, dairy, fat content, soy, and salt. Total consumption of red meat has been found to be directly associated with lung cancer risk (Alavanja et al., 2001; Deneo-Pellegrini, DeStefani, Ronco, Mendilaharsu, & Carzoglio, 1996; DeStefani, Brennan, Ronco, et al., 2002; Mao, 2001). A significant increase in relative risk has been found when red meats are cooked at high temperatures, particularly fried, deep-fried, roasted, or grilled (Alavanja et al.; Sinha et al., 1998). The risk is not seen with white meat (DeStefani, Brennan, Boffetta, et al., 2002). Most of the effect of red meat is attributable to its fat content (DeStefani, Brennan, Boffetta, et al., 2002). In general, total fat intake is associated with an increased lung cancer risk. All other dietary lipids and dietary cholesterol have been associated with significantly increased risks of lung cancer as well (Deneo-Pellegrini et al.). Total, saturated, monounsaturated, and polyunsaturated fats are positively associated with lung cancer risk (DeStefani, Brennan, Boffetta, et al.). Results are conflicting for dairy products, which may be attributed to the varying fat content of milk (Axelsson et al., 1996; Knekt et al., 1991). Higher intake of soy foods significantly reduces the risk of lung cancer, independent of other dietary intake (Seow et al., 2002; Takezaki et al., 2001). Cooked or raw fish lowers the risk of lung cancer (Takezaki et al.).

The literature is increasingly suggesting that alcohol may increase risk of lung cancer, after controlling for cigarette smoking, in a dose-response fashion (Bandera, Freudenheim, & Vena, 2001). Variability in reports of risk has been attributed to differences in "recall of consumption" (Bandera, 2001). The risk is most notably seen with heavy consumption of beer and liquor, whereas consumption of wine may be protective (DeStefani, Correa, et al., 2002). Light or occasional consumption of beer and wine also may be protective (Djousse et al., 2002; Prescott, Gronbaek, Becker, & Sorensen, 1999). Bandera postulates that limited consumption may be indicative of people who lead an overall healthier lifestyle.

The association between alcohol and cancer is stronger for women than men. Men have more gastric alcohol dehydrogenase than do females for a given amount of alcohol ingested, thus increasing alcohol metabolism and lowering blood alcohol levels (Longnecker, 1999). The impact of cigarette smoking and alcohol is synergistic (Rachtan, 2002). Alcohol may change the capacity of liver enzymes to metabolize tobacco carcinogens. Heavy alcohol consumption also may alter the absorption of nutrients, particularly antioxidants, such as alpha and beta carotene, increasing the risk of cancer. In addition, alcohol metabolism is associated with production of free radicals, which have been implicated in carcinogenesis (Longnecker).

Primary and Secondary Prevention

Primary prevention remains the best approach to control lung cancer. Most lung cancers could be prevented by the elimination of smoking. If smoking were completely eradicated, an estimated 85% of lung cancers would be eliminated (Doll & Peto, 1981). Efforts to prevent smoking focus on antismoking education, legislation, and taxation. Antismoking legislation began in 1964 with the release of the U.S. Surgeon General's Report on the dangers of smoking. Laws were passed requiring health warnings on cigarette packaging (Doll, 1981). In 1995, the U.S. Food and Drug Administration (FDA) began to restrict advertising targeted at minors and to reduce access to cigarettes (Johnson & Ballin, 1995). In the following years, legislation for a national comprehensive tobacco control plan was initiated but halted in June 1998 because of a strong tobacco lobby. Almost all states have passed legislation prohibiting the sale of tobacco to minors and have imposed high excise taxes on cigarettes. These strategies are thought to be the most effective in reducing both the number of adolescents who smoke and the recruitment of new smokers (Aisner & Belani, 1993).

Although primary prevention is the most effective means of controlling lung cancer, the elimination of all smoking is unrealistic. Smoking cessation as a secondary goal can reduce the risk of lung cancer in a smoker. Cessation strategies will be reviewed more thoroughly later.

Chemoprevention (Tertiary Prevention)

The fact that fewer than 20% of heavy smokers develop lung cancer suggests that other factors may play a role in causation (Bilello, Murin, & Matthay, 2002). Chemoprevention agents are being investigated as a means of preventing primary or secondary cancer development after carcinogen exposure.

Cancer chemoprevention is a rapidly growing field that approaches carcinogenesis from a different perspective. Although preventing cancer may not be possible, interfering with the process of carcinogenesis may be possible. This entails the use of specific natural chemicals, which are pharmacologically active agents, to reverse, suppress, or prevent carcinogenesis (Goodman, 1993; Goodman et al., 1993; Huber, Lee, & Hong, 1993; Lippman, Spitz, Trizna, Benner, & Hong, 1994). Researchers are looking at two major areas of chemoprevention: (a) dietary micronutrients and their synthetic analogs and (b) synthetic agents, such as nonsteroidal anti-inflammatory drugs (NSAIDs) and retinoids.

Several large intervention trials initiated in the 1990s examined the effects of retinoid supplementation on reducing the subsequent risk for lung cancer. None of these trials showed a chemoprotective effect. The two largest and most publicized trials were the Alpha-Tocopherol, Beta-Carotene (ATBC) trial in Finland and the Beta-Carotene and Retinol Efficacy Trial (CARET). The ATBC trial was a primary prevention study of 29,133 males who smoked an average of one pack per day for 36 years. Patients were treated with beta carotene and/or alpha tocopherol (vitamin E) at a 5.5-fold higher dose than median dietary intake for 6.5 years. Vitamin E did not reduce the incidence of lung cancer, and participants receiving beta carotene alone or in combination with alpha-tocopherol had an 18% increase in incidence and mortality (Albanes et al., 1996; "The Effect of Vitamin E," 1994). The increased risk was most pronounced in participants who smoked more than 20 cigarettes per day ("The Effect of Vitamin E"). The CARET trial randomized 18,314 high-risk participants, male and female, to receive beta carotene and vitamin A (Thornquist et al., 1993). No benefit was found, and a 28% increased incidence and mortality was found in the treatment arm beginning 24 months after randomization (Hennekens et al., 1996; Omenn, 1998; Omenn et al., 1996). Although both of these studies found an overwhelming increase in cancer incidence, the mechanism is not yet understood. Beta carotene supplementation does increase the production of cytochrome P450 enzymes, which can activate carcinogens in the lung (Albanes et al., 1996). Beta carotene also was found to increase the conversion of carcinogens found in cigarette smoke to their carcinogenic form (Lippman & Spitz, 2001).

Although vitamin supplementation has not been shown to prevent lung cancer (Patterson, White, Kristal, Neuhouser, & Potter, 1997), certain foods have some preventive effect. A report of pooled data from two large cohort studies showed a 20%–25% lower risk of cancer in participants who consumed diets high in beta carotene and lycopene (Michaud et al., 2000).

Several biomarkers currently are under investigation, including epidermal growth factor receptor (EGFR), *HER2/neu, HER3, HER4,* and cyclooxygenase (COX)-inhibitors. Attractive pharmacologic targets include receptor and nonreceptor kinases, growth factor receptors, and enzymes (especially those of signal transduction pathways) (Dragnev, Stover, & Dmitrovsky, 2003).

COX-2 regulates the synthesis of prostaglandins that promote tumorigenesis. COX-2 overexpression inhibits apoptosis, and COX-2 is linked to regulation of angiogenesis. Overexpression of COX-2 occurs in lung cancer (Hosomi et al., 2000; Soslow et al., 2000). Increased expression of COX-2 has a negative prognostic impact on early stage lung cancer (Khuri et al., 2001). COX-2 inhibitors currently are being evaluated for cancer prevention (Hong & Sporn, 1997). Preliminary studies already have been reported on NSAIDs. NSAIDs have been shown to inhibit the development of lung cancer in animal models. Regular use of NSAIDs three times per week or more for one year suggests a possible chemoprotective benefit (Muscat et al., 2003). In a case-control study of 489 patients with lung cancer and 978 control subjects, daily intake of NSAIDs for at least two years prior to the study was associated with a 68% reduction in relative risk of lung cancer. The results suggest that regular NSAID intake may prevent tobacco carcinogenesis through COX-2 blockade (Harris, Padilla, Koumas, Ray, & Phipps, 2002).

EGFR activation plays a role in cell division and differentiation. EGFR abnormalities have been found in patients with lung cancer (Brabender et al., 2001). EGFR inhibitors may be used to oppose cell growth. They also may be helpful targets for receptor blockade. Although much remains to be explored, chemoprevention is the most promising area of exploration in lung cancer prevention. Biomarkers may be used in both risk assessment and as markers for response to therapy (Hong & Yang, 1997).

The Challenge of Tobacco Control

Lung cancer is believed to be the leading cause of cancer mortality in the United States. Epidemiologic evidence documents that almost 90% of lung cancers are attributable to a single cause—cigarette smoking. Although considerable strides have been made in detection and treatment of lung cancer, overall survival is dismal. Clearly, smoking avoidance or preventing people from starting to smoke and smoking cessation for current smokers would result in significantly decreased mortality. Prevention, specifically the primary prevention of avoiding tobacco smoke carcinogens, is a number-one target for public health advocates.

Tobacco smoke contains more than 4,000 chemicals, including carbon monoxide, formaldehyde, arsenic, and lead. It also contains several known carcinogens. The most notable carcinogen classes in tobacco include polycyclic aromatic hydrocarbons (PAHs) and N-nitrosamines. Of the PAHs, benzo(a)pyrene is the most extensively studied lung carcinogen. Metabolic activation of PAHs and N-nitrosamines can prompt DNA adduct formation, gene mutation, and a sequence of events that can lead to cancer (Koh, Kannler, & Geller, 2001).

Cigarette marketing and smoking practices have changed to a great extent since the U.S. Surgeon General first acknowledged the health consequences of smoking in 1964 in the now-famous Surgeon General's Report. When the first warning label "Caution: Cigarette smoking may be hazardous to your health" was placed on cigarette packaging in 1965, 42% of Americans smoked cigarettes. Today, approximately 25% of American adults continue to smoke. The combination of mounting information about the health risks of tobacco use and the development of related public policy have contributed to this decrease in the smoking population in the United States.

Public policy events have had an impact on smoking, including use of increasingly larger and stronger warning labels on cigarette advertising and packaging and the ban of tobacco ads on television and radio. In 1972, the Surgeon General warned of the increased risk from exposure to secondhand or environmental smoke, and the Environmental Protection Agency classified environmental tobacco smoke as a class A carcinogen. As a result, state and federal legislation began to restrict smoking in public places, including in airplanes and workplaces. Twenty years later, the Joint Commission on Accreditation of Healthcare Organizations required hospitals to be smoke free. Staff and patients alike are required to abstain from smoking inside hospitals.

A pivotal event occurred in 1998 when the attorneys general of 46 states sued the tobacco industry to recover the Medicaid health costs of treating tobacco-related illnesses. The states settled the suit to collectively receive $206 billion dollars paid out over 25 years. This settlement, known as the Master Tobacco Settlement, redresses the harm the tobacco industry caused by withholding information about the risks and dangers of smoking. In return for the settlement monies, states cannot file additional lawsuits against the tobacco companies, although individuals can.

Data about why people continue to smoke despite clear warnings about the consequences of smoking point to the highly addictive nature of nicotine found in tobacco products. Nicotine is the initial source of tobacco pleasure and continued source of tobacco dependence. It is as addictive as heroin and cocaine. Nicotine activates receptors in the brain to release neurotransmitters that cause pleasurable mood-altering effects. Neurotransmitter-induced effects of nicotine are listed in Table 3-1. Unfortunately, like other addictive substances, the body becomes tolerant of the nicotine and requires more and more of it to achieve the same effect. The user also experiences withdrawal symptoms when the substance is taken away, so that the continued use of the nicotine is perpetuated. To help those trying to quit smoking, one must view the cigarette as a nicotine delivery device and understand the role of nicotine in tobacco dependence (Cooley, 2003).

Historically, nursing as a profession always has been in the forefront of advocacy and action concerning public health issues. Individual nurses can take positive action toward tobacco control on a variety of levels (Gallagher & Holm, 1996). The

Table 3-1. Neurotransmitter-Induced Effects of Nicotine

Neurotransmitter	Physiologic Effect
Acetylcholine	Increase stimulation Increase cognitive performance
Beta-endorphin	Decrease anxiety and tension
Dopamine	Increase pleasure Decrease appetite
Norepinephrine	Increase stimulation Increase alertness and vigilance Decrease appetite
Serotonin	Increase relaxation Decrease stress Decrease appetite

Note. From "Understanding and Treating Tobacco Dependence in Adults With Lung Cancer" (p. 243) by M.E. Cooley in M. Hass (Ed.), *Contemporary Issues in Lung Cancer: A Nursing Perspective,* 2002, Sudbury, MA: Jones and Bartlett. Copyright 2002 by Jones and Bartlett. Reprinted with permission.

first level is to become aware of the problem related to tobacco use. Oncology nurses, because of their extensive involvement in the treatment of cancer, management of symptoms, and support of patients, may overlook the overwhelming harm caused by tobacco and the necessary work of prevention.

The second level of participation in tobacco control is initiation of personal action. Nurses are in a unique position to foster smoking cessation because nurses are viewed as a credible source of health information and have access to large numbers of smokers who may be ready to attempt to quit. Effective treatment for tobacco dependence exists, and the first step in this process is screening for tobacco use and advising smokers to quit. Tobacco-dependence treatment guidelines are described in a subsequent section.

Personal action also includes individual nurses expressing opinions about tobacco-related health policy or regulation. Elected representatives and other government officials view nurses as credible and trustworthy. Communication from a nurse who is a voter can be powerful. Nurses can provide valuable information about the impact of tobacco use on health and public safety. One avenue for advocacy on tobacco issues is through the Oncology Nursing Society's (ONS) online Legislative Action Center (LAC) (www.ons.org/xp6/ONS/News.xml/LAC.xml). ONS issues "Action Alerts" when federal initiatives come up for discussion and vote. Nurses who indicate willingness to be contacted receive electronic messages about the issue, including advice and direction to contact their legislators. Nurses also can check the LAC on their own and learn of pending issues. Often, this form of advocacy takes very little time in the age of electronic communication, but it can have a strong impact on a legislator who is forming an opinion or deciding how to vote on a particular issue.

The third level of participation entails nurses joining together to initiate or support public action. Nurses can make the largest impact on lung cancer through involvement in community, state, and national programs to deter smoking and to protect nonsmokers from environmental tobacco smoke. The tobacco industry has enormous resources to market products and to gather political support to avoid interference in business activities. Community strategies to counter the tobacco industry's efforts include restricting minors' access to tobacco; widely disseminating effective school-based tobacco programs; reducing the appeal of tobacco products through advertising restrictions; and raising the cost of tobacco products.

Nurses also can take action against the international epidemic of tobacco use through organizational support for the World Health Organization's Framework Convention on Tobacco Control (FCTC). The FCTC is a treaty that calls for international cooperation to curb tobacco advertising, apply health warning labels on cigarette packaging, protect nonsmokers in public places from exposure to tobacco smoke, mark tobacco products to eliminate smuggling, and discourage duty-free sale of tobacco.

Lastly, nursing as a discipline must pursue additional research and evidence in the areas of tobacco cessation and prevention of tobacco use. Researchers should be encouraged to consider tobacco use as a variable potentially affecting outcomes in other research studies. Nursing research about tobacco, although increasing, has been limited and appears to lag behind other scientific contributions to the field. This may be related to such factors as the interdisciplinary nature of tobacco dependence and care, but a call has been made to increase nursing research contributions to this public health issue (Sarna & Lillington, 2002).

Tobacco Dependence Treatment

A key feature of the updated Public Health Service's (PHS's) Clinical Practice Guideline *Treating Tobacco Use and Dependence* (Fiore et al., 2000) is the conceptualization of tobacco use as a chronic illness rather than a "bad habit." The focus of the guideline is the aggressive combat of a life-threatening disease process through the use of medication, counseling, and social intervention. The guideline is evidence-based, broad in scope, and intended to help clinicians overcome obstacles in addressing this problem. Reasons that clinicians most frequently cite for failure to assess and treat tobacco dependence include a relative lack of familiarity with the specialized assessment of nicotine dependence or the efficacy of available treatments, inadequate institutional sup-

port for such interventions, or the time restraints of patient care (Ahuja, Weibel, & Leone, 2003).

Screening

Screening for tobacco use at every visit is the single most important step in addressing tobacco use. Systematic procedures that query and document tobacco use are recommended. The PHS's practice guidelines suggest expanding the vital sign assessment to designate a patient as a "current, former, or never" smoker (Fiore et al., 2000). This first step—asking every patient about tobacco use at every visit—separates patients into three treatment categories: patients willing to quit, patients unwilling to quit, and patients who have recently quit. Brief clinician interventions aimed explicitly at each category then can be delivered.

Brief Clinical Intervention

A brief message or advice from a clinician (nurse or physician) can be critical in emphasizing and personalizing the importance of smoking cessation. Smoking cessation is a dynamic process involving several stages through which current smokers move back and forth before finally achieving sustained cessation (Risser, 1996). Different counseling approaches are indicated for smokers at different stages in the process of quitting (see Table 3-2). The brief intervention strategy from the PHS Clinical Practice Guideline (Fiore et al., 2000) centers around the "5 A's" (see Figure 3-1) for those

Table 3-2. The Stage of Change	
Stages of Change	**Therapeutic Task of the Clinician**
Precontemplation: No intent of quitting	Discuss benefits of quitting and reasons for not smoking.
Contemplation: Aware of need but ambivalent	Motivate by giving personally relevant feedback.
Planning: Movement toward decision	Establish quit date, and build plan to overcome barriers.
Action: Initial cessation	Provide support, and assess adequacy of plan.
Maintenance: Establish non-smoking over months to years	Continue vigilant relapse preventive efforts, and reinforce benefits of quitting.
Termination: No urges to smoke	Track years since quitting.

Note. From "Prevention of Lung Cancer: The Key Is to Stop Smoking," by N.L. Risser, 1996, *Seminars in Oncology Nursing, 12,* p. 263. Copyright 1996 by W.B. Saunders. Reprinted with permission.

Figure 3-1. The 5 A's for Brief Intervention

Ask about tobacco use at every visit.

Advise smokers to quit (i.e., "I think it is important for you to quit smoking now, and I can help you.").

Assess readiness to make a quit attempt (e.g., within the next 30 days).

Assist in the quit attempt.
- Set a quit date.
- Encourage specific plans.
- Recommend the use of approved pharmacotherapy, except in special circumstances.
- Help patient obtain extra treatment or social support.
- Provide supplemental materials.

Arrange follow-up contact, preferably within the first week after the quit date.

Note. From *Treating Tobacco Use and Dependence* [Clinical Practice Guideline] (p. 26), by M.C. Fiore, W.C. Bailey, S.J. Cohen, S.F. Dorfman, M.G. Goldstein, E.R. Gritz, et al., 2000, Rockville, MD: U.S. Department of Health and Human Services, Public Health Service.

---

patients who indicate desire to quit and the "5 R's" (see Figure 3-2) for patients who use tobacco but are unwilling to quit at this time. Relapse prevention for a recent tobacco quitter can take the form of discussion regarding threats to or problems encountered during abstinence. These interventions are meant to be short, often requiring less than three minutes of clinician time.

Intensive Clinical Intervention

Smoking cessation treatment provided by specialists offers more opportunity for behavioral modification, stresses long-term relapse prevention, and explores smoking-related behavioral triggers. Sessions may include individual or group counseling in addition to aggressive pharmacotherapy. A strong dose-response relationship exists between counseling intensity and cessation success (Ahuja et al., 2003). Referral to intensive smoking-cessation programs is especially efficacious and cost effective. Smoking-cessation treatment should be included as a paid or covered benefit by health benefit plans (Fiore et al., 2000).

Nicotine Replacement Therapy

Nicotine withdrawal symptoms and cravings often cause early relapses within the first week after quitting. Acute withdrawal symptoms experienced with nicotine abstinence are irritability, anxiety, difficulty concentrating, restlessness, increased appetite, and depressed affect. Nicotine replacement products are intended to relieve nicotine cravings and withdrawal symptoms. Nicotine replacement therapy (NRT) is designed to deliver nicotine more slowly and usually at a lower dosage level than a patient normally achieves from smoking. After the initial abstinence period, nicotine replacement products should be gradually withdrawn and used only to prevent relapse. Table 3-3 describes the five forms of NRT currently available: nicotine patch, gum, lozenge, spray, and inhaler. The nicotine inhaler and spray are available by prescription only; the patch, gum, and lozenge can be obtained without a prescription.

Combination NRT uses a passive-dosing system of nicotine (i.e., the patch) in concert with an as-needed delivery product (i.e., gum, inhaler, lozenge, or spray) that allows for self-titrated dosing based on the patient's perceived need. Limited data are available about this combination strategy; however, the PHS Clinical Practice Guideline recommends that patients be encouraged to use combined treatments if they are unable to quit using a single type of first-line pharmacotherapy (Fiore et al., 2000).

Bupropion SR

Bupropion sustained release (SR) is the first FDA-approved non-nicotine medication for smoking cessation. Analysis of two large, multicenter trials showed that bupropion SR approximately doubled long-term abstinence rates when compared to placebo. Its mechanism of action is presumed to be mediated by its capacity to block neural re-uptake of dopamine and/or norepinephrine. It is contraindicated in patients with a seizure disorder or a prior diagnosis of bulimia or anorexia nervosa, those who have used a monoamine oxidase inhibitor within the past 14 days, or those on another medication that contains bupropion (Fiore et al., 2000).

Patients should begin taking bupropion SR one to two weeks before they quit smoking. Initially, patients are instructed to take 150 mg every morning for three days. Then,

---

Figure 3-2. The 5 R's for Enhancing Motivation to Quit Tobacco

---

Relevance: Make quitting personally relevant. Connect tobacco to patient's disease status or social situation (e.g., having children at home).

Risks: Ask the patient to identify potential risks of tobacco.

Rewards: Ask the patient to identify potential benefits of quitting.

Roadblocks: Ask patient to identify barriers to quitting, and note elements of therapy to address barriers.

Repetition: Repeat motivational message with every encounter.

Note. From *Treating Tobacco Use and Dependence* [Clinical Practice Guideline] (pp. 32–33), by M.C. Fiore, W.C. Bailey, S.J. Cohen, S.F. Dorfman, M.G. Goldstein, E.R. Gritz, et al., 2000, Rockville, MD: U.S. Department of Health and Human Services, Public Health Service.

Table 3-3. Nicotine Replacement Therapy

Product	Dose	Duration	Adverse Effects
Nicotine patch	For 1–25 cigarettes per day 21 mg per 24 hours 14 mg per 24 hours 7 mg per 24 hours More than 25 cigarettes per day: can start with 21–42 mg per 24 hours Less than 10 cigarettes per day: should start with 7 mg per 24 hours	 4 weeks 2 weeks 2 weeks	Local skin reaction, insomnia
Nicotine gum	For 1–25 cigarettes per day: 2 mg gum (up to 24 pieces) More than 25 cigarettes per day: 4 mg gum (up to 24 pieces)	Up to 12 weeks	Mouth soreness, dyspepsia
Nicotine inhaler	6–16 cartridges per day	Up to 6 months	Local irritation of mouth and throat, nasal irritation
Nicotine nasal spray	8–40 doses per day	3–6 months	Nasal irritation
Nicotine lozenge*	9–15 lozenges per day For less than 30 minutes until first cigarette of day: 4 mg lozenge For 30 minutes or greater until first cigarette of day: 2 mg lozenge	6 weeks then taper	Nausea, hiccups, coughing, heartburn

* Based on information from Foulds, 2003.

Note. From "Lung Cancer: The Oncologist's Role in Smoking Cessation," by R. Ahuja, S.B. Weibel, and F.T. Leone, 2003, *Seminars in Oncology, 30*, p. 98. Copyright 2003 by Elsevier. Adapted with permission.

the dosage should be increased to 150 mg twice a day and continued until 7–12 weeks after the patient's quit date. For maintenance therapy, patients may be instructed to take 150 mg twice a day for up to six months. If insomnia is marked, taking the second dose earlier in the day (i.e., in the afternoon, at least eight hours after the first dose) may be helpful.

Second-Line Therapy

Nortriptyline and clonidine are two other medications that can be used for smoking cessation, although the FDA has not approved either for this use. The PHS's Clinical Practice Guideline suggests these two agents be considered under a physician's direction for patients who are unable to use first-line medications or who are unable to quit using first-line therapy (Fiore et al., 2000). Limited data are available, but a few studies do show efficacy for both agents compared to placebo in increasing abstinence rates.

Summary

Clinicians can have a significant impact on patients who smoke or who recently quit smoking by making smoking cessation a priority message in the course of healthcare con-

sultation. The updated PHS Clinical Practice Guideline *Treating Tobacco Use and Dependence* offers specific evidence-based information in full text and a "Quick Reference Guide for Clinicians" for reference on this important topic. It is available online at www.surgeongeneral.gov/tobacco/default.htm. A consumer version, "You Can Quit Smoking," is available at www.ahrq.gov/consumer/tobacco/quits.htm or by calling the Agency for Healthcare Research and Quality toll free at 800-358-9295. Primary prevention (helping people avoid the carcinogens in tobacco smoke) is the key to decreasing lung cancer's morbidity and mortality.

Screening and Early Detection

Overall five-year survival from lung cancer, regardless of stage, is approximately 14%. However, surgical resection of early-stage disease can produce cures, with five-year survival from resected stage I lung cancers as high as 70%. Unfortunately, less than 16% of lung cancers are localized at the time of diagnosis (Jemal et al., 2004). Most lung cancers are diagnosed in advanced stages, and five-year survival of locally advanced and metastatic disease is less than 10%. Advanced lung cancer accounts for more cancer deaths in the United

States than the combination of the next three most common causes of death from cancer: colorectal, breast, and prostate. Yet, lung cancer is the only one of these cancers for which no screening recommendations exist (Jett, 2000; Joyce & Houlihan, 2001).

Effective early detection of a disease requires a preclinical phase of the disease, the technology to detect the disease in the preclinical stage, and the ability to employ effective interventions during the "period of opportunity" (Kennedy, Miller, & Prindiville, 2000). Ample evidence exists to support a preclinical phase of lung cancer. Accumulation of genetic mutations of endobronchial cells leading to progressive malignancies and invasion have been well identified. The earlier a lung cancer is identified, the better are the patient's chances for survival (Naruke, Tsuchiya, Kondo, Asamura, & Nakayama, 1997). Research, however, has failed to produce the definitive technology required for systematic surveillance of high-risk individuals. Recent advances in technology and understanding have produced studies that offer an encouraging vision for the value of early detection and effective treatment (Kennedy et al., 2000).

Elements of Screening Tests

Henschke, Yankelevitz, Libby, and Kimmel (2002) defined screening as the pursuit of presymptomatic, early diagnosis for the purpose of effective early intervention that incorporates specific regimens, diagnostic distributions, and curability. The benefit of a screening test is assessed according to two main criteria. The first is that the test must increase life expectancy by detecting the disease earlier so that the usual course can be altered through treatment. The second criterion is that the test should not cause pain or harm to the individual or society. Harm should not occur directly from the test or indirectly, as a result of false positives, which lead to undue anxiety and unnecessary, invasive, and dangerous procedures. In addition, society should not be affected unnecessarily by vast appropriation of resources nor interference in the provision of care to others (Bach, Kelley, Tate, & McCrory, 2003).

Efficacy of screening tests is evaluated through randomized clinical trials, population-based studies, and observational studies in selected cohorts (see Table 3-4). In randomized trials, individuals undergo varying intensities of treatment, and disease-specific mortality is observed. In population-based studies, the impact of a disease-specific screening program implemented across a broad population is evaluated through changes in the disease-related mortality rate in the population. Finally, the observational study of screening a specific cohort is evaluated on the frequency with which the test can detect early stages of the disease and the impact it has on disease-specific mortality. This is determined by data on outcomes of study participants with early-stage disease and documentation of survival (Bach, Niewoehner, Black, & the American College of Chest Physicians, 2003).

Screening programs for lung cancer aimed at increasing the detection of early-stage disease have been the targets of investigation for the last 50 years. Despite the evidence that specific screening tests can detect cancers earlier, no complementary decline in mortality has resulted, and the new technological advances have led to confusion in interpretation and treatment. Studies continue to examine whether traditional methods, including sputum cytology and chest x-ray (CXR), have merit while newer studies test the efficacy of low radiation dose computed tomography (LDCT) scanning and molecular, genetic, and cellular characteristic relevance (Bach, Kelley, et al., 2003). The following is a review of screening program research and the tests currently used for early detection of lung cancer (see Figure 3-3).

Chest Radiography

Chest radiography or x-ray is the most commonly used screening test for lung cancer based on its usefulness in detecting lung cancers in symptomatic patients (Bach, Niewoehner, et al., 2003). However, CXR has variable sensitivity for identifying malignant lesions depending on the size and location of the lesion, quality of the image, and skill of the interpreting physician. As a screening tool, use of CXR has not led to a reduction in mortality (Ginsberg, Vokes, & Rosenzweig, 2001).

Three large, randomized controlled trials of CXR were conducted during the 1960s and 1970s in the United States,

Table 3-4. Evaluation of Screening Tests

Method	Description	Outcome Criteria
Randomized clinical trials	Random assignment to different screening technique for comparison	Disease-specific mortality rate in trial arms
Population-based studies	Implement screening program to a population and observe for change	Disease-specific mortality rate in population
Observation-based studies	Frequency of detection in select cohorts (early stage)	Disease-specific mortality rate in cohort or documentation of survival in study participants

Figure 3-3. Screening Tests for Lung Cancer

- Sputum cytology
- Chest radiography
- Low radiation dose computed tomography
- Fluorescence bronchoscopy

England, and Czechoslovakia. These trials compared the benefit of regular CXR with less-frequent x-ray (Berlin, Buncher, Fontana, Frost, & Melamed, 1984; Fontana et al., 1984; Kubick & Polak, 1990). The NCI-sponsored Mayo Lung Project focused on the combined impact of regular sputum cytology in conjunction with CXR. In all three studies, lung cancer was detected more often in the screened group with an increased number at earlier stages. However, no difference was found in cumulative mortality (Bach, Niewoehner, et al., 2003).

NCI has included CXR in the current Prostate, Lung, Colorectal, and Ovarian Cancer Screening Trial, a national trial examining whether screening will reduce the number of deaths from these four cancers (Prorok et al., 2000). The advantage of the lung cancer portion of this trial over previous trials is that a randomized control group is assigned to no screening, providing a better comparison. In addition, women are included for the first time in a lung cancer screening trial (Kosco & Held-Warmkessel, 2000). Results of this trial may provide more definitive information about the usefulness of CXR for lung cancer screening.

Sputum Cytology

Sputum cytology as a screening test for lung cancer has been studied extensively in conjunction with CXR. The rationale for use of sputum samples for a screening test is that many individuals with lung cancer have cancerous cells in their sputum at the time of diagnosis (Bach, Niewoehner, et al., 2003). NCI funded two randomized studies combining sputum cytology and CXR. The Johns Hopkins Lung Project and the Memorial Sloan-Kettering Cancer Center Lung Cancer Screening Program randomized patients to CXR alone or CXR plus sputum cytology. Individuals were assigned to regular CXR with or without sputum samples at four-month intervals for five years. These studies primarily were designed to test the incremental benefit of sputum cytology in a CXR-screened cohort. The results of both studies showed no difference in the number of lung cancers detected, the percentage that were resectable, or the lung cancer mortality rates, although this may have been related to the study design and insensitivity of sputum cytology (Bach, Kelley, et al., 2003).

New techniques to increase the sensitivity of sputum analysis now are under investigation. Identification of molecular abnormalities in sputum epithelial cells has led to beginning clinical trials for screening purposes. Two monoclonal anti-

bodies are being used on archived sputum samples from the Johns Hopkins study on subjects who developed lung cancer after moderate dysplasia (Kennedy et al., 2000). Other study targets include evidence of aberrant protein overexpression and specific genetic changes in proto-oncogenes (Ras family), tumor suppressor genes (*p53, 3p, 9p*), and microsatellite gene alterations (Tockman, 2000). These enhanced techniques in sputum analysis offer the potential for determining a molecular diagnosis of lung cancer far in advance of clinical presentation.

Low Radiation Dose Computed Tomography

In the 1970s, the availability of computed tomography (CT) introduced a major advance in the ability to detect and stage lung cancer without invasive techniques (Jett, 2000). LDCT scanning, also known as helical or spiral CT, is a new technique that produces a low-resolution image of the entire thorax obtained in a single breath-hold. LDCT offers the advantages of a lower radiation exposure, no IV contrast injection, and lower cost than a standard chest CT (Henschke et al., 1999). The scan is very sensitive and capable of detecting nodules as small as 2–3 mm at their greatest diameter. In addition, data obtained in LDCT can be used to construct three-dimensional images from sequential scans to assess for change in size and appearance of nodules and can avoid invasive procedures for benign lesions. These two factors, the ability to identify very small lesions and to prevent unnecessary procedures, support its usefulness as a screening tool (Bach, Niewoehner, et al., 2003).

Multiple international trials of LDCT in Japan, the United States, and Germany were conducted during the 1990s. The results of these observational studies revealed that LDCT detected noncalcified pulmonary nodules, malignant tumors,

Figure 3-4. Picture of Low-Dose Computed Tomography for Screening

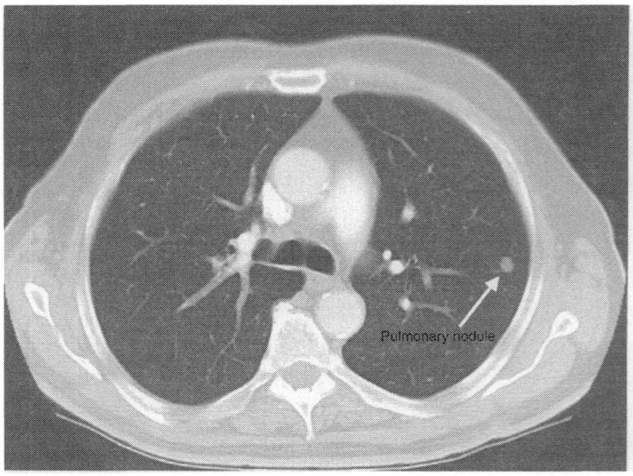

and stage I tumors more often when compared with chest ra-diography (Henschke et al., 1999, 2001). Large observational and randomized trials are under way to further examine the usefulness of LDCT. The New York–based Early Lung Can-cer Action Project (ELCAP) study targets 10,000 current or former smokers for annual screening and should yield infor-mation on the frequency of abnormal test results, the diag-nostic workup of abnormalities, and the frequency of unnec-essary procedures and interval-diagnosed cancers. The Inter-national ELCAP coordinates many trial activities, setting stan-dard protocols for future data pooling. NCI is conducting a randomized trial of 50,000 individuals with a smoking his-tory comparing CXR with LDCT. These projects are expected to take years but should provide answers to many of the ques-tions surrounding the usefulness of LDCT as a screening tool (Bach, Niewoehner, et al., 2003). Recommendations for in-terested high-risk individuals should include referral to cen-ters offering clinical trials of LDCT. To locate these centers see www.nyelcap.org/, www.cancer.gov/NLST, or www.cancer.gov/nlst/screeningcenters or call 800-4-CAN-CER.

Concerns exist about the impact of LDCT as a screening tool. The sensitivity of the increasingly improving scan tech-nology results in discovery of many abnormalities that require monitoring but do not require treatment. The risk of unnec-essary procedures and overdiagnosis and the associated anxi-ety for individuals present a potential source of harm. In ad-dition, the cost of mass screening with LDCT for high-risk individuals and the subsequent follow-up scanning, consul-tation, and other testing may not prove to be cost-effective if mortality is not impacted. Trials of CXR and sputum cytol-ogy described previously have identified earlier stage cancers that were resectable but did not produce improvement in mortality. The effectiveness of LDCT for screening is prom-ising but still must be determined (Bach, Kelly, et al., 2003).

Fluorescence Bronchoscopy

Lung imaging fluorescence endoscopy (LIFE) bronchos-copy is another method for detecting early malignant lesions. Conventional bronchoscopy, which uses white light for vi-sualization of bronchial tissues, can be ineffective in diagnos-ing carcinoma in situ and micro-invasive tumors. LIFE bron-choscopy systems deliver blue light to the bronchial surface, which can more clearly identify areas of dysplasia, carcinoma in situ, and invasive carcinoma. Clinical trials have docu-mented that this technique greatly enhances the ability to lo-calize early and otherwise invisible lesions in current and past smokers. Other trials have employed LIFE bronchoscopy for diagnosing lesions in those with dysplastic sputum cytology (Lam et al., 1998). However, application of this technique for screening has yet to be determined for several reasons. Bron-choscopy only can highlight areas in the large central airways (hilar) and is, therefore, not useful for identifying the more

common peripheral lesions (Kennedy, Lam, & Hirsch, 2001). The procedure is invasive and expensive and may lead to unnecessary procedures and post-procedure complications (Kennedy et al., 2001). Finally, classification systems and treatment strategies for metaplasia and dysplasia are still un-der development (Kosco & Held-Warmkessel, 2000).

LIFE bronchoscopy is of value in acquiring tissue for molecular biology studies of lung carcinogenesis. Bronchial mucosal cells that appear histologically normal in high-risk individuals have been found to be littered with genetic abnor-malities. Fluorescence bronchoscopy can identify areas of preneoplastic tissue for studies defining progression to neo-plasia. Studies also have indicated a correlation between ab-normal fluorescence and angiogenic dysplasia, a key step in the transition of intraepithelial preneoplasia to submucosal invasion.

Although much work is needed to define the significance of these changes, development of chemoprevention strategies and preoperative evaluation of disease in resectable patients may be relevant (Kennedy et al., 2001).

Future Challenges

Recent advances have renewed the hope that early detec-tion of lung cancer is possible and may improve survival. These advances include a better definition of risk groups, better chest imaging, better localization of endobronchial le-sions, and better local treatment modalities. Kennedy et al. (2000) outlined the future challenges and areas of research that will continue to address these issues.
- Advancing sputum sensitivity
- Improving definitions of risk factors to narrow the risk group and target screening
- Improving fluorescence bronchoscopy to be more sensi-tive and localize more distal lesions
- Validating LDCT as an inexpensive, safe, fast, sensitive, and specific screening tool
- Evaluating positron emission technology scans as an ad-junct to LDCT
- Developing and validating localized therapies for early lesions to include advances in brachytherapy, photody-namic therapy, cryotherapy, and laser therapy

In addition, population-based studies of all of these techniques are needed for national screening recommendations to be made.

Early detection and treatment is the only strategy other than smoking cessation than can affect the epidemic and death rates from lung cancer. An estimated 50 million people in the United States currently smoke, and another 50 million are past smokers. The numbers of new lung cancer cases and deaths increase each year. For many political and financial reasons, lung cancer has not been able to attract the research funding devoted to other cancers and diseases despite its epidemic rates and public health threat. Only recently have advocacy programs been developed to increase awareness about the need to address lung cancer so that more research dollars are devoted to this important health concern. Continued research is vital to reduce mortality and save the many victims who would otherwise perish, perhaps unnecessarily (Kennedy et al., 2000).

References

Adami, H.O., Persson, I., Hoover, R., Schairer, C., & Bergkvist, L. (1989). Risk of cancer in women receiving hormone replacement therapy. *International Journal of Cancer, 44,* 833–839.

Ahuja, R., Weibel, S.B., & Leone, F.T. (2003). Lung cancer: The oncologist's role in smoking cessation. *Seminars in Oncology, 30,* 94–103

Aisner, J., & Belani, C.P. (1993). Lung cancer: Recent changes and expectations of improvements. *Seminars in Oncology, 20,* 383–393.

Alavanja, M.C., Field, R.W., Sinha, R., Brus, C.P., Shavers, V.L., Fisher, E.L., et al. (2001). Lung cancer risk and red meat consumption among Iowa women. *Lung Cancer, 34*(1), 37–46.

Albanes, D., Heinonen, O.P., Taylor, P.R., Virtamo, J., Edwards, B.K., Rautalahti, M., et al. (1996). Alpha-tocopherol and beta-carotene supplements and lung cancer incidence in the alpha-tocopherol, beta-carotene cancer prevention study: Effects of baseline characteristics and study compliance. *Journal of the National Cancer Institute, 88,* 1560–1570.

Alberg, A.J., & Samet, J.M. (2003). Epidemiology of lung cancer. *Chest, 123*(Suppl. 1), 21S–49S.

Axelson, O., Andersson, K., Desai, G., Fagerlund, I., Jansson, B., Karlsson, C., et al. (1988). Indoor radon exposure and active and passive smoking in relation to the occurrence of lung cancer. *Scandinavian Journal of Work, Environment and Health, 14,* 286–292.

Axelsson, G., Liljeqvist, T., Andersson, L., Bergman, B., & Rylander, R. (1996). Dietary factors and lung cancer among men in west Sweden. *International Journal of Epidemiology, 25*(1), 32–39.

Bach, P.B., Cramer, L.D., Warren, J.L., & Begg, C.B. (1999). Racial differences in the treatment of early-stage lung cancer. *New England Journal of Medicine, 341,* 1198–1205.

Bach, P.B., Kattan, M.W., Thornquist, M.D., Kris, M.G., Tate, R.C., Barnett, M.J., et al. (2003). Variations in lung cancer risk among smokers. *Journal of the National Cancer Institute, 95,* 470–478.

Bach, P.B, Kelley, M.J., Tate, R.C., & McCrory, D.C. (2003). Screening for lung cancer: A review of the current literature. *Chest, 123*(Suppl. 1), 72S–82S.

Bach, P.B., Niewoehner, D.E., Black, W.C., & the American College of Chest Physicians. (2003). Screening for lung cancer: The guidelines. *Chest, 123*(Suppl. 1), 83S–88S.

Baker, F., Ainsworth, S.R., Dye, J.T., Crammer, C., Thun, M.J., Hoffmann, D., et al. (2000). Health risks associated with cigar smoking. *JAMA, 284,* 735–740.

Bandera, E.V. (2001). Re: Diet and lung cancer mortality: A 1987 National Health Interview Survey cohort study. *Cancer Causes and Control, 12,* 577–578.

Bandera, E.V., Freudenheim, J.L., & Vena, J.E. (2001). Alcohol consumption and lung cancer: A review of the epidemiologic evidence. *Cancer Epidemiology, Biomarkers and Prevention, 10,* 813–821.

Benhamou, S., & Benhamou, E. (1994). The effect of age at smoking initiation on lung cancer risk. *Epidemiology, 5,* 560.

Benhamou, S., Benhamou, E., Auquier, A., & Flamant, R. (1994). Differential effects of tar content, type of tobacco and use of a filter on lung cancer risk in male cigarette smokers. *International Journal of Epidemiology, 23,* 437–443.

Berlin, N., Buncher, C.R., Fontana, R.S., Frost, J.K., & Melamed, M.R. (1984). The National Cancer Institute Cooperative Lung Cancer Detection Program. Results of the initial screen (prevalence). Early lung cancer detection: Introduction. *American Review of Respiratory Disease, 130,* 545–549.

Bilello, K.S., Murin, S., & Matthay, R.A. (2002). Epidemiology, etiology, and prevention of lung cancer. *Clinics in Chest Medicine, 23*(1), 1–25.

Blot, W.J., Xu, Z.Y., Boice, J.D., Jr., Zhao, D.Z., Stone, B.J., Sun, J., et al. (1990). Indoor radon and lung cancer in China. *Journal of the National Cancer Institute, 82,* 1025–1030.

Boffetta, P., Pershagen, G., Jockel, K.H., Forastiere, F., Gaborieau, V., Heinrich, J., et al. (1999). Cigar and pipe smoking and lung cancer risk: A multicenter study from Europe. *Journal of the National Cancer Institute, 91,* 697–701.

Boffetta, P., Ye, W., Boman, G., & Nyren, O. (2002). Lung cancer risk in a population-based cohort of patients hospitalized for asthma in Sweden. *European Respiratory Journal, 19*(1), 127–133.

Brabender, J., Danenberg, K.D., Metzger, R., Schneider, P.M., Park, J., Salonga, D., et al. (2001). Epidermal growth factor receptor and HER2-neu mRNA expression in non-small cell lung cancer is correlated with survival. *Clinical Cancer Research, 7,* 1850–1855.

Brownson, R.C., & Alavanja, M.C. (2000). Previous lung disease and lung cancer risk among women (United States). *Cancer Causes and Control, 11,* 853–858.

Buring, J.E., & Hennekens, C.H. (1995). Beta-carotene and cancer chemoprevention. *Journal of Cellular Biochemistry Supplement, 22,* 226–230.

Burns, D.M. (2000). Primary prevention, smoking, and smoking cessation: Implications for future trends in lung cancer prevention. *Cancer, 89*(Suppl. 11), 2506–2509.

Byers, T., & Perry, G. (1992). Dietary carotenes, vitamin C, and vitamin E as protective antioxidants in human cancers. *Annual Review of Nutrition, 12,* 139–159.

Caputi, M., Esposito, V., Mancini, A., & Giordano, A. (2002). Air pollution and respiratory pathology: Lung cancer. *Monaldi Archives for Chest Disease, 57,* 177–179.

Caputi, M., Groeger, A.M., Esposito, V., De Luca, A., Masciullo, V., Mancini, A., et al. (2002). Loss of pRb2/p130 expression is associated with unfavorable clinical outcome in lung cancer. *Clinical Cancer Research, 8,* 3850–3856.

Cardenas, V.M., Thun, M.J., Austin, H., Lally, C.A., Clark, W.S., Greenberg, R.S., et al. (1997). Environmental tobacco smoke and lung cancer mortality in the American Cancer Society's Cancer Prevention Study II. *Cancer Causes and Control, 8,* 57–64.

Clinton, S.K., Emenhiser, C., Schwartz, S.J., Bostwick, D.G., Williams, A.W., Moore, B.J., et al. (1996). Cis-trans lycopene isomers, carotenoids, and retinol in the human prostate. *Cancer Epidemiology, Biomarkers and Prevention, 5,* 823–833.

Colbert, L.H., Hartman, T.J., Tangrea, J.A., Pietinen, P., Virtamo, J., Taylor, P.R., et al. (2002). Physical activity and lung cancer risk in male smokers. *International Journal of Cancer, 98,* 770–773.

Cooley, M.E. (2002). Understanding and treating tobacco dependence in adults with lung cancer. In M. Haas (Ed.), *Contemporary issues in lung cancer: A nursing perspective* (pp. 241–253). Sudbury, MA: Jones and Bartlett.

Cooper, D.A., Eldridge, A.L., & Peters, J.C. (1999). Dietary carotenoids and lung cancer: A review of recent research. *Nutrition Reviews, 57*(5 Pt. 1), 133–145.

Deneo-Pellegrini, H., DeStefani, E., Ronco, A., Mendilaharsu, M., & Carzoglio, J.C. (1996). Meat consumption and risk of lung cancer: A case-control study from Uruguay. *Lung Cancer, 14*(2–3), 195–205.

DeStefani, E., Brennan, P., Boffetta, P., Mendilaharsu, M., Deneo-Pellegrini, H., Ronco, A., et al. (2002). Diet and adenocarcinoma of the lung: A case-control study in Uruguay. *Lung Cancer, 35*(1), 43–51.

DeStefani, E., Brennan, P., Ronco, A., Fierro, L., Correa, P., Boffetta, P., et al. (2002). Food groups and risk of lung cancer in Uruguay. *Lung Cancer, 38*(1), 1–7.

DeStefani, E., Correa, P., Deneo-Pellegrini, H., Boffetta, P., Gutierrez, L.P., Ronco, A., et al. (2002). Alcohol intake and risk of lung cancer: A case control study in Uruguay. *Lung Cancer, 38*(1), 9–14.

Djousse, L., Dorgan, J.F., Zhang, Y., Schatzkin, A., Hood, M., D'Agostino, R.B., et al. (2002). Alcohol consumption and risk of lung cancer: The Framingham Study. *Journal of the National Cancer Institute, 94,* 1877–1882.

Doll, R. (1976). Epidemiology of cancer: Current perspectives. *American Journal of Epidemiology, 104,* 396–404.

Doll, R. (1981). Relevance of epidemiology to policies for the prevention of cancer. *Journal of Occupational Medicine, 23,* 601–609.

Doll, R., & Hill, A.B. (1952). A study of the etiology of carcinoma of the lung. *British Medical Journal, 2,* 1271.

Doll, R., & Peto, R. (1981). The causes of cancer: Quantitative estimates of avoidable risks of cancer in the United States today. *Journal of the National Cancer Institute, 66,* 1191–1308.

Dragnev, K.H., Stover, D., & Dmitrovsky, E. (2003). Lung cancer prevention: The guidelines. *Chest, 123*(Suppl. 1), 60S–71S.

Dresler, C.M., Fratelli, C., Babb, J., Everley, L., Evans, A.A., & Clapper, M.L. (2000). Gender differences in genetic susceptibility for lung cancer. *Lung Cancer, 30*(3), 153–160.

Dwyer, T., Blizzard, L., Shugg, D., Hill, D., & Ansari, M.Z. (1994). Higher lung cancer rates in young women than young men: Tasmania, 1983 to 1992. *Cancer Causes and Control, 5,* 351–358.

Ebbert, J.O., Yang, P., Vachon, C.M., Vierkant, R.A., Cerhan, J.R., Folsom, A.R., et al. (2003). Lung cancer risk reduction after smoking cessation: Observations from a prospective cohort of women. *Journal of Clinical Oncology, 21,* 921–926.

The effect of vitamin E and beta carotene on the incidence of lung cancer and other cancers in male smokers. The Alpha-Tocopherol, Beta Carotene Cancer Prevention Study Group. (1994). *New England Journal of Medicine, 330,* 1029–1035.

Fearon, E.R. (1997). The smoking gun and the damage done: Genetic alterations in the lungs of smokers. *Journal of the National Cancer Institute, 89,* 834–836.

Feskanich, D., Ziegler, R.G., Michaud, D.S., Giovannucci, E.L., Speizer, F.E., Willett, W.C., et al. (2000). Prospective study of fruit and vegetable consumption and risk of lung cancer among men and women. *Journal of the National Cancer Institute, 92,* 1812–1823.

Fiore, M.C., Bailey, W.C., Cohen, S.J., Dorfman, S.F., Goldstein, M.G., Gritz, E.R., et al. (2000). *Treating tobacco use and dependence* [Clinical Practice Guideline]. Rockville, MD: U.S. Department of Health and Human Services, Public Health Service.

Fontana, R., Sanderson, D.R., Taylor, W.F., Woolner, L.B., Miller, W.E., Muhm, J.R., et al. (1984). Early lung cancer detection: Results of the initial (prevalence) radiologic and cytologic screening in the Mayo Clinic study *American Review of Respiratory Disease, 130,* 561–563.

Gallagher, J., & Holm, L. (1996). Power of one: Nurses and tobacco control. *Seminars in Oncology Nursing, 27,* 270–275.

Garshick, E., Schenker, M.B., Munoz, A., Segal, M., Smith, T.J., Woskie, S.R., et al. (1988). A retrospective cohort study of lung cancer and diesel exhaust exposure in railroad workers. *American Review of Respiratory Disease, 137,* 820–825.

Garte, S. (1998). The role of ethnicity in cancer susceptibility gene polymorphisms: The example of CYP1A1. *Carcinogenesis, 19,* 1329–1332.

Gilbert, E.S., Stovall, M., Gospodarowicz, M., Van Leeuwen, F.E., Andersson, M., Glimelius, B., et al. (2003). Lung cancer after treatment for Hodgkin's disease: Focus on radiation effects. *Radiation Research, 159*(2), 161–173.

Gilliland, F.D., & Samet, J.M. (1994). Lung cancer. *Cancer Surveys, 20,* 175–195.

Ginsberg, R., Vokes, E., & Rosenzweig, K. (2001). Non small cell lung cancer. In V.T. DeVita, S. Hellman, & S.A. Rosenberg (Eds.), *Cancer: Principles and practice of oncology* (6th ed., pp. 925–975). Philadelphia: Lippincott Williams & Wilkins.

Giovannucci, E. (1999a). Insulin-like growth factor-I and binding protein-3 and risk of cancer. *Hormone Research, 51*(Suppl. 3), 34–41.

Giovannucci, E. (1999b). Tomatoes, tomato-based products, lycopene, and cancer: Review of the epidemiologic literature. *Journal of the National Cancer Institute, 91,* 317–331.

Goodman, G.E. (1993). Cancer prevention: Chemoprevention vs dietary modifications. *Preventive Medicine, 22,* 689–692.

Goodman, G.E., Omenn, G.S., Thornquist, M.D., Lund, B., Metch, B., & Gylys-Colwell, I. (1993). The Carotene and Retinol Efficacy Trial (CARET) to prevent lung cancer in high-risk populations: Pilot study with cigarette smokers. *Cancer Epidemiology, Biomarkers and Prevention, 2,* 389–396.

Goodman, J.I., & Watson, R.E. (2002). Altered DNA methylation: A secondary mechanism involved in carcinogenesis. *Annual Review of Pharmacology and Toxicology, 42,* 501–525.

Greenwald, H.P., Polissar, N.L., Borgatta, E.F., McCorkle, R., & Goodman, G. (1998). Social factors, treatment, and survival in early-stage non-small cell lung cancer. *American Journal of Public Health, 88,* 1681–1684.

Guengerich, F.P., & Turvy, C.G. (1991). Comparison of levels of several human microsomal cytochrome P-450 enzymes and epoxide hydrolase in normal and disease states using immunochemical analysis of surgical liver samples. *Journal of Pharmacology and Experimental Therapeutics, 256,* 1189–1194.

Hackshaw, A.K., Law, M.R., & Wald, N.J. (1997). The accumulated evidence on lung cancer and environmental tobacco smoke. *British Medical Journal, 315*(7114), 980–988.

Halpern, M.T., Gillespie, B.W., & Warner, K.E. (1993). Patterns of absolute risk of lung cancer mortality in former smokers. *Journal of the National Cancer Institute, 85,* 457–464.

Hammond, E.C., Selikoff, I.J., Lawther, P.L., & Seidman, H. (1976). Inhalation of benzpyrene and cancer in man. *Annals of the New York Academy of Sciences, 271,* 116–124.

Harris, S.G., Padilla, J., Koumas, L., Ray, D., & Phipps, R.P. (2002). Prostaglandins as modulators of immunity. *Trends in Immunology, 23*(3), 144–150.

Hart, C.L., Hole, D.J., Gillis, C.R., Smith, G.D., Watt, G.C., & Hawthorne, V.M. (2001). Social class differences in lung cancer mortality: Risk factor explanations using two Scottish cohort studies. *International Journal of Epidemiology, 30,* 268–274.

Hegmann, K.T., Fraser, A.M., Keaney, R.P., Moser, S.E., Nilasena, D.S., Sedlars, M., et al. (1993). The effect of age at smoking initiation on lung cancer risk. *Epidemiology, 4,* 444–448.

Hein, H.O., Suadicani, P., & Gyntelberg, F. (1992). Lung cancer risk and social class. The Copenhagen Male Study—17-year follow up. *Danish Medical Bulletin, 39*(2), 173–176.

Hennekens, C.H., Buring, J.E., Manson, J.E., Stampfer, M., Rosner, B., Cook, N.R., et al. (1996). Lack of effect of long-term supplementation with beta carotene on the incidence of malignant neoplasms and cardiovascular disease. *New England Journal of Medicine, 334,* 1145–1149.

Henschke, C.I., McCauley, D.I., Yankelevitz, D.F., Naidich, D.P., McGuinness, G., Miettinen, O.S., et al. (1999). Early lung cancer action project: Overall design and findings from baseline screening. *Lancet, 354*(9173), 99–105.

Henschke, C.I., McCauley, D.I., Yankelevitz, D.F., Naidich, D.P., McGuinness, G., Miettinen, O.S., et al. (2001). Early lung cancer action project: A summary of the findings on baseline screening. *The Oncologist, 6*, 147–152.

Henschke, C.I., Yankelowitz, D.F., Libby, D., & Kimmel, M. (2002). CT screening for lung cancer: The first ten years. *The Cancer Journal, 8*(Suppl. 1), S47–S54.

Holick, C.N., Michaud, D.S., Stolzenberg-Solomon, R., Mayne, S.T., Pietinen, P., Taylor, P.R., et al. (2002). Dietary carotenoids, serum beta-carotene, and retinol and risk of lung cancer in the alpha-tocopherol, beta-carotene cohort study. *American Journal of Epidemiology, 156*, 536–547.

Hong, J.Y., & Yang, C.S. (1997). Genetic polymorphism of cytochrome P450 as a biomarker of susceptibility to environmental toxicity. *Environmental Health Perspectives, 105*(Suppl. 4), 759–762.

Hong, W.K., & Sporn, M.B. (1997). Recent advances in chemoprevention of cancer. *Science, 278*(5340), 1073–1077.

Hosomi, Y., Yokose, T., Hirose, Y., Nakajima, R., Nagai, K., Nishiwaki, Y., et al. (2000). Increased cyclooxygenase 2 (COX-2) expression occurs frequently in precursor lesions of human adenocarcinoma of the lung. *Lung Cancer, 30*(2), 73–81.

Howe, H.L., Wingo, P.A., Thun, M.J., Ries, L.A., Rosenberg, H.M., Feigal, E.G., et al. (2001). Annual report to the nation on the status of cancer (1973 through 1998), featuring cancers with recent increasing trends. *Journal of the National Cancer Institute, 93*, 824–842.

Hu, J., Mao, Y., Dryer, D., & White, K. (2002). Risk factors for lung cancer among Canadian women who have never smoked. *Cancer Detection and Prevention, 26*(2), 129–138.

Huber, M.H., Lee, J.S., & Hong, W.K. (1993). Chemoprevention of lung cancer. *Seminars in Oncology, 20*, 128–141.

Iribarren, C., Tekawa, I.S., Sidney, S., & Friedman, G.D. (1999). Effect of cigar smoking on the risk of cardiovascular disease, chronic obstructive pulmonary disease, and cancer in men. *New England Journal of Medicine, 340*, 1773–1780.

Janerich, D.T., Thompson, W.D., Varela, L.R., Greenwald, P., Chorost, S., Tucci, C., et al. (1990). Lung cancer and exposure to tobacco smoke in the household. *New England Journal of Medicine, 323*, 632–636.

Jemal, A., Tiwari, R.C., Murray, T., Ghafoor, A., Samuels, A., Ward, E., et al. (2004). Cancer statistics, 2004. *CA: A Cancer Journal for Clinicians, 54*, 8–29.

Jett, J.R. (2000). Screening for lung cancer in high risk groups: Current status of low-dose spiral CT scanning and sputum markers. *Seminars in Respiratory Critical Care Medicine, 21*, 385–392.

Johnson, J., & Ballin, S. (1995). The power to regulate tobacco. *Circulation, 92*, 2021.

Joyce, M., & Houlihan, N. (2001). Current strategies in the diagnosis and treatment of lung cancer. *Oncology Nursing Updates, 8*(1), 1–15.

Kabat, G.C., Ng, S.K., & Wynder, E.L. (1993). Tobacco, alcohol intake, and diet in relation to adenocarcinoma of the esophagus and gastric cardia. *Cancer Causes and Control, 4*(2), 123–132.

Kennedy, T.C., Lam, S., & Hirsch, F.R. (2001). Review of recent advances in fluorescence bronchoscopy in early localization of central airway lung cancer. *The Oncologist, 6*, 257–262.

Kennedy, T., Miller, Y., & Prindiville, S. (2000). Screening for lung cancer revisited and the role of sputum cytology and fluorescence bronchoscopy in a high-risk group. *Chest, 117*(4 Suppl. 1), 72S–79S.

Khuri, F.R., Wu, H., Lee, J.J., Kemp, B.L., Lotan, R., Lippman, S.M., et al. (2001). Cyclooxygenase-2 overexpression is a marker of poor prognosis in stage I non-small cell lung cancer. *Clinical Cancer Research, 7*, 861–867.

King, T.E., Jr., & Brunetta, P. (1999). Racial disparity in rates of surgery for lung cancer. *New England Journal of Medicine, 341*, 1231–1233.

Kishi, K., Gurney, J.W., Schroeder, D.R., Scanlon, P.D., Swensen, S.J., & Jett, J.R. (2002). The correlation of emphysema or airway obstruction with the risk of lung cancer: A matched case-controlled study. *European Respiratory Journal, 19*, 1093–1098.

Knekt, P., Jarvinen, R., Seppanen, R., Hellovaara, M., Teppo, L., Pukkala, E., et al. (1997). Dietary flavonoids and the risk of lung cancer and other malignant neoplasms. *American Journal of Epidemiology, 146*, 223–230.

Knekt, P., Seppanen, R., Jarvinen, R., Virtamo, J., Hyvonen, L., Pukkala, E., et al. (1991). Dietary cholesterol, fatty acids, and the risk of lung cancer among men. *Nutrition and Cancer, 16*(3–4), 267–275.

Koh, H.K., Kannler, C., & Geller A.C. (2001). Cancer prevention: Preventing tobacco- related cancers. In V.T. DeVita, S. Hellman, & S.A. Rosenberg (Eds.), *Cancer: Principles and practice of oncology* (6th ed., pp. 617–626). Philadelphia: Lippincott Williams & Wilkins.

Koo, L.C. (1988). Dietary habits and lung cancer risk among Chinese females in Hong Kong who never smoked. *Nutrition and Cancer, 11*(3), 155–172.

Kosco, P., & Held-Warmkessel, J. (2000). Lung cancer: Can early detection become a reality in the 21st century. *American Journal of Nursing, 100*(Suppl. 4), 13–17, 52–54.

Koskinen, K., Pukkala, E., Martikainen, R., Reijula, K., & Karjalainen, A. (2002). Different measures of asbestos exposure in estimating risk of lung cancer and mesothelioma among construction workers. *Journal of Occupational and Environmental Medicine, 44*, 1190–1196.

Kreuzer, M., Gerken, M., Kreienbrock, L., Wellmann, J., & Wichmann, H.E. (2001). Lung cancer in lifetime nonsmoking men: Results of a case-control study in Germany. *British Journal of Cancer, 84*(1), 134–140.

Kreuzer, M., Heinrich, J., Kreienbrock, L., Rosario, A.S., Gerken, M., & Wichmann, H.E. (2002). Risk factors for lung cancer among nonsmoking women. *International Journal of Cancer, 100*, 706–713.

Kubick, A., & Polak, J. (1990). Lack of benefit from semi-annual screening for cancer of the lung: Follow-up report of a randomized controlled trial on population of high risk males in Czechoslovakia. *International Journal of Oncology, 45*, 26–33.

Kure, E.H., Ryberg, D., Hewer, A., Phillips, D.H., Skaug, V., Baera, R., et al. (1996). p53 mutations in lung tumours: Relationship to gender and lung DNA adduct levels. *Carcinogenesis, 17*, 2201–2205.

Lam, S., Kennedy, T., Unger, M., Miller, Y.E., Gelmont, D., Rusch, V., et al. (1998). Localization of bronchial intraepithelial neoplastic lesions by fluorescence bronchoscopy. *Chest, 113*, 696–672.

Lee, I.M., Sesso, H.D., & Paffenbarger, R.S., Jr. (1999). Physical activity and risk of lung cancer. *International Journal of Epidemiology, 28*, 620–625.

Lee, P.N. (2001). Relation between exposure to asbestos and smoking jointly and the risk of lung cancer. *Occupational and Environmental Medicine, 58*(3), 145–153.

Le Marchand, L., Yoshizawa, C.N., Kolonel, L.N., Hankin, J.H., & Goodman, M.T. (1989). Vegetable consumption and lung cancer risk: A population-based case-control study in Hawaii. *Journal of the National Cancer Institute, 81*, 1158–1164.

Levin M.L., & Gerhardt P.R. (1950). Cancer and tobacco smoking: A preliminary report. *JAMA, 143*, 336.

Liao, M.L., Wang, J.H., Wang, H.M., Ou, A.Q., Wang, X.J., & You, W.Q. (1996). A study of the association between squamous cell carcinoma and adenocarcinoma in the lung, and history of menstruation in Shanghai women, China. *Lung Cancer, 14*(Suppl. 1), S215–S221.

Lippman, S.M., Spitz, M., Trizna, Z., Benner, S.E., & Hong, W.K. (1994). Epidemiology, biology, and chemoprevention of aerodigestive cancer. *Cancer, 74*(Suppl. 9), 2719–2725.

Lippman, S.M., & Spitz, M.R. (2001). Lung cancer chemoprevention: An integrated approach. *Journal of Clinical Oncology, 19*(Suppl. 18), 74S–82S.

London, S.J., Yuan, J.M., Travlos, G.S., Gao, Y.T., Wilson, R.E., Ross, R.K., et al. (2002). Insulin-like growth factor I, IGF-binding protein 3, and lung cancer risk in a prospective study of men in China. *Journal of the National Cancer Institute, 94*, 749–754.

Longnecker, M.P. (1999). The Framingham results on alcohol and breast cancer. *American Journal of Epidemiology, 149*(2), 102–104.

Lubin, J.H. (1984). Modifying risk of developing lung cancer by changing habits of cigarette smoking. *British Medical Journal, 289*(6449), 921.

Lubin, J.H., & Boice, J.D., Jr. (1989). Estimating Rn-induced lung cancer in the United States. *Health Physics, 57*, 417–427.

Lubin, J.H., & Boice, J.D., Jr. (1997). Lung cancer risk from residential radon: Meta-analysis of eight epidemiologic studies. *Journal of the National Cancer Institute, 89*, 49–57.

Lubin, J.H., Boice, J.D., Jr., Edling, C., Hornung, R.W., Howe, G., Kunz, E., et al. (1995). Radon-exposed underground miners and inverse dose-rate (protraction enhancement) effects. *Health Physics, 69*, 494–500.

Mansson, J., Marklund, B., Bengtsson, C., & Oden, A. (1995). Differences in cancer incidence between parts with different socioeconomic structure within a Swedish big-city area. *Neoplasma, 42*(4), 149–153.

Mao, L. (2001). Molecular abnormalities in lung carcinogenesis and their potential clinical implications. *Lung Cancer, 34*(Suppl. 2), S27–S34.

Mao, L., Lee, J.S., Kurie, J.M., Fan, Y.H., Lippman, S.M., Lee, J.J., et al. (1997). Clonal genetic alterations in the lungs of current and former smokers. *Journal of the National Cancer Institute, 89*, 857–862.

Mayne, S.T., Buenconsejo, J., & Janerich, D.T. (1999). Previous lung disease and risk of lung cancer among men and women nonsmokers. *American Journal of Epidemiology, 149*(1), 13–20.

Mayne, S.T., Handelman, G.J., & Beecher, G. (1996). Beta-carotene and lung cancer promotion in heavy smokers—a plausible relationship? *Journal of the National Cancer Institute, 88*, 1513–1515.

McDuffie, H.H. (1991). Clustering of cancer in families of patients with primary lung cancer. *Journal of Clinical Epidemiology, 44*(1), 69–76.

Michaud, D.S., Feskanich, D., Rimm, E.B., Colditz, G.A., Speizer, F.E., Willett, W.C., et al. (2000). Intake of specific carotenoids and risk of lung cancer in 2 prospective U.S. cohorts. *American Journal of Clinical Nutrition, 72*, 990–997.

Miller, R.A. (1993). Aging and cancer: Another perspective. *Journal of Gerontology, 48*(1), B8–9.

Muscat, J.E., Chen, S.Q., Richie, J.P., Jr., Altorki, N.K., Citron, M., Olson, S., et al. (2003). Risk of lung carcinoma among users of nonsteroidal antiinflammatory drugs. *Cancer, 97*, 1732–1736.

Naruke, T., Tsuchiya, R., Kondo, H., Asamura, H., & Nakayama, H. (1997). Implications of staging in lung cancer. *Chest, 112*(Suppl. 4), 242S–248S.

Neugut, A.I., Weinberg, M.D., Ahsan, H., & Rescigno, J. (1999). Carcinogenic effects of radiotherapy for breast cancer. *Oncology, 13*, 1245–1256.

Nomura, A., Stemmermann, G.N., Chyou, P.H., Marcus, E.B., & Buist, A.S. (1991). Prospective study of pulmonary function and lung cancer. *American Review of Respiratory Disease, 144*, 307–311.

Omenn, G.S. (1998). Chemoprevention of lung cancer: The rise and demise of beta-carotene. *Annual Review of Public Health, 19*, 73–99.

Omenn, G.S., Goodman, G.E., Thornquist, M.D., Balmes, J., Cullen, M.R., Glass, A., et al. (1996). Effects of a combination of beta carotene and vitamin A on lung cancer and cardiovascular disease. *New England Journal of Medicine, 334*, 1150–1155.

Ooi, W.L., Elston, R.C., Chen, V.W., Bailey-Wilson, J.E., & Rothschild, H. (1986). Familial lung cancer: Correcting an error in calculation. *Journal of the National Cancer Institute, 77*, 990.

Patterson, R.E., White, E., Kristal, A.R., Neuhouser, M.L., & Potter, J.D. (1997). Vitamin supplements and cancer risk: The epidemiologic evidence. *Cancer Causes and Control, 8*, 786–802.

Pearce, N., & Bethwaite, P. (1997). Social class and male cancer mortality in New Zealand, 1984–7. *New Zealand Medical Journal, 110*(1045), 200–202.

Peto, R., Darby, S., Deo, H., Silcocks, P., Whitley, E., & Doll, R. (2000). Smoking, smoking cessation, and lung cancer in the UK since 1950: Combination of national statistics with two case-control studies. *British Medical Journal, 321*(7257), 323–329.

Pohlabeln, H., Jockel, K.H., Bruske-Hohlfeld, I., Mohner, M., Ahrens, W., Bolm-Audorff, U., et al. (2000). Lung cancer and exposure to man-made vitreous fibers: Results from a pooled case-control study in Germany. *American Journal of Industrial Medicine, 37*, 469–477

Prescott, E., Gronbaek, M., Becker, U., & Sorensen, T.I. (1999). Alcohol intake and the risk of lung cancer: Influence of type of alcoholic beverage. *American Journal of Epidemiology, 149*, 463–470.

Prorok, P.C., Andriole, G.L., Bresalier, R.S., Buys, S.S., Chia, D., Crawford, E.D., et al. (2000). Design of the Prostate, Lung, Colorectal and Ovarian (PLCO) Cancer Screening Trial. *Control Clinical Trials, 21*(Suppl. 6), 273S–309S.

Rachtan, J. (2002). Alcoholic beverages consumption and lung cancer cell types among women in Poland. *Lung Cancer, 35*(2), 119–127.

Radzikowska, E., Glaz, P., & Roszkowski, K. (2002). Lung cancer in women: Age, smoking, histology, performance status, stage, initial treatment and survival. Population-bases study of 20,561 cases. *Annals of Oncology, 13*, 1087–1093.

Ratnasinghe, D.L., Yao, S.X., Forman, M., Qiao, Y.L., Andersen, M.R., Giffen, C.A., et al. (2003). Gene-environment interactions between the codon 194 polymorphism of XRCC1 and antioxidants influence lung cancer risk. *Anticancer Research, 23*(1B), 627–632.

Reid, M.E., Duffield-Lillico, A.J., Garland, L., Turnbull, B.W., Clark, L.C., & Marshall, J.R. (2002). Selenium supplementation and lung cancer incidence: An update of the nutritional prevention of cancer trial. *Cancer Epidemiology, Biomarkers and Prevention, 11*, 1285–1291.

Risch, H.A., Howe, G.R., Jain, M., Burch, J.D., Holowaty, E.J., & Miller, A.B. (1993). Are female smokers at higher risk for lung cancer than male smokers? A case-control analysis by histologic type. *American Journal of Epidemiology, 138*, 281–293.

Risser, N.L. (1996). Prevention of lung cancer: The key is to stop smoking. *Seminars in Oncology Nursing, 12*, 260–289.

Rubino, C., de Vathaire, F., Diallo, I., Shamsaldin, A., Grimaud, E., Labbe, M., et al. (2002). Radiation dose, chemotherapy and risk of lung cancer after breast cancer treatment. *Breast Cancer Research and Treatment, 75*(1), 15–24.

Samet, J.M. (1992). The health benefits of smoking cessation. *Medical Clinics of North America, 76*, 399–414.

Samet, J.M. (1993). The epidemiology of lung cancer. *Chest, 103*(Suppl. 1), 20S–29S.

Samet, J.M., Humble, C.G., & Pathak, D.R. (1986). Personal and family history of respiratory disease and lung cancer risk. *American Review of Respiratory Disease, 134*, 466–470.

Samet, J.M., Kutvirt, D.M., Waxweiler, R.J., & Key, C.R. (1984). Uranium mining and lung cancer in Navajo men. *New England Journal of Medicine, 310,* 1481–1484.

Sarna, L., & Lillington, L. (2002). Tobacco: An emerging topic in nursing research. *Nursing Research, 51,* 245–253.

Schottenfeld, D. (1996). Epidemiology of lung cancer. In H.I. Pass, J.B. Mitchell, D.H. Johnson, & A.T. Turrisi (Eds.), *Lung cancer: Principles and practice* (pp. 305–321). Philadelphia: Lippincott Williams & Wilkins.

Seow, A., Poh, W.T., Teh, M., Eng, P., Wang, Y.T., Tan, W.C., et al. (2002). Diet, reproductive factors and lung cancer risk among Chinese women in Singapore: Evidence for a protective effect of soy in nonsmokers. *International Journal of Cancer, 97,* 365–371.

Simonato, L., Agudo, A., Ahrens, W., Benhamou, E., Benhamou, S., Boffetta, P., et al. (2001). Lung cancer and cigarette smoking in Europe: An update of risk estimates and an assessment of inter-country heterogeneity. *International Journal of Cancer, 91,* 876–887.

Sinha, R., Kulldorff, M., Curtin, J., Brown, C.C., Alavanja, M.C., & Swanson, C.A. (1998). Fried, well-done red meat and risk of lung cancer in women (United States). *Cancer Causes and Control, 9,* 621–630.

Smith, G.D., Hart, C., Blane, D., & Hole, D. (1998). Adverse socioeconomic conditions in childhood and cause specific adult mortality: Prospective observational study. *British Medical Journal, 316*(7145), 1631–1635.

Soslow, R.A., Dannenberg, A.J., Rush, D., Woerner, B.M., Khan, K.N., Masferrer, J., et al. (2000). COX-2 is expressed in human pulmonary, colonic, and mammary tumors. *Cancer, 89,* 2637–2645.

Speizer, F.E., Colditz, G.A., Hunter, D.J., Rosner, B., & Hennekens, C. (1999). Prospective study of smoking, antioxidant intake, and lung cancer in middle-aged women (USA). *Cancer Causes and Control, 10,* 475–482.

Steinmetz, K.A., & Potter, J.D. (1991). Vegetables, fruit, and cancer. I. Epidemiology. *Cancer Causes and Control, 2,* 325–357.

Steinmetz, K.A., Potter, J.D., & Folsom, A.R. (1993). Vegetables, fruit, and lung cancer in the Iowa Women's Health Study. *Cancer Research, 53,* 536–543.

Stewart, A.K., Bland, K.I., McGinnis, L.S., Jr., Morrow, M., & Eyre, H.J. (2000). Clinical highlights from the National Cancer Data Base, 2000. *CA: A Cancer Journal for Clinicians, 50,* 171–183.

Taioli, E., & Wynder, E.L. (1994). Re: Endocrine factors and adenocarcinoma of the lung in women. *Journal of the National Cancer Institute, 86,* 869–870.

Takezaki, T., Hirose, K., Inoue, M., Hamajima, N., Yatabe, Y., Mitsudomi, T., et al. (2001). Dietary factors and lung cancer risk in Japanese: With special reference to fish consumption and adenocarcinomas. *British Journal of Cancer, 84,* 1199–1206.

Thornquist, M., Omenn, G.S., Goodman, G.E., Grizzle, J., Rosenstock, L., Barnhart, S., et al. (1993). Statistical design of the Carotene and Retinol Efficacy Trial (CARET). *Controlled Clinical Trials, 14,* 308–324.

Thun, M.J. (1998). Mixed progress against lung cancer. *Tobacco Control, 7*(3), 223–226.

Thune, I., & Lund, E. (1997). The influence of physical activity on lung-cancer risk: A prospective study of 81,516 men and women. *International Journal of Cancer, 70,* 57–62.

Tockman, M.S. (2000). Advances in sputum analysis for screening and early detection of lung cancer. *Cancer Control: Journal of the Moffitt Cancer Center, 7*(1), 19–24.

Tockman, M.S., Anthonisen, N.R., Wright, E.C., & Donithan, M.G. (1987). Airways obstruction and the risk for lung cancer. *Annals of Internal Medicine, 106,* 512–518.

Tredaniel, J., Boffetta, P., Saracci, R., & Hirsch, A. (1994). Exposure to environmental tobacco smoke and risk of lung cancer: The epidemiological evidence. *European Respiratory Journal, 7,* 1877–1888.

Ulvestad, B., Kjaerheim, K., Martinsen, J.I., Damberg, G., Wannag, A., Mowe, G., et al. (2002). Cancer incidence among workers in the asbestos-cement producing industry in Norway. *Scandinavian Journal of Work Environment and Health, 28,* 411–417.

Vagero, D., & Persson, G. (1986). Occurrence of cancer in socioeconomic groups in Sweden: An analysis based on the Swedish Cancer Environment Registry. *Scandinavian Journal of Social Medicine, 14,* 151–160.

van Loon, A.J., Goldbohm, R.A., & van den Brandt, P.A. (1995). Lung cancer: Is there an association with socioeconomic status in The Netherlands? *Journal of Epidemiology and Community Health, 49*(1), 65–69.

Willett, W.C., & Trichopoulos, D. (1996). Nutrition and cancer: A summary of the evidence. *Cancer Causes and Control, 7,* 178–180.

Wynder, E.L., & Kabat, G.C. (1988). The effect of low-yield cigarette smoking on lung cancer risk. *Cancer, 62,* 1223–1230.

Zablotska, L.B., & Neugut, A.I. (2003). Lung carcinoma after radiation therapy in women treated with lumpectomy or mastectomy for primary breast carcinoma. *Cancer, 97,* 1404–1411.

Zang, E.A., & Wynder, E.L. (1992). Cumulative tar exposure: A new index for estimating lung cancer risk among cigarette smokers. *Cancer, 70,* 69–76.

Zang, E.A., & Wynder, E.L. (1996). Differences in lung cancer risk between men and women: Examination of the evidence. *Journal of the National Cancer Institute, 88*(3–4), 183–192.

Ziegler, R.G., Mason, T.J., Stemhagen, A., Hoover, R., Schoenberg, J.B., Gridley, G., et al. (1986). Carotenoid intake, vegetables, and the risk of lung cancer among white men in New Jersey. *American Journal of Epidemiology, 123,* 1080–1093.

Ziegler, R.G., Mayne, S.T., & Swanson, C.A. (1996). Nutrition and lung cancer. *Cancer Causes and Control, 7,* 157–177.

CHAPTER 4

Patient Assessment

Leslie B. Tyson, MS, ANP-C, OCN®

Introduction

Lung cancer is not only a prevalent disease but a lethal one: a predicted 160,440 people will die from the disease in 2004 (Jemal et al., 2004). Because of this, clinicians must be aware of the different clinical presentations of lung cancer, including oncologic emergencies and paraneoplastic syndromes, and astute in the assessment of patients with potential or suspected lung cancer. The clinical presentation of lung cancer varies widely. In fewer than 5% of patients with lung tumors, cancer is found incidentally on routine exam (e.g., chest x-ray performed for unrelated preoperative testing) (Kraut & Wozniak, 2000). Others may present with symptoms related to local or distant effects of the lung cancer that have been present for varying amounts of time. Signs and symptoms of oncologic emergencies and paraneoplastic syndromes prompt others to see their physicians or go to the emergency room. The first part of this chapter will focus on the clinical presentations of lung cancer, including signs and symptoms of oncologic emergencies and paraneoplastic syndromes. The second part of this chapter will provide a summary of the diagnostic tests used to determine the presence of lung cancer.

Clinical Presentation

Lung cancer may be present for several years before symptoms develop. Typically, lung cancer has a delayed presentation; signs and symptoms of lung cancer develop once the tumor is large enough to interfere with normal lung function or the tumor has spread to distant areas and causes problems, such as pain from bone metastases. Signs and symptoms of lung cancer depend on the area of involvement; more than 90% of patients are estimated to have symptoms at presentation (Beckles, Spiro, Colice, & Rudd, 2003). Once signs and symptoms develop, the malignancy usually is advanced and resection may not be possible. Signs and symptoms usually are categorized as those from local-regional effects of tumor,

extrathoracic spread of tumor, or systemic symptoms. See Table 4-1 for the clinical manifestations of lung cancer.

Local-Regional Effects of Tumor

Cough is the most common presenting symptom and occurs in 50%–75% or more of all patients diagnosed with lung cancer (Ingle, 2000; Patel & Peters, 1993). In patients who are current smokers, subtle changes may occur in the cough. For many, the cough initially is attributed to smoking. In others, it may be attributed to an upper respiratory tract infection, and one or more courses of empiric antibiotics are given before additional testing is performed. A new or worsening cough or cough lasting more than seven days in a patient with a significant smoking history should indicate need for a chest radiograph. Patients who present with signs or symptoms of pneumonia (e.g., cough, fever, pleuritic chest pain) also should have a chest radiograph regardless of smoking history.

Dyspnea is the second most common symptom of lung cancer, occurring in an estimated 40%–60% of patients (Kraut & Wozniak, 2000; Maddus & Ginsberg, 2002). Dyspnea has many different causes in patients with lung cancer. It may be related to underlying lung disease, such as chronic obstructive pulmonary disease, asthma, or cardiac disease. In patients with centrally located tumors or disease in hilar lymph nodes, dyspnea is usually the result of bronchial obstruction, partial or complete. With airway obstruction, atelectasis can occur, and this, too, can contribute to dyspnea. Dyspnea may be caused by pleural effusion as a direct result of tumor, lymphangitic spread of tumor, alveolar spread of tumor, or, rarely, as a result of pneumothorax from invasion of the visceral pleura (Maddus & Ginsberg). In patients with peripheral tumors, dyspnea may or may not be present.

Bronchorrhea is the abnormally abundant production of mucous secretions produced by coughing. It often is associated with bronchoalveolar carcinoma of the lung (Fraser, Paré, Fraser, & Paré, 1994b). Hemoptysis is defined as blood that is coughed up; it may be mixed with sputum. In 25%–35% of patients, hemoptysis is present at diagnosis (Kraut & Wozniak, 2000). It usually occurs in patients who have centrally located tumors as a result of tumor-invading blood vessels or tumor necrosis. The amount of blood varies from small streaks or tinges of blood mixed with sputum to massive amounts of frank, red blood. Massive hemoptysis is rare but can occur when a major pulmonary vessel is invaded by tumor; this is often fatal. Hemoptysis can occur in patients with chronic bronchitis, infections such as pneumonia or tuberculosis, and congestive heart failure. It often is attributed to bronchitis, and antibiotics are prescribed. Recurrent or persistent hemoptysis requires further evaluation.

Wheezing, a whistling or sighing sound, also occurs in patients with lung cancer, and is, in some instances, the presenting symptom. Wheezing is the result of the vibration of a narrowed airway as air passes through it. In patients with lung cancer, wheezing often is caused by a lesion in the mainstem bronchi. The wheezing is localized and may be associated with a cough. This should be differentiated from generalized wheezing, which usually is caused by bronchospasm (e.g., asthma). Stridor is a type of wheeze that is caused by partial obstruction of the larynx or trachea. It primarily occurs on inspiration and tends to be high pitched.

Chest pain is another common presenting symptom, estimated to occur in 30%–50% of patients at diagnosis (Ingle, 2000; Kraut & Wozniak, 2000). Chest pain most often is seen in patients with peripheral tumors, although the etiology of chest pain is not always clear (Ingle). In some patients, chest pain may be directly related to chest wall or pleural invasion. For example, patients with superior sulcus tumors (apical tumors) commonly present with shoulder pain. This pain may be present for six months or more prior to diagnosis (Warren, 2000). With growth of the apical tumor, shoulder pain progresses to pain and numbness in the arm (Warren). In others, the pain may be inexplicable, and it can occur in patients with early-stage disease (Kraut & Wozniak). Established methods of pain control should be used in these patients, regardless of the etiology of the pain.

Hoarseness is caused by tumor impingement or invasion of the left recurrent laryngeal nerve and is the result of locally advanced disease. The laryngeal nerves supply the vocal cords and allow humans to perform three basic functions: swallow (by sealing the trachea), breathe (by opening the cords over the airway), and speak (Hiebert, Liebermann-Meffert, & Kraus, 2002) (see Table 4-2). Anatomically, the left recurrent laryngeal nerve passes through the aortic arch; hoarseness is caused by lymphadenopathy in the anterior mediastinum or aortopulmonary window that invades or impinges the recurrent laryngeal nerve. In patients with lung cancer, the left recurrent laryngeal nerve most often is damaged because of its anatomic location. Paralysis or poor function of the left recurrent laryngeal nerve from tumor also can result in aspiration and poor cough reflex. These patients need to be carefully evaluated if pulmonary dysfunction (i.e., poor cough reflex, aspiration, and dysphagia) is suspected. Hoarseness indicates locally advanced disease, and surgery is usually not an option for these patients (Kraut & Wozniak, 2000). Permanent damage to the recurrent laryngeal nerve from the tumor cannot be corrected with systemic treatment, even if the tumor responds. In patients with pulmonary dysfunction, the current treatment of choice is open medialization of the vocal chord (Hiebert et al.). This procedure involves inserting a wedge-shaped Silastic® (Dow Corning, Midland, MI) implant placed in a pocket created on the deep surface of the thyroid cartilage (Hiebert et al.). The Silastic wedge moves the vocal chord to the midline, thereby promoting proper or near proper functioning of the vocal cords.

Table 4-1. Clinical Manifestations Associated With Lung Cancer

Category	Signs and Symptoms
Local-regional manifestations	Cough Dyspnea Hemoptysis Wheezing Chest pain Stridor Hoarseness Hiccups Atelectasis Pneumonia Pancoast syndrome Horner's syndrome Pleural effusion Pericardial effusion Superior vena cava syndrome Bone pain
Manifestations of extrathoracic involvement	Headache Central nervous system disturbances Gastrointestinal disturbances Jaundice Hepatomegaly Abdominal pain
Systemic symptoms	Weakness Fatigue Anorexia Cachexia Weight loss Anemia Symptoms associated with paraneoplastic syndromes

Note. From "Lung Cancers" (p. 1308) by R.J. Ingle in C.H. Yarbro, M.H. Frogge, M. Goodman, and S.L. Groenwald (Eds.), *Cancer Nursing: Principles and Practice* (5th ed.), 2000, Sudbury, MA: Jones and Bartlett. Copyright 2000 by Jones and Bartlett. Reprinted with permission.

Table 4-2. Overview of Laryngeal Functions

Cord Position	Primary Use	Secondary Uses
Abducted (open)	Breathing Airway protection while swallowing	Huffing Whispering Gargling Whistling Blowing out a candle Sniffing a rose
Adducted (sealed)	Coughing	Straining to initiate urination or defecation Parturition
Adducted (loosely)	Speaking Singing Humming	Laughing Crying Clearing phlegm Groaning Moaning Shouting Gasping

Note. From "Laryngeal Nerve Palsy" (p. 332) by C.A. Hiebert, D. Liebermann-Meffert, and D.H. Kraus in F.G. Pearson, J.D. Cooper, J. Deslauriers, R.J. Ginsberg, C.A. Hiebert, G.A. Patterson, et al. (Eds.), *Thoracic Surgery* (2nd ed.), 2002, New York: Churchill Livingstone. Copyright 2002 by Churchill Livingstone. Reprinted with permission.

Dysphagia and paralysis of the phrenic nerve are the result of locally advanced disease. Dysphagia can occur in patients with bulky mediastinal adenopathy, which causes pressure on the esophagus. Paralysis of the phrenic nerve (likely from aortopulmonary window lymphadenopathy) most commonly results in elevation of the left hemidiaphragm or hiccups. These signs and symptoms are not common in patients with lung cancer.

Pancoast syndrome is the result of nerve (brachial plexus), chest wall, and rib involvement by tumor located in the apex of the lung. It is named after Henry Pancoast, who was among the first to describe this tumor in the 1920s (Krebs & Williams, 1997). These tumors also are referred to as superior sulcus tumors, because of their location in the apex of the lung. Because of this location, nearly all patients are symptomatic at the time of diagnosis. Classically, patients present with shoulder pain, usually located at the medial (paraspinal) aspect of the scapula (Warren, 2000). As the tumor enlarges, patients typically have arm pain and headache and can develop Horner's syndrome. Horner's syndrome is usually a mani-festation of late disease and implies involvement of the nerves of or alongside the vertebral column (Warren). Horner's syndrome is caused by tumor invasion of the cervical sympathetic nerves and is characterized by ptosis and miosis.

Lymphangitic spread of tumor throughout the lung parenchyma is characterized by increasing dyspnea, cough, and hypoxia. Radiographically, it is associated with an enlarging infiltrate (Kraut & Wozniak, 2000). Specifically, lymphangitic spread refers to a tumor that grows along or is spread through the lymphatic channels. In the lung, it often mimics interstitial lung disease, such as idiopathic pulmonary fibrosis, infection, or radiation pneumonitis, and, as a result, often is difficult to diagnose (Grossman & Niroumand, 2002; Kraut & Wozniak). Chest radiographs have been reported to be normal in up to 50% of patients with biopsy-proven disease (Grossman & Niroumand). High-resolution computed tomography (CT) scan often is required to support the diagnosis (Grossman & Niroumand). Firm diagnosis is made pathologically, through bronchoscopy with bronchoalveolar lavage or open lung biopsy (Kraut & Wozniak). In patients who are unable to tolerate these procedures, empiric use of high-dose corticosteroids and antibiotics is recommended and may provide some relief of symptoms (Kraut & Wozniak). Lymphangitic spread of tumor is an ominous sign that often leads to rapid decline (Kraut & Wozniak).

Local-regional effects of the tumor also can cause pleural effusion, pericardial effusion, and superior vena cava syndrome (see Table 4-1). These are addressed in detail in Chapter 5.

Extrathoracic Spread of Tumor

Extrathoracic effects of tumor occur when the cancer spreads beyond the lungs. Signs and symptoms depend on the organ or system affected. Extrathoracic effects can include central nervous system symptoms, gastrointestinal symptoms, and pain.

Brain metastases are reported to occur in up to 50% of patients with small cell lung cancer (SCLC) and, to a lesser degree, in patients with non-small cell lung cancer (NSCLC) (Kraut & Wozniak, 2000). As many as 90% of these patients have signs or symptoms of metastases (Ingle, 2000). Signs and symptoms depend on the location of the tumor and the degree of accompanying swelling or bleeding. With increased intracranial pressure, patients may experience headache, nausea, and vomiting. Additionally, patients may experience changes in personality or level of consciousness. Focal weakness and seizures also can occur in patients with central nervous system metastases.

Gastrointestinal symptoms can be caused by local effects of the tumor or systemic effects, such as anorexia. Hepatic metastases, which are common in patients with lung cancer, can cause nausea, vomiting, jaundice, and pain. However, most patients with hepatic metastases are asymptomatic. Gastrointestinal obstruction also can occur as a direct result of metastatic disease, but this is uncommon.

Adrenal metastases usually are asymptomatic, including in patients with bilateral adrenal disease. Even bilateral adrenal metastases rarely result in adrenal insufficiency (Maddus & Ginsberg, 2002). Although rare, large adrenal metastatic tumors can cause flank pain.

Pain is not an uncommon symptom in patients with lung cancer, and it can have many causes. Pain caused by bone metastases is a common symptom, as bone metastases are frequent in patients with lung cancer; this symptom is seen in approximately 37% of patients (Ingle, 2000). Management of bone metastases often requires aggressive treatment with analgesics. Pain from bone metastases can improve with systemic treatment. Radiotherapy often is needed when chemotherapy fails to control pain or a weight-bearing bone is affected (Kraut & Wozniak, 2000).

Back pain with neurologic symptoms such as weakness, sensory loss, and autonomic dysfunction is indicative of spinal cord compression. In some patients, this may be the initial manifestation of lung cancer. Spinal cord compression is addressed in more detail in Chapter 5.

Systemic Symptoms

Systemic symptoms may or may not be present on initial evaluation of the patient with lung cancer. The incidence of systemic symptoms is similar in both NSCLC and SCLC. The etiology of the symptoms is not well understood (Ingle, 2000). Paraneoplastic syndromes are the result of remote effects of the tumor and are not related to metastatic spread of tumor. They can be the cause of a variety of systemic symptoms in patients with lung cancer. Overall, paraneoplastic syndromes in cancer are rare, but they are seen in 10%–20% of patients with lung cancer (Kraut & Wozniak, 2000). Some paraneoplastic syndromes characteristically are seen in patients with SCLC (e.g., Lambert-Eaton myasthenic syndrome), while others are more prevalent in those with NSCLC (e.g., hypertrophic osteoarthropathy). The hypercoagulable state is seen in patients with either type of lung cancer. The most common paraneoplastic syndromes in patients with lung cancer are discussed in Chapter 6.

Oncologic Urgencies and Emergencies and Paraneoplastic Syndromes

The initial manifestation of disease in patients with NSCLC and SCLC can include signs and symptoms of oncologic emergencies and paraneoplastic syndromes. As a result, clinicians must be familiar with the different emergent situations and paraneoplastic syndromes. In patients with lung cancer, the oncologic urgencies and emergencies include superior vena cava syndrome, cardiac tamponade, pleural or pericardial effusion, and malignant spinal cord compression. The most common paraneoplastic syndromes are humoral hypercalcemia of malignancy, ectopic adrenocorticotropic hormone syndrome, syndrome of inappropriate antidiuretic hormone (SIADH), Lambert-Eaton myasthenic syndrome, anti-Hu antibody–associated paraneoplastic cerebellar degeneration, Trousseau's syndrome, clubbing, and hypertrophic pulmonary osteoarthropy. Tables 4-3 and 4-4 outline the more common oncologic urgencies and emergencies and paraneoplastic syndromes, their incidence in patients with lung cancer, and the most common presenting signs and symptoms. More information regarding oncologic urgencies and emergencies and paraneoplastic syndromes can be found in later chapters.

Diagnostic Tests

History and Physical Exam

Findings on patient history and physical exam in many cases will guide diagnostic testing. Additionally, a careful history and physical exam may prevent unnecessary surgery (Lau & Harpole, 2000). If symptoms suggest metastatic disease, additional testing can confirm this and thus avoid surgery. Table 4-5 outlines the clinical and laboratory findings that suggest metastatic disease (Silvestri, Tanoue, Margolis, Barker, & Detterbeck, 2003).

The initial part of the patient history will include the chief complaint (the reason the patient sought medical care). The main symptoms should be fully explored and described in terms of location, quality, severity, timing, aggravating and alleviating factors, and other associated factors (Bates & Hoekelman, 1991). Past history may reveal hospitalization or treatment for pneumonia or other respiratory illnesses. A thorough tobacco history should be elicited, including type and amount of tobacco smoked per day and duration of smoking history. Additionally, the history should include exposure to passive smoking or other known carcinogens (e.g., radon). Family history may reveal other family members who have been diagnosed with lung cancer. The remainder of the patient history should focus on a review of systems, including the presence of constitutional symptoms, such as fatigue, weight change, weakness, and fever. Physical exam may or may not reveal abnormal findings. Inspection of the head and neck may show nasal flaring if shortness of breath or, possibly, cyanosis is present. Palpation of the neck may reveal enlarged cervical or supraclavicular lymph nodes. If superior vena cava obstruction is present, swelling of the face and neck may be observed. Additionally, redness or flushing of the face (plethora) may be present. Inspection of the chest may reveal use of accessory muscles (retraction and bulging) if the patient is having difficulty breathing. The presence of prominent vascular markings on the chest wall should raise suspicion for superior vena cava syndrome or a blood clot. Swelling of the extremities may be present with thrombosis. Digital clubbing may be noted on examination of the hands and feet. A thorough exam of the chest should include palpation, percussion, and auscultation.

Table 4-3. Oncologic Emergencies Associated With Lung Cancer		
Oncologic Urgency or Emergency	Incidence (%)	Selected Signs and Symptoms
Superior vena cava syndrome	6–7	Dyspnea; head fullness; chest pain; facial, neck, and arm swelling; stridor; positive distension of superficial veins of chest, neck, and upper arms
Cardiac effusion and tamponade	5–10	Dyspnea, cough, anxiety, jugular vein distension, tachycardia, pulsus paradoxis, and substernal chest pain
Pleural effusion	15–20	Dyspnea, dry cough, pleuritic chest pain, dullness on chest percussion, and tracheal deviation
Malignant spinal cord compression	5–10*	Radicular or band-like back pain, neurologic symptoms, motor and sensory weakness, and autonomic dysfunction

* This represents the incidence of malignant spinal cord compression in all patients with cancer, but the most common cause is lung cancer (Sullivan, 1996).

Findings indicative of the need for further evaluation include signs of pleural effusion (e.g., decreased breath sounds, dullness on percussion, egophony), pericardial effusion (i.e., muffled heart sounds), wheezing, stridor, or elevation of the hemidiaphragm (i.e., phrenic nerve paralysis). A screening neurologic exam, including assessment of cranial nerves, will determine the presence of focal weakness, other signs suggestive of central nervous system metastases, or findings consistent with Horner's syndrome. Although unusual, liver enlargement (from metastatic disease) may be found on abdominal exam.

Noninvasive Diagnostic Testing

In addition to the history and physical exam, diagnostic testing for patients with suspected lung cancer consists of laboratory testing, radiography, and sampling of tissue or fluid to determine definitive diagnosis and cell type. The results of these tests will determine tumor type, help to determine clinical stage, and assist the clinician in developing an individual treatment plan. Radiographic findings, in addition to symptom assessment, can even lead to a presumptive differentiation between SCLC and NSCLC (Rivera, Detterbeck, & Mehta, 2003). SCLC is more likely to present as a hilar or centrally located mass and may be associated with a paraneoplastic syndrome (Rivera et al.). Additionally, the results of these tests can help clinicians to estimate individual prognoses. Laboratory testing most often includes an assessment of the hematologic and metabolic systems. A complete blood count and comprehensive metabolic profile, including electrolytes, liver enzymes, and renal function tests, are usually the initial laboratory tests performed. Abnormal results may provide clues about metastatic disease. Anemia may represent a paraneoplastic syndrome or the presence of chronic disease. An elevation in serum calcium

or alkaline phosphatase may be indicative of bone metastasis, whereas abnormalities in electrolytes may occur in patients with SIADH. At present no blood tests (e.g., serum markers) are available to identify patients with lung cancer (Lau & Harpole, 2000). In fact, the results of these laboratory tests may be completely normal despite the presence of lung cancer.

Often the first radiographic test to be performed is the chest x-ray. Both posterior-anterior and lateral views should be obtained. Chest x-ray can reveal the primary tumor as well as the presence of pleural or pericardial effusions. In general, malignant lesions may be differentiated from benign lesions on chest radiograph. Characteristics suggestive of malignant lesions include size greater than 3 cm, irregular or spiculated border, distortion of surrounding vascular markings, and thick, irregular-walled cavitary lesions (Lau & Harpole, 2000). Benign lesions also may share some of these characteristics; any lesion with the aforementioned characteristics should be considered malignant until proven otherwise (Lau & Harpole). If an earlier chest radiograph is available, it should be used for comparative purposes. Pericardial effusion may present as an enlarged cardiac silhouette on chest film; pleural effusion is suspected with blunting of the costophrenic angle. Additionally, elevation of a hemidiaphragm can be detected on chest radiograph, which may indicate phrenic nerve involvement. A chest CT scan usually is the next diagnostic test obtained, and it is considered to be standard for evaluating patients with suspected or documented lung cancer (Maddus & Ginsberg, 2002). High-resolution or conventional CT is the modality used to image the lung parenchyma (Novelline, 1997b). With this technique, very thin slices (1.0–1.5 mm) are obtained. Helical CT scans (high speed or spiral) are now available in some centers; these high-speed scans yield 1-mm thick images with only one breath hold by the patient and take only seconds to perform (McLoud, 2002; Novelline,

Table 4-4. Paraneoplastic Syndromes Associated With Lung Cancer

Paraneoplastic Syndrome[a]	Selected Signs and Symptoms
Humoral hypercalcemia of malignancy	Nausea, fatigue, lethargy, constipation, altered mental status, and dehydration
Ectopic adrenocorticotropic hormone	Muscle weakness, hypokalemia, metabolic alkalosis, glucose intolerance, and hypertension
Syndrome of inappropriate antidiuretic hormone	Fatigue, headache, weakness, muscle cramps, nausea, vomiting, lethargy, and loss of deep tendon reflexes
Lambert-Eaton myasthenic syndrome	Proximal muscle weakness, muscle fatigue with exercise, constipation, and postural hypotension
Anti-hu antibody cerebellar degeneration	Multifocal neurologic disease including severe ataxia, dysarthria, dysphagia, diplopia, and sensory neuropathy
Trousseau's syndrome	Deep vein thrombosis: Asymmetrical limb edema, pain, and redness Pulmonary embolism: Acute dyspnea, pleuritic chest pain, and cough
Hypertrophic pulmonary osteoarthropy	Symmetrical joint pain, joint effusions, joint swelling and erythema
Clubbing	Characteristic appearance of fingers and toes

[a] Paraneoplastic syndromes are clinically apparent in 10%–20% of patients with lung cancer (Kraut & Wozniak, 2000).

1997a). CT scan with IV contrast is valuable in the assessment of the primary tumor, mediastinal lymph nodes, bony involvement, and tumor invasion of other structures. The use of IV contrast helps to differentiate lymph nodes from vessels and also aids in determining the extent of the primary tumor (Quint, Francis, Wahl, & Gross, 2000). Pagani (1984) demonstrated liver metastases in 3%–6% of patients and adrenal metastases in 3%–7%. Therefore, all CT scans of the chest should routinely include the upper abdomen to identify adrenal and liver metastases.

The CT scan also is used to assess tumor involvement with mediastinal lymph nodes. The most common criterion used to evaluate malignant involvement of a mediastinal lymph node is the short axis lymph node diameter; malignancy is suspected if the measurement is 1 cm or more on a transverse CT scan (Silvestri et al., 2003). Quint, Glazer, Orringer, Francis, and Booksta (1986) found that in evaluating mediastinal lymph node involvement, the short axis diameter of the lymph node is a more accurate predictor of actual size than the longitudinal axis by CT scan. A CT scan with "positive" lymph node involvement is only predictive of actual involvement 70% of the time (Maddus & Ginsberg, 2002). Lymph node enlargement also can be caused by inflammation, infection, and reactive hyperplasia (Quint et al., 2000). Patients require histologic diagnosis and should not be denied surgery based on results of CT scan alone (Maddus & Ginsberg; Silvestri et al.). Magnetic resonance imaging (MRI) is an imaging technique that does not use ionizing radiation. MRI of the chest is not used routinely in the staging or diagnosis

of lung cancer for several reasons. It does not offer significantly more information than chest CT (Maddus & Ginsberg); it is a longer test, typically taking 30–45 minutes to produce images; and it is affected by respiratory motion, which creates motion artifact on the images (Novelline, 1997a).

In some specific circumstances, MRI does provide more information than chest CT. MRI is helpful in evaluation of a lung mass that may be invading either a vertebral body or the spinal canal. In these situations, MRI has been found to be better than CT because it provides exceptional detail of the spinal canal and can detect changes in the bone marrow (Maddus & Ginsberg, 2002). MRI is better at imaging soft tissues than CT scan, and it offers multiplanar capability (Patz, 2000). Additionally, MRI is superior at determining if a tumor has invaded vessels (Maddus & Ginsberg). MRI is more beneficial than CT in patients with superior sulcus tumors, in which chest wall invasion, brachial plexus invasion, and subclavian vessels and vertebral body involvement exist (Patz; Quint et al., 2000). Heelan et al. (1989) found that MRI was accurate 94% of the time (compared with 63% with chest CT) in evaluating superior sulcus tumors that have invaded other structures. CT scan and MRI also are useful in determining the presence of metastatic disease. The search for metastatic disease usually is suggested by the results of the history and physical exam and by the results of laboratory data. In patients suspected of having brain metastases, either modality can be used. At initial staging in patients with NSCLC, routine use of these tests is controversial in patients with no symptoms suggestive of brain metastases, as asymptomatic brain metastases are observed only in 3%–9% of patients overall (Olak & Ferguson, 2000; Patz). In contrast, evaluation of the head with MRI or CT is recommended in patients with SCLC, who commonly present with brain metastases (Patz). As noted previously, adrenal and hepatic metastases usually are visualized on a CT of the chest with upper abdomen, making separate scans of the abdomen unnecessary. Patients with bone metastases usually are symptomatic and may have laboratory abnormalities (elevated serum alkaline phosphatase or calcium). In patients with these findings, further testing may include bone radiograph, radionuclide bone scan, or MRI (Patz).

Positron emission tomography (PET) with radiopharmaceutical F-2-deoxy-D-glucose (FDG) is becoming recognized as a valuable tool in imaging thoracic tumors (Erasmus & Patz, 1999). FDG-PET is a noninvasive imaging technique that can provide additional information with conventional radiographs, CT, and MRI scans. Clinical trials have shown PET scans to be an important imaging modality in the preoperative staging of NSCLC (Pieterman et al., 2000). The recent American College of Chest Physicians *Diagnosis and Management of Lung Cancer: Evidence-Based Practice Guidelines* recommended that PET scanning be used to evaluate the mediastinum in patients who are potential candidates for surgery (Silvestri et al., 2003). With an abnormal PET scan, biopsy of mediastinal lymph nodes should be performed prior to surgery when possible (Silvestri et al.). FDG (a glucose analog) is the preferred radiopharmaceutical agent in imaging tumors, because tumor cells have increased glucose metabolism and thus readily absorb FDG (Ginsberg, Erasmus, Patz, & Herman, 2002). The amount of FDG uptake in tumor cells has been shown to correlate with both tumor aggressiveness and tumor growth rates (Duhaylongsod et al., 1995). Most insurance companies now approve reimbursement for PET scans used for staging patients with lung cancer. PET scans provide quantitative information regarding the amount of glucose use in selected tissue (Goldsmith & Kostakoglu, 2000). Increased glucose metabolism will appear as a "hot spot" on the scan. These "hot spots" can be measured as a standard uptake value (SUV) or standard uptake ratio (SUR). A lesion is considered to be abnormal if the SUV is more than 2.5 (Silvestri). Non-neoplastic conditions, such as inflammation, infection, and granulomatous diseases, also can appear as "hot spots" on PET scans. Thus, a positive PET scan does not always imply malignant disease; tissue will need to be obtained to determine malignancy. Additionally, tumors with low metabolic activity, such as carcinoid or bronchoalveolar tumors, may appear as false-negative PET scans (Goldsmith & Kostakoglu). Whole-body PET scanning also can be valuable in the detection of metastatic disease and can be accomplished with no additional radiation exposure (Goldsmith & Kostakoglu). Patients are required to fast prior to undergoing PET scan, because increased serum glucose levels may interfere with FDG uptake by the tumor. Similarly, this can be a concern in patients with diabetes who have elevated serum

glucose levels. Although some researchers have not found this to be a major problem in patients with lung cancer, others suggest that for more meaningful imaging, serum glucose levels should not exceed 250–300 mg/dl (Goldsmith & Kostakoglu; Lowe & Naunheim, 1998).

Sputum cytology is a noninvasive method of diagnosing lung cancer. Clinical trials have found that sputum cytology is more likely to diagnose patients who have centrally located tumors than those who have peripheral tumors (Schreiber & McCrory, 2003). Additionally, studies have found that sputum cytology is more likely to diagnose lung cancer when three or more sputum cytology specimens per patient are produced and the samples are of adequate material (Bocking, Biesterfeld, Chatelain, Gien-Gerlach, & Esser, 1992). Diagnostic sensitivity has been shown to be high in patients who provide multiple specimens (Travis, Linder, & Mackay, 2000). Patients with squamous cell lung cancers, tumors larger than 2.4 cm, and bloody sputum also are more likely to have positive diagnosis by sputum cytology (Risse, van't Hof, Vooijs, 1987). Because lung cancer diagnosis by sputum cytology depends on the quality of the specimen, patients must be given specific instructions (Fraser, Paré, Fraser, & Paré, 1994a). The best samples are those that are collected first thing in the morning. Instruct the patient to rinse the mouth with water and then cough deeply and expectorate a sample into a collecting jar.

Table 4-5. Clinical Findings Suggesting Metastatic Disease	
Testing	**Finding**
Symptoms elicited in history	Constitutional: Weight loss (> 10 lb) Musculoskeletal: Focal skeletal pain Neurologic: Headaches, syncope, seizures, extremity weakness, recent change in mental status
Signs found on physical examination	Lymphadenopathy (> 1 cm) Hoarseness, superior vena cava syndrome Bone tenderness Hepatomegaly (> 13-cm span) Focal neurologic signs, papilledema Soft-tissue mass
Routine laboratory tests	Hematocrit (< 40% in men and < 35% in women) Elevated alkaline phosphatase, GGT, SGOT, and calcium levels

Note. From "The Non-Invasive Staging of Non-Small Cell Lung Cancer: The Guidelines," by G.A. Silvestri, L.T. Tanoue, M.L. Margolis, J. Barker, and F. Detterbeck, 2003, *Chest, 12*(Suppl. 1), p. 1535. Copyright 2003 by American College of Chest Physicians. Reprinted with permission.

Invasive Diagnostic Testing

Needle aspiration is an important tool in the cytologic diagnosis of lung cancer. Transthoracic needle aspiration (TTNA) taken through the chest wall, transbronchial aspiration at the time of bronchoscopy, and intraoperative needle aspiration at the time of mediastinoscopy are techniques that provide highly reliable samples with little discomfort or complications for patients (Fraser et al., 1994a). TTNA is more likely to yield a diagnosis in patients who have peripheral lesions that cannot be reached by bronchoscopy (Rivera et al., 2003). TTNA is technically easier in patients with peripheral lesions; studies show that lesions greater than 1.5 cm resulted in a trend toward higher diagnostic yield (94%) as compared to lesions less than 1.5 cm (78%) (Schreiber & McCrory, 2003). Very often, CT scanning, ultrasound, or fluoroscopy is used to help localize lesions at the time of aspiration. CT localization in an interventional radiology setting is used more often than the other modalities. The use of CT-guided TTNA has allowed for biopsy of lesions as small as 0.5 cm (Schreiber & McCrory).

Fine needles (22–25 gauge) for aspiration provide samples for cytology. Use of fine needles also is known as fine needle aspiration (FNA). FNA commonly is used to aspirate palpable lymph nodes as well, such as supraclavicular or cervical lymph nodes.

Bronchoscopy with or without transbronchial needle aspiration (TBNA) and bronchoalveolar lavage (BAL) also are used in diagnosing and staging lung cancer. Bronchoscopy is the most common procedure performed to diagnose lung cancer (Travis et al., 2000). Flexible bronchoscopy is most useful in patients with centrally located tumors (Rivera et al., 2003). Bronchoscopy allows for direct visualization of endobronchial abnormalities and direct sampling by brushing or washing of the abnormalities to yield a cytologic diagnosis. Endobronchial biopsy (using forceps) can provide histologic samples. Additionally, TBNA can be performed through the bronchoscope to sample lymph nodes in the mediastinum and peribronchial areas. It is also the standard method for sampling submucosal disease (Mazzone, Jain, Arroliga, & Matthay, 2002). Bronchoscopy with transbronchial biopsy and fluoroscopic guidance can be used to sample peripheral lesions (Mazzone et al.).

TBNA with flexible bronchoscopy is a good alternative to mediastinoscopy. It is less invasive and does not require the use of general anesthesia, and some lymph node stations not accessible by mediastinoscopy (aortopulmonary window nodes) can be sampled with this procedure (Mazzone et al., 2002). In general, this is a safe procedure with a low rate of complications. Complications include pneumothorax and bleeding, but these are rare (Mazzone et al.). BAL is a technique used with bronchoscopy that uses fluid to collect cells from the lung (Travis et al., 2000). In this procedure, a narrow bronchoscope is passed to the fifth- or sixth-order bronchi, saline is instilled through the scope, and cells are "washed" out and collected (Travis et al.). This fluid then can be examined to determine if malignant cells are present. BAL can provide diagnosis in 60% of patients who have lung carcinoma and is especially valuable in patients who have peripheral lesions that cannot be reached by washing or brushing methods (Travis et al.). It is also valuable in the diagnosis of bronchoalveolar carcinoma, in which tumor cells can be easily washed out of the alveoli for cytologic diagnosis (Greco et al., 1986). In some instances, BAL cytologic results may be difficult to interpret if infection (e.g., pneumonia) or inflammation exists (Mazzone et al.).

Mediastinoscopy is an invasive method used to evaluate the mediastinum in patients with lung cancer; it is considered to be the "gold standard" for evaluation of mediastinal lymph nodes (Detterbeck, DeCamp, Kohman, & Silvestri, 2003). This procedure is performed under general anesthesia in the operating room. Patients usually are discharged from the hospital the same day as the procedure, if stable. Mediastinoscopy is performed by making a small incision at the suprasternal notch. The mediastinoscope then is passed alongside the trachea, allowing biopsy of mediastinal lymph nodes. The sensitivity of this procedure in documenting cancer is 80%–85% (Detterbeck et al.). Most mediastinal lymph nodes can be sampled with this procedure. Routinely, one node from five lymph node stations should be sampled. Supraclavicular lymph nodes (e.g., ipsilateral scalene nodes) also can be sampled by mediastinoscopy (Lee & Ginsberg, 1996). Lymph nodes not accessible with mediastinoscopy include posterior subcarinal, inferior mediastinal, aortopulmonary window, and anterior mediastinal nodes (Detterbeck et al.).

Aortopulmonary lymph nodes can be assessed using the Chamberlain procedure, also known as an anterior mediastinotomy (Detterbeck et al., 2003). The Chamberlain procedure involves making a small incision in the second or third intercostal space just to the left of the sternum. When used in addition to mediastinoscopy, the sensitivity of this procedure is estimated at 87% (Detterbeck et al.). Thoracoscopy (also known as video-assisted thoracic surgery [VATS]) can be used to assess lymph nodes not accessible by mediastinoscopy. This procedure provides access to the hemithorax, like thoracotomy, but is less invasive (Mentzer, DeCamp, Harpole, & Sugarbaker, 1995). As a result, VATS is especially useful with older patients or those with comorbid problems (Mentzer et al.). Through a left-sided VATS, the aortopulmonary window lymph nodes can be sampled. VATS also provides the ability to assess chest wall lesions and other lung parenchymal abnormalities (Mentzer et al.). Additionally, VATS can assess pleural effusions.

Most lung cancers (95%) can be diagnosed and staged using the other procedures discussed previously (Maddus & Ginsberg, 2002). Thoracotomy usually is reserved for patients with a high probability of lung cancer but for whom other diagnostic measures have failed to provide a diagnosis.

Excisional or Tru-Cut biopsies are performed for tissue diagnosis. If a lung cancer diagnosis is made by thoracotomy, staging of the mediastinum with lymph node sampling should be performed at the same time. Accurate diagnosis and staging of lung cancer is paramount. Once a tissue diagnosis is made, accurate staging will help to determine the treatment plan and also can make an estimate of the prognosis. Staging separates patients who are surgical candidates from those who are candidates for chemotherapy, radiotherapy, or a combination of therapies. Staging is more complicated in patients with NSCLC; for these patients, surgery may be an option depending on disease stage. Staging for SCLC is not as complicated, because this disease usually is not considered to be operable. Staging for both types of lung cancer is addressed in Chapters 7 and 8.

References

Bates, B., & Hoekelman, R.A. (1991). Interviewing and the health history. In B. Bates (Ed.), *A guide to physical examination and history taking* (pp. 1–33). Philadelphia: Lippincott.

Beckles, M.A., Spiro, S.G., Colice, G.L., & Rudd, R.M. (2003). Initial evaluation of the patient with lung cancer: Symptoms, signs, laboratory tests, and paraneoplastic syndromes. *Chest, 123*(Suppl. 1), 97S–104S.

Bocking, A., Biesterfeld, S., Chatelain, R., Gien-Gerlach, G., & Esser, E. (1992). Diagnosis of bronchial carcinoma on sections of paraffin-embedded sputum: Sensitivity and specificity of an alternative to routine cytology. *Acta Cytologica, 36,* 37–47.

Detterbeck, F.C., DeCamp, M.M., Kohman, L.J., & Silvestri, G.A. (2003). Lung cancer: Invasive staging: The guidelines. *Chest, 123*(Suppl. 1), 167S–175S.

Duhaylongsod, F.G., Lowe, V.J., Patz, E.F., Vaughn, A.L., Coleman, R.E., & Wolfe, W.G. (1995). Lung tumor growth correlates with glucose metabolism measured by fluoride-18-fluorodeoxy-glucose positron emission tomography. *Annals of Thoracic Surgery, 60,* 1348–1352.

Erasmus, J.J., & Patz, E.F. (1999). Positron emission tomography imaging in the thorax. *Clinics in Chest Medicine, 20,* 715–724.

Fraser, R.S., Paré, J.A.P., Fraser, R.G., & Paré, P.D. (1994a). Methods of roentgenologic and pathologic investigation. In R.S. Fraser, J.A.P. Paré, R.G. Fraser, & P.D. Paré (Eds.), *Synopsis of diseases of the chest* (pp. 117–140). Philadelphia: Saunders.

Fraser, R.S., Paré, J.A.P., Fraser, R.G., & Paré, P.D. (1994b). Neoplastic disease of the lungs. In R.S. Fraser, J.A.P. Paré, R.G. Fraser, & P.D. Paré (Eds.), *Synopsis of diseases of the chest* (pp. 445–538). Philadelphia: Saunders.

Ginsberg, M.S., Erasmus, J.J., Patz, E.R., & Herman, S.J. (2002). Imaging of the lung. In F.G. Pearson, J.D. Cooper, J. Deslauriers, R.J. Ginsberg, C.A. Hiebert, G.A. Patterson, et al. (Eds.), *Thoracic surgery* (2nd ed., pp. 443–498). New York: Churchill Livingstone.

Goldsmith, S.J., & Kostakoglu, L. (2000). Nuclear medicine imaging of lung cancer. *Radiologic Clinics of North America, 38,* 511–524.

Greco, R.J., Steiner, R.M., Goldman, S., Cotler, H., Patchefsky, A., & Cohn, H.E. (1986). Bronchoalveolar cell carcinoma of the lung. *Annals of Thoracic Surgery, 41,* 652–656.

Grossman, R.F., & Niroumand, M. (2002). Interstitial lung disease. In F.G. Pearson, J.D. Cooper, J. Deslauriers, R.J. Ginsberg, C.A. Hiebert, G.A. Patterson, et al. (Eds.), *Thoracic surgery* (2nd ed., pp. 662–684). New York: Churchill Livingstone.

Heelan, R.T., Demas, B.E., Caravelli, J.F., Martini, N., Bains, M.S., McCormack, P.M., et al. (1989). Superior sulcus tumors: CT and MR imaging. *Radiology, 170,* 673–681.

Hiebert, C.A., Liebermann-Meffert, D., & Kraus, D.H. (2002). Laryngeal nerve palsy. In F.G. Pearson, J.D. Cooper, J. Deslauriers, R.J. Ginsberg, C.A. Hiebert, G.A. Patterson, et al. (Eds.), *Thoracic surgery* (2nd ed., pp. 331–340). New York: Churchill Livingstone.

Ingle, R.J. (2000). Lung cancers. In C.H. Yarbro, M.H. Frogge, M. Goodman, & S.L. Groenwald (Eds.), *Cancer nursing: Principles and practice* (5th ed., pp. 1298–1328). Sudbury, MA: Jones and Bartlett.

Jemal, A., Tiwari, R.C., Murray, T., Ghafoor, A., Samuels, A., Ward, E., et al. (2004). Cancer statistics, 2004. *CA: A Cancer Journal for Clinicians, 54,* 8–29.

Kraut, M., & Wozniak, A. (2000). Clinical presentation. In H.L. Pass, J.B. Mitchell, D.H. Johnson, A.T. Turissi, & J.D. Minna (Eds.), *Lung cancer: Principles and practice* (2nd ed., pp. 521–534). Philadelphia: Lippincott Williams & Wilkins.

Krebs, L.U., & Williams, P. (1997). Lung cancer. In R.A. Gates & R.M. Fink (Eds.), *Oncology nursing secrets* (pp. 189–195). Philadelphia: Hanley & Belfus, Inc.

Lau, C.L., & Harpole, D.H. (2000). Noninvasive clinical staging modalities for lung cancer. *Seminars in Surgical Oncology, 18,* 116–123.

Lee, J.D., & Ginsberg, R.J. (1996). Lung cancer staging: The value of ipsilateral scalene lymph node biopsy performed at mediastinoscopy. *Annals of Thoracic Surgery, 62,* 338–341.

Lowe, V.J., & Naunheim, K.S. (1998). Positron emission tomography in lung cancer. *Annals of Thoracic Surgery, 65,* 1821–1829.

Maddus, M.A., & Ginsberg, R.J. (2002). Clinical features, diagnosis, and staging of lung cancer. In F.G. Pearson, J.D. Cooper, J. Deslauriers, R.J. Ginsberg, C.A. Hiebert, G.A. Patterson, et al. (Eds.), *Thoracic surgery* (2nd ed., pp. 813–836). New York: Churchill Livingstone.

Mazzone, P., Jain, P., Arroliga, A.C., & Matthay, R.A. (2002). Bronchoscopy and needle biopsy techniques for diagnosis and staging of lung cancer. *Clinics in Chest Medicine, 23,* 137–158.

McLoud, T.C. (2002). Imaging techniques for diagnosis and staging of lung cancer. *Clinics in Chest Medicine, 23,* 123–136.

Mentzer, S.J., DeCamp, M.M., Harpole, D.H., & Sugarbaker, D.J. (1995). Thoracoscopy and video-assisted thoracic surgery in the treatment of lung cancer. *Chest, 107*(Suppl. 6), 298S–301S.

Novelline, R.A. (1997a). The imaging techniques. In R.A. Novelline (Ed.), *Squires fundamentals of radiology* (pp. 12–41). Cambridge, MA: Harvard University Press.

Novelline, R.A. (1997b). The lung. In R.A. Novelline (Ed.), *Squires fundamentals of radiology* (pp. 92–111), Cambridge, MA: Harvard University Press.

Olak, J., & Ferguson, M.K. (2000). Surgical management of second primary and metastatic lung cancer. In H.L. Pass, J.B. Mitchell, D.H. Johnson, A.H. Turrisi, & J.D. Minna (Eds.), *Lung cancer: Principles and practice* (2nd ed., pp. 730–741). Philadelphia: Lippincott Williams & Wilkins.

Pagani, J.J. (1984). Non-small cell lung carcinoma adrenal metastases: Computed tomography and percutaneous needle biopsy in their diagnosis. *Cancer, 53,* 1058–1060.

Patel, A.M., & Peters, S.G. (1993). Clinical manifestations of lung cancer. *Mayo Clinic Proceedings, 68,* 273–277.

Patz, E.F. (2000). Imaging bronchogenic carcinoma. *Chest, 117*(Suppl. 1), 90S–95S.

Pieterman, R., vanPutten, J., Meuzelar, J., Moogaart, E., Vaalburg, W., Koeter, G., et al. (2000). Preoperative staging of non small cell lung cancer with positron emission tomography. *New England Journal of Medicine, 343,* 254–261.

Quint, L., Glazer, G., Orringer, M., Francis, I.R., & Booksta, F.L. (1986). Mediastinal lymph node detection and sizing at CT and autopsy. *American Journal of Roentgenology, 147,* 469–472.

Quint, L.E., Francis, I.R., Wahl, R.L, & Gross, B.H. (2000). Imaging. In H.L. Pass, J.B. Mitchell, D.H. Johnson, A.T. Turrisi, & J.D. Minna. (Eds.), *Lung cancer: Principles and practice* (2nd ed., pp. 535–578). Philadelphia: Lippincott Williams & Wilkins.

Risse, E.K., van't Hof, M.A., & Vooijs, G.P. (1987). Relationship between patient characteristics and the sputum cytologic diagnosis of lung cancer. *Acta Cytologica, 31,* 159–165.

Rivera, M.P., Detterbeck, F., & Mehta, A.C. (2003). Diagnosis of lung cancer. The guidelines. *Chest, 123*(Suppl. 1), 129S–136S.

Schreiber, G., & McCrory, D.C. (2003). Performance characteristics of different modalities for diagnosis of suspected lung cancer. Summary of published evidence. *Chest, 123*(Suppl. 1), 115S–128S.

Silvestri, G.A., Tanoue, L.T., Margolis, M.L., Barker, J., & Detterbeck, F. (2003). The non-invasive staging of non-small cell lung cancer: The guidelines. *Chest, 123*(Suppl. 1), 147S–156S.

Sullivan, F. (1996). Palliative radiotherapy for lung cancer. In H.L. Pass, J.B. Mitchell, D.H. Johnson, & A.T. Turrisi (Eds.). *Lung cancer: Principles and practice* (pp. 775–789). Philadelphia: Lippincott Williams & Wilkins.

Travis, W.D., Linder, J., & Mackay, B. (2000). Classification, histology, cytology, and electron microscopy. In H.L. Pass, J.B. Mitchell, D.H. Johnson, A.T. Turrisi, & J.D. Minna (Eds.), *Lung cancer: Principles and practice* (2nd ed., pp. 453–495). Philadelphia: Lippincott Williams & Wilkins.

Warren, W.H. (2000). Chest wall involvement including Pancoast tumors. In H.L. Pass, J.B. Mitchell, D.H. Johnson, A.T. Turrisi, & J.D. Minna (Eds.), *Lung cancer: Principles and practice* (2nd ed., pp. 716–729). Philadelphia: Lippincott Williams & Wilkins.

CHAPTER 5

Oncologic Urgencies and Emergencies

Leslie B. Tyson, MS, ANP-C, OCN®

Introduction

Initial manifestations of non-small cell lung cancer (NSCLC) can include signs and symptoms of oncologic emergencies. Because of this, clinicians must be familiar with the different emergent situations. In patients with lung cancer, oncologic urgencies and emergencies include superior vena cava syndrome (SVCS), cardiac tamponade, pleural effusion, and malignant spinal cord compression (MSCC). The following section will review the pathophysiology, presenting signs and symptoms, and treatment of these conditions.

Superior Vena Cava Syndrome

Introduction

SVCS is caused by an obstruction of the superior vena cava from tumor, thrombosis, radiation fibrosis, or infection. When Hunter first described this syndrome in the mid 1700s, it most commonly was caused by infection from syphilis-induced aortic aneurysm or fibrosis from tuberculosis (Haapoja & Blendowski, 1999). With the development of antibiotics and the successful treatment of infections, the most common cause of SVCS today is malignancy.

SVCS usually is caused by external compression on the vessel by tumor or enlargement of mediastinal lymph nodes from tumor. Less commonly, it can be caused by invasion of the superior vena cava by tumor and thrombus within the vessel. Iatrogenic SVCS is caused by a clot associated with a central venous catheter, implanted venous access port, or pacemaker. Although many still consider SVCS an oncologic emergency, most symptoms develop gradually. Malignancy is the cause in more than 95% of all cases of SVCS (Mack, 1997), and 60%–95% of those cases are a result of lung cancer (Stewart, 1996). Despite this, SVCS is still a fairly rare occurrence in patients with any type of cancer; overall incidence is estimated at only 3%–4% (Mack; Sitton, 2000).

SCLC is the most frequent histology for SVCS, and squamous cell lung cancer is the second most common histology (Mack; Stewart). Both of these tumor types are more commonly central in location as opposed to other types of lung cancer, which tend to grow in peripheral areas of the lungs. SVCS is still an uncommon complication in lung cancer, with only 6%–7% of all patients developing the syndrome (Mack). Non-Hodgkin's lymphoma is the second most common cause of SVCS.

Pathophysiology

The superior vena cava is located in the right side of the chest in the anterior mediastinum, making it more vulnerable to compression or invasion from a mass in the right side of the chest. It is surrounded by rigid structures, including the sternum and vertebrae, trachea, right bronchus, aorta, pulmonary artery, and lymph nodes (right hilar, right paratracheal, and subcarinal groups). The superior vena cava is the vessel that is responsible for drainage of venous blood from the head, neck, upper extremities, and upper thorax to the heart. The vessel is thin-walled and carries low pressure. Obstruction of the superior vena cava results in diminished venous return to the right atrium and, accordingly, an increase in venous pressure behind the obstruction (Mack, 1997). The increase in venous pressure leads to venous stasis in the head, neck, upper arms, and upper chest with subsequent engorgement of the superficial vessels in the area. If occlusion occurs gradually, then collateral circulation can develop, which may lead to relief of some of the obstructive symptoms (Mack). In patients with acute onset of SVCS, the cause is usually complete obstruction from thrombus, whereas a more gradual onset of symptoms usually is caused by extrinsic compression of the vessel from tumor or enlarged lymph nodes (Haapoja & Blendowski, 1999). SVCS is rarely life threatening, and most patients have symptoms for at least a week. A definitive diagnosis should be made prior to treatment because treatments differ depending on the cause.

Signs and Symptoms

Signs and symptoms of SVCS depend on how rapidly the obstruction develops, the degree of obstruction, and the presence or absence of collateral circulation (Haapoja & Blendowski, 1999). Dyspnea is the most common presenting symptom, occurring in more than 60% of patients (Pinover & Coia, 1998; Yahalom, 2001). The next most common symptom is facial swelling or head fullness, which has been reported in 50% of patients (Pinover & Coia). Patients also report cough, arm swelling, facial redness (plethora), dysphagia, and chest pain. Physical exam may reveal distention of the superficial veins of the upper chest and arms; facial, periorbital, neck, and arm swelling; plethora; mental status changes; and lethargy. Some patients report that symptoms worsen on bending forward, stooping, or lying down (Yahalom).

Assessment and Diagnosis

In addition to notation of signs and symptoms, clinicians must assess for relevant past medical history, which would include history of cancer. Diagnostic tests include chest x-ray, computed tomography (CT) scan, magnetic resonance imaging (MRI), and contrast venography. The initial diagnostic test usually is a chest radiograph. Chest x-ray may demonstrate mediastinal widening or right hilar mass. More than 60% of patients who have SVCS have mediastinal widening (Pinover & Coia, 1998). Right-sided pleural effusion from venous hypertension and obstruction of thoracic lymphatics also may be present (Sitton, 2000).

Chest CT with contrast or thoracic MRI will provide more information regarding the thoracic anatomy. CT scan is 100% accurate in determining whether the cause of SVCS is mass or thrombus (Haapoja & Blendowski, 1999). It also can determine if a mass is present, the size and position of the mass, and the extent of collateral circulation. Additionally, these tests can determine the degree of obstruction of the superior vena cava.

Contrast venography can be performed to locate the area and degree of occlusion of the superior vena cava in patients who are candidates for stent placement or surgery (Haapoja & Blendowski, 1999; Sitton, 2000). Disadvantages of this procedure are that it is invasive and it requires the use of contrast material. CT can provide similar information. MRI also is being investigated as a noninvasive approach to evaluate the chest (Yahalom, 2001). Diagnostic tests must be performed on patients without a diagnosis, as emergent radiotherapy before diagnosis can interfere with diagnosis and further treatment. These tests include mediastinoscopy, sputum cytology, bronchoscopy, or fine-needle biopsy to obtain pathology for diagnosis. Initially, an increased risk of hemorrhage during diagnostic procedures in patients with SVCS was theorized; however, Ahmann (1984) demonstrated that this risk was small and without life-threatening complications. In situations that are not life-threatening, diagnosis should be made for all patients to ensure appropriate treatment.

Treatment

In general, treatment depends on the underlying problem. Patients with SVCS caused by thrombus from implanted venous access devices are treated with anticoagulants and antithrombolytics. Antithrombolytics are used to lyse the thrombus, whereas anticoagulants (heparin and warfarin) are used to prevent further clot formation and progression. A catheter-related thrombus occasionally results in removal of the catheter. Warfarin prophylaxis (1 mg per day) has been shown to prevent catheter-related thrombus formation (Bern et al., 1990).

In patients with tumor-induced SVCS, conservative management with steroids and diuretics often is used in patients with minimal symptoms or in those who are acutely ill and unable to tolerate more aggressive therapy. The use of both steroids and diuretics is controversial because of the absence of clinical trials showing efficacy. Theoretically, steroids are used to decrease inflammation, although inflammation is usually not associated with SVCS (Mack, 1997). Steroids may be useful in situations in which respiratory distress is present or to decrease edema associated with radiation therapy (Haapoja & Blendowski, 1999; Mack). Use of diuretics is thought to decrease edema, although their efficacy has not been proven (Mack).

In patients with SCLC, chemotherapy or radiotherapy is usually the preferred initial treatment. These tumors are generally sensitive and have been shown to respond with similar frequency (> 90%) to both modalities (Yahalom, 2001). Resolution or reduction of symptoms usually occurs within 7–10 days of treatment (Mack, 1997; Sitton, 2000). Combination treatment with chemotherapy and radiation therapy sometimes is used, but the incidence of toxicity is greater with combined modalities. SCLC responds to combinations of chemotherapy such as etoposide and cisplatin or cytoxan, Adriamycin® (Pfizer, New York, NY), and vincristine. Chemotherapy is the choice of treatment for those who have previously received chest radiotherapy. Extreme care must be used when administering chemotherapy to patients with SVCS. Because of swelling and venous stasis from SVCS, some practitioners recommend not using the involved upper extremities because local accumulation of drug, vein irritation, and poor absorption of drug may occur (Sitton, 2000). SVCS is not considered to be a poor prognostic sign in patients with SCLC (Mack; Yahalom).

Radiotherapy and chemotherapy also are used to treat SVCS associated with NSCLC. Radiotherapy usually is the initial treatment because NSCLC generally is not recognized to be a chemosensitive tumor (Sitton, 2000; Yahalom, 2001). In general, this tumor is not as sensitive to treatment as SCLC. In contrast, SVCS usually is a poor prognostic sign for patients with NSCLC (Mack, 1997). Overall prognosis in patients with SVCS depends on many factors, including the underlying disease and stage of disease, previous treatment, the responsiveness of the tumor to the chemotherapy or radiotherapy, and the patient's performance status.

If histologic diagnosis cannot be determined and the status of the patient is deteriorating, radiation therapy is the recommended treatment (Yahalom, 2001). Different fractionation schedules have been investigated, but no current data support one fractionation scheme over another. Symptoms usually abate by two weeks, with maximum effect seen at three weeks (Sitton, 2000). Intravascular stent placement is a newer option in patients with SVCS. The stents are placed by an interventional radiologist. Three types of stents commonly are used: the Wallstent® (Boston Scientific Corp, Natick, MA), the Gianturco Z-Stent® (Wilson Cook Inc., Winston-Salem, NC), and the Palmaz® stent (Cordis Endovascular, Warren, NJ). The Wallstent is the most commonly used of the three (Schindler & Vogelzang, 1999; Yahalom). No prospective randomized trials support the use of one stent over another (Schindler & Vogelzang). Success rates are reported to be in the range of 68%–100% (Sitton, 2000). Symptom improvement is immediate for some, with most patients experiencing symptom improvement within 12 hours; peripheral edema usually improves within 1–7 days (Sitton, 2000). The use of anticoagulants in patients with stents has not been resolved (Schindler & Vogelzang).

Conclusions

Overall, SVCS is an uncommon complication in patients with malignancy. It is most often seen in patients with SCLC, NSCLC with squamous cell histology, or non-Hodgkin's lymphoma. For most patients, symptoms are present for one or more weeks and it rarely presents as a life-threatening complication. Healthcare providers must be aware of the signs and symptoms of SVCS so that treatment can be initiated before complete obstruction occurs. Chemotherapy and radiotherapy are the most commonly employed treatments; however, stent placement represents a new option for some.

Pericardial Effusion and Cardiac Tamponade

Introduction

Pericardial effusion is an abnormal increase in fluid within the pericardial sac. It can lead to cardiac tamponade, in which the heart is compromised from increased pericardial pressure. Cardiac tamponade is a medical emergency and is most commonly caused by malignant disease (Beauchamp, 1998; Knoop & Willenberg, 1999). The malignancies most often associated with pericardial effusion and tamponade are lung and breast cancers (Knoop & Willenberg). Other malignancies that can cause effusion include malignant mesothelioma, leukemia, and lymphoma. The incidence of pericardial effusion is highest in patients with lung cancer, and has been reported to occur in 40%–80% of patients (Kaplow, 2000; Shelton, 2000). In one retro-

spective study, cardiac tamponade was the initial presentation of NSCLC in 30% of patients (Wang et al., 2000). For most patients, cardiac tamponade is a late manifestation of metastatic disease and long-term survival for these patients is limited (Ewer, Durand, Swafford, & Yusuf, 2002). Cough and dyspnea are common symptoms and often are attributed to the patient's underlying malignancy, especially in patients with thoracic malignancies.

Pathophysiology

In healthy people, the pericardial sac contains 15–50 ml of fluid, which provides lubrication. Pericardial effusion is an abnormally large accumulation of fluid within the pericardial sac; the amount of fluid can range from as little as 200 ml to as much as 1,800 ml (Beauchamp, 1998). Effusions can be caused by metastatic disease, pericarditis from radiation therapy, or increased capillary permeability caused by high-dose chemotherapy or biotherapy (Shelton, 2000). Metastatic disease or direct tumor extension may block venous or lymphatic drainage, leading to increased fluid around the heart (Knoop & Willenberg, 1999). Other causes include infection, hemorrhage, and myocardial infarction. Additionally, some reports have documented the development of tamponade following improper placement of central venous catheters (Knoop & Willenberg).

Development of tamponade depends on the compliance of the pericardium and the rate and amount of fluid accumulation (Kaplow, 2000). The body can compensate if fluid accumulates slowly; however, compensatory mechanisms fail if fluid accumulates quickly. Cardiac tamponade results when the heart is compromised from this increased pericardial pressure and can no longer function normally. Specifically, pressure is exerted on all four chambers of the heart, resulting in decreased cardiac output and stroke volume, increased intracardiac pressure, and decreased ventricular diastolic filling (Beauchamp, 1998). As a result of decreased cardiac output, the body compensates with adrenergic stimulation, which leads to tachycardia and peripheral vasoconstriction (Knoop & Willenberg, 1999). Cardiovascular collapse can ensue when the body is no longer able to compensate for the increased intrapericardial volume and pressure.

Signs and Symptoms

The development of signs and symptoms of cardiac tamponade depend on the rate at which fluid accumulates within the pericardial space and the patient's baseline cardiac function. In general, if fluid accumulates slowly, patients may be asymptomatic or have vague symptoms. In contrast, if fluid accumulates rapidly, patients may quickly decompensate and become critically ill. Patients with compromised cardiac function from comorbid conditions are likely to experience increased symptoms earlier in the course.

With slow accumulation of pericardial fluid, patients may experience mild symptoms, such as fatigue, mild dyspnea, orthopnea, and cough. Dyspnea and cough are the most common symptoms in patients with pericardial effusion (Zwischenberger & Bradford, 1996). Patients also may experience vague retrosternal chest pain and palpitations (Knoop & Willenberg, 1999). Chest pain usually is more severe when the patient is in the supine position (Camp-Sorrell, 1997). As the fluid increases within the pericardial sac, symptoms become more pronounced and include worsening dyspnea and cough, peripheral edema, and, less likely, low-grade fever. With severe tamponade, patients may have anxiety or become restless and confused (Kaplow, 2000).

Physical exam may be normal or abnormal and also depends on the amount of fluid and how rapidly fluid accumulates within the pericardial sac. Signs of tachycardia, muffled heart sounds, hypotension, jugular venous distension, and edema may be present. Paradoxical pulse (pulsus paradoxus) and narrowed pulse pressure also are common findings on exam. Pulsus paradoxus is best determined with a sphygmomanometer. Normally on inspiration, systolic pressure drops 10 mm/Hg. With pulsus paradoxus, the drop in systolic pressure is greater than 10 mmHg and is accompanied by diminution or disappearance of pulse (Knoop & Willenberg, 1999). Paradoxical pulse is a classic finding in cardiac tamponade but also may occur in patients with other lung disease, such as chronic obstructive pulmonary disease (Ewer et al., 2002). It is not diagnostic of effusion and tamponade.

Assessment and Diagnosis

The gold standard for diagnosis of cardiac tamponade is the two-dimensional echocardiogram. This test is noninvasive and specific and may be done at the bedside if needed. It also is useful in determining hemodynamic stability of the heart (Ewer et al., 2002). Common findings on echocardiography include right atrial compression, diastolic collapse of the right ventricle, and cardiac "rocking" (Ewer et al.). The right side of the heart is more likely to be affected by the pressure of pericardial fluid because it contains less muscle than the left side of the heart (Beauchamp, 1998). Echocardiography also is useful in patients who require pericardiocentesis or placement of a drainage catheter. Other tests include chest x-ray, CT, and electrocardiogram. Chest x-ray may reveal an enlarged heart or the classic "water-bottle cardiac silhouette" and a widened mediastinum (Schrump & Nguyen, 2001). CT is not the test of choice because it is both time-consuming and is no more accurate than echocardiogram. The main advantage of chest CT is that it can detect very small amounts of pericardial fluid and help to identify the type of effusion (Schrump & Nguyen). Electrocardiogram is not diagnostic but may support the diagnosis if low-voltage QRS complexes and electrical alternans are seen. Additionally, one may see elevated ST segments and nonspecific T wave changes (Camp-Sorrell, 1997).

Pericardial fluid should be analyzed to help confirm the diagnosis of malignant effusion. In patients with malignant effusions, the fluid can be sanguineous or serosanguineous and have an increased lactic dehydrogenase (LDH) (Camp-Sorrell, 1997). A recent retrospective study demonstrated that serous pericardial effusions are as likely to be associated with malignancy as bloody effusions (Chiu, Atar, & Siegel, 2001). Fluid also should be analyzed for the presence of malignant cells, although in patients with NSCLC with cardiac tamponade, the most likely cause of effusion is the cancer whether or not malignant cells are present in the fluid (Wang et al., 2000).

Treatment

The initial goal of treatment in tamponade is fluid removal. Several different methods are used to treat pericardial effusion and tamponade. Patient considerations that must be taken into account to determine the best method for fluid removal include the initial presenting symptoms, the diagnosis and stage of disease, prognosis, patient age and physical condition, and hemodynamic stability (Kaplow, 2000). Goals of care also should include restoration of cardiac function, prevention of fluid reaccumulation, and prevention of complications (Kaplow). Overall, the best way to control or prevent cardiac tamponade is to control the tumor. Pericardiocentesis is indicated in patients who have life-threatening tamponade and are unable to undergo surgery. This procedure can be performed at the bedside with cardiac monitoring (Kaplow; Shelton, 2000). A pericardial catheter often is left in place to drain the remaining fluid. The catheter is removed when the total 24-hour drainage is between 50–100 ml (Shelton). The disadvantage to this procedure is that fluid will reaccumulate in most patients unless a more definitive procedure is performed. Pericardiocentesis with intrapericardial sclerosis is a more definitive procedure for prevention of recurrent effusions. In this procedure, fluid is drained as previously described. When the drainage is less than 50–100 ml in a 24-hour period, a sclerosing agent is instilled within the pericardial sac. Instillation of the agent creates an inflammatory response within the pericardial sac, which eventually leads to obliteration of the pericardial space, thus preventing reaccumulation of fluid. Commonly used sclerosing agents include, but are not limited to, thiotepa, doxycycline, bleomycin, and minocycline (Kaplow; Zwischenberger & Bradford, 1996).

A retrospective study examining 93 patients with malignant pericardial effusion demonstrated that patients who had drainage of pericardial effusion and sclerosis had lower morbidity, mortality, and recurrence rates as compared to those who had drainage alone (Maher, Shephard, & Todd, 1996). In another retrospective study, pericardiocentesis with intrapericardial sclerosis was as effective as open surgical drainage for malignant pericardial effusions (Girardi,

Ginsberg, & Burt, 1997). Additionally, the costs associated with surgery far exceeded those of pericardiocentesis with sclerosis. One disadvantage to pericardial sclerosis is that it can be a painful procedure and generally requires the use of narcotic analgesics, depending on the agent used. Additionally, some agents will cause a febrile reaction. Thiotepa is the choice of sclerosing agent at one institution as it generally does not cause pain or a febrile reaction (Girardi et al.) Surgical management involves either formation of a pericardial window or a pericardiectomy. Both procedures are performed in the operating room with general anesthesia, although, in selected cases, pericardial window may be performed with local anesthesia and IV sedation (Moores et al., 1995). In general, both procedures should only be performed in those who are expected to have a longer survival (Beauchamp, 1998). Formation of a pericardial window involves removal of a section of pericardium and insertion of mesh, which allows fluid to drain into the surrounding tissue (Shelton, 2000). Pericardiectomy involves removing or striping of the pericardial membrane. This procedure rarely is performed because other options are readily available (Shelton).

Conclusions

In conclusion, cardiac tamponade is a life-threatening complication seen in patients with pericardial effusion. The majority of patients with tamponade are those with a diagnosis of bronchogenic cancer. Prompt recognition and treatment (evacuation of pericardial fluid) are required to prevent hemodynamic collapse and possible death. Healthcare providers should be aware of this complication. Several treatment options are available, and the best option takes into account patient physical health, prognosis, and diagnosis.

Pleural Effusion

Introduction

Pleural effusion, an excess accumulation of fluid within the pleural space, is a common complication of cancer. It is estimated to occur in about half of all patients with lung cancer, and lung and breast cancers cause up to 75% of all pleural effusions (Stretton, Edmonds, & Marrinan, 1999; Taubert, 2001). Malignant pleural effusion most commonly is caused by lung cancer, and it may be the initial presentation in those patients. Symptoms depend on the amount of fluid present and the rate at which the fluid accumulates. Patients with small effusions may be relatively asymptomatic, whereas those with large amounts of fluid may have severe symptoms. Although rare, pleural effusions become emergent when a large amount of fluid is present and an associated opacification of the hemithorax with mediastinal shift exists, which can lead to hemodynamic compromise.

Pathophysiology

The pleural surface is made up of a single layer of mesothelial cells that line the lungs (visceral pleura), chest wall, diaphragm, and mediastinum (parietal pleura) (Erasmus, Goodman, & Patz, 2000). The theoretical space between the parietal and visceral layers (the pleural space) normally contains 10–20 ml of fluid. However, over a 24-hour period, as much as 100–200 ml of fluid may pass through this space (Mayo, 1999). This fluid acts as a lubricant during respiration. Fluid within the pleural space is regulated by five processes: capillary permeability, oncotic pressure, hydrostatic pressure, negative intrapleural pressure, and lymphatic drainage. One or more of these processes is disrupted in the patient with lung cancer, which results in the accumulation of abnormal amounts of fluid within the pleural space. Alteration of lymphatic drainage from the pleural space is usually the cause with malignancy (Baciewicz, 2000). Accumulation of large amounts of fluid within the pleural space can lead to restriction of lung function and affect the patient's ability to breathe. Pleural effusions are classified as transudates or exudates. Characteristically, exudates in people over 60 years of age most commonly are caused by malignancy (Erasmus et al.). Exudates usually are caused by local problems that have an effect on the formation and absorption of pleural fluid, such as malignancy, pneumonia, or tuberculosis (Hayes, 2001). Characteristically, an exudate contains white blood cells, red blood cells, and protein, resulting in fluid that appears to be cloudy or serosanguineous. Alternatively, if the exudate is caused by infection, it will have a purulent appearance (empyema). Transudates result from systemic problems, such as cirrhosis or left-ventricular failure. Essentially, they are devoid of plasma proteins and white cells and, thus, are watery or straw colored (Hayes).

Signs and Symptoms

The severity of symptoms is related to the amount of pleural fluid and the rate at which the fluid accumulates. The majority (77%) of patients with malignant pleural effusion have symptoms (Baciewicz, 2000), which usually include shortness of breath, dry cough, and pleuritic chest pain. As the amount of pleural fluid increases, patients also may experience orthopnea. With involvement of the diaphragmatic parietal pleura, ipsilateral shoulder pain or discomfort may exist (Baciewicz). In patients with lung cancer, these symptoms are common as a result of the underlying disease; they can be exacerbated by the development of a malignant pleural effusion. As a result, not all symptoms may be relieved with treatment of the pleural effusion. Most signs found on physical exam are attributable to fluid in the pleural space that separates the air-filled lung from the chest wall. Signs include dullness to percussion over the fluid and decreased or absent tactile fremitus on palpation. With a large effusion with mediastinal shift, the trachea may be deviated to the opposite side (away from the effusion). Auscultation reveals decreased or absent breath sounds, and egophony or a pleural rub may be heard.

Assessment and Diagnosis

When pleural effusion is suspected, usually the first test to be performed is a chest radiograph, with posterior-anterior and lateral views. If fluid is evident on the radiograph (seen as blunting of the costophrenic angle), a lateral decubitus film should be performed. As little as 175 ml of fluid may be detected on an upright chest film, and smaller amounts may be seen on the lateral decubitus view (Baciewicz, 2000). A lateral decubitus film will determine if the fluid is free-flowing or loculated. This is important because it will help to determine treatment. With large pleural effusions, chest film may demonstrate complete opacification of the hemithorax and mediastinal shift. Often, chest CT also is performed. CT will definitively determine effusion, atelectasis, or pleural-based tumor (Baciewicz). CT also can help to determine loculated effusions. Mediastinal adenopathy and tumors also may be seen on CT. CT is an important test, especially if pleural effusion is the presenting sign of malignancy. However, this test will not determine the etiology of the effusion.

Thoracentesis with examination of the pleural fluid is often the next step in determining the cause of the pleural effusion. This test will help to determine whether the cause is cancer related. Typically, malignant pleural fluid will appear grossly bloody and as an exudate. Not all bloody effusions are malignant. Malignant effusions usually are characterized as exudates, and 85% of malignant effusions are exudates (Baciewicz, 2000). Characteristics of an exudate include pleural-to-serum protein ratio greater than 0.5, total protein greater than 3 g/dl, pleural LDH-to-serum ratio greater than 0.6, and pleural fluid LDH level greater than 200 international units (Baciewicz; Stretton et al., 1999). Very often, the effusion has a leukocyte count of 1,000–10,000. In general, the white cells are mostly lymphocytes; however, if the predominant cell type is a neutrophil, inflammation should be considered (Baciewicz). Fluid also needs to be examined for cytology because 70% of malignant pleural effusions will demonstrate positive cytology (Works & Maxwell, 2000). Occasionally, a malignant effusion will present as a transudate; this can happen early in the malignant process and usually is related to mediastinal adenopathy with impaired lymphatic drainage (Baciewicz). Figure 5-1 shows an algorithm for diagnosis and management of malignant pleural effusion.

Treatment

Patients with small asymptomatic malignant effusions usually do not require local treatment. Depending on the tumor type, the effusions may resolve with systemic treatment of the tumor. In patients who are symptomatic and have a larger effusion, goals of treatment include fluid removal for both symptom control and diagnosis. Thoracentesis often may be the first procedure, especially if a diagnosis needs to be established. Thoracentesis also is effective for short-term control of symptoms associated with pleural effusion, but repeated thoracentesis may lead to risk of infection; loculated effusion and recurrence is frequent.

Pleurodesis offers a more definitive outcome and should be considered unless the prognosis is poor and the patient is too ill to tolerate the procedure. This procedure is performed under local anesthesia. Pleurodesis involves placement of a chest tube (tube thoracoscopy) to drain the effusion. When this is

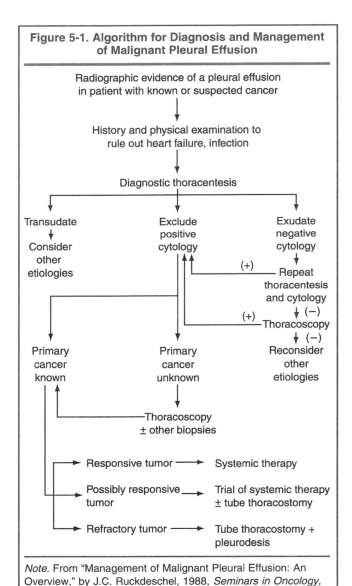

Figure 5-1. Algorithm for Diagnosis and Management of Malignant Pleural Effusion

Note. From "Management of Malignant Pleural Effusion: An Overview," by J.C. Ruckdeschel, 1988, *Seminars in Oncology, 15*(3 Suppl. 3), p. 26. Copyright 1988 by W.B. Saunders. Reprinted with permission.

accomplished, a sclerosing agent is instilled through the chest tube into the pleural space. The agent causes irritation of the pleural cavity, which leads to an inflammatory reaction. This inflammatory reaction causes the parietal and visceral pleura to adhere, thus eliminating the pleural space and preventing fluid reaccumulation. Three factors contribute to successful pleurodesis: the pleural space must be completely drained of fluid, the lung needs to reexpand, and the sclerosing agent must be adequately distributed (Stretton et al., 1999).

Alternatively, in patients who need a diagnosis, video-assisted thoracoscopy (VATS) may be used. At the time of VATS, a chest tube is placed and sclerosis can be performed at the conclusion of the procedure (Baciewicz, 2000). This is a surgical procedure and requires general anesthesia.

Over the years, many different agents have been used for sclerosis. Tetracycline was the sclerosing agent of choice for many years; however, this agent is no longer available (Works & Maxwell, 2000). Most commonly, bleomycin and sterilized talc are used (Works & Maxwell). Talc is considered to be the agent of first choice because success rates have been reported in 90%–96% of procedures (Baciewicz, 2000). It is inexpensive and offers no risk of the systemic side effects associated with bleomycin. Complications of talc pleurodesis include respiratory distress syndrome and pneumonitis. Pain and fever also may occur with pleural sclerosis.

Pleuroperitoneal shunting is the recommended procedure in recurrent effusions or in patients who have nonexpansion of the lung (trapped-lung syndrome) (Baciewicz, 2000; Stretton et al., 1999). A pleuroperitoneal shunt can be placed using local anesthesia (Stretton et al.). Patients must be able to operate the shunt for 10 minutes (pressing the pump 100 times in each 10-minute period) four to six times each day (Works & Maxwell, 2000). Disadvantages include shunt malfunction and clotting of the device.

Placement of an indwelling pleural catheter with intermittent drainage is another treatment approach for patients with recurrent malignant pleural effusions. The catheter can be placed at the bedside or in the outpatient setting under local anesthesia. The catheter has a one-way valve, allowing outflow of pleural fluid but preventing air and fluid from entering the catheter (Taubert, 2001). Pleural fluid usually is drained every one to two days. "Mechanical pleurodesis" occurs in many patients because the catheter acts as an irritant in the pleural cavity and drains the pleural cavity dry, essentially the same process as with chemical pleurodesis (Taubert). This procedure offers a great advantage to many patients and caregivers. It allows the patient to be at home with symptom control maintained by draining the fluid every one or two days. This is especially important as the life expectancy in patients with recurrent malignant pleural effusion is limited. The Pleurex® (Denver Biomedical, Golden, CO) pleural catheter is a type of small-bore silicone tube placed for long-term drainage of malignant pleural effusions (Brubacher & Gobel, 2003). The manufacturer provides special kits con-

taining vacuum bottles and dressing supplies. Spontaneous pleurodesis has been reported to occur in some cases with the catheter alone (Brubacher & Gobel). This catheter is placed in an outpatient setting with local anesthesia and conscious sedation as necessary. It is used primarily in patients with symptomatic, recurrent pleural effusions, those in whom pleurodesis has failed, and those unable to tolerate more invasive procedures.

Pleurectomy is another option for managing effusions. This is a surgical procedure that must be performed in the operating room under general anesthesia. In this procedure, a thoracotomy is performed and the parietal pleura removed, causing a mechanical pleurodesis (Taubert, 2001). This procedure is reserved for patients with recurrent malignant pleural effusions who have a good performance status and life expectancy.

Conclusions

Malignant pleural effusion is a common complication in patients with lung cancer. Pleural effusions may be the initial presentation or may occur later in the course of the disease. In rare cases, when a large effusion is present, pleural effusion may present as an emergent situation, with opacification of the hemithorax, mediastinal shift, and hemodynamic compromise. In this case, immediate removal of fluid is required. For most patients, goals of treatment include palliation of symptoms and maintenance of quality of life. Small effusions, in patients who are not symptomatic, may not require intervention. In some, systemic treatment of the tumor may lead to resolution of the effusion. Larger effusions and patients who are symptomatic require intervention by one of the procedures outlined herein. In this case, the goals of treatment are obliteration of the pleural space and palliation of symptoms.

Malignant Spinal Cord Compression

Introduction

Spinal cord compression is the second most common neurologic complication from cancer. Lung cancer is the leading cause of spinal cord compression (Sullivan, 1996). Other causes of malignant spinal cord compression include breast cancer, prostate cancer, and multiple myeloma. Overall, 5%–10% of patients with cancer will develop spinal cord compression during the course of their illness (Peterson-Rivera & Watters, 1997; Rades, Karstens, & Alberti, 2002). In the majority of cases, spinal cord compression is a later manifestation of malignancy; however, it is estimated to be the initial manifestation of malignancy in 8%–35% of cases (Labovich, 1994).

Spinal cord compression is a true neurologic emergency. Successful outcomes depend on early recognition of signs and symptoms of spinal cord compression and early intervention. Without prompt diagnosis and intervention, patients may become irreversibly paralyzed and experience sensory loss and sphincter incontinence. In patients with a loss of function at diagnosis of spinal cord compression, treatment is not likely to reverse damage. However, early treatment is estimated to be effective in 90% of patients (Fuller, Heiss, & Oldfield, 2001).

Pathophysiology

The spinal cord, a portion of the central nervous system, is protected by the vertebral column. It consists of nervous tissue that connects the brain and the body (Sunderland, 1994). The spinal column extends from the brain to the first two lumbar vertebrae (Flaherty, 2000; Sunderland). Below this, extending through the remaining vertebral column (lumbar, sacral, and coccygeal areas) is the cauda equina (a collection of nerve roots) (Flaherty; Flounders & Ott, 2003). The spinal cord and brain are protected by three membranes (the meninges), the dura mater, the arachnoid membrane, and the pia mater (Sunderland). The dura mater is the outermost layer closest to the vertebrae and skull; the pia mater lies closest to the brain and spinal cord. The arachnoid membrane lies in between the dura and pia mater. The epidural or extradural space lies between the vertebrae or skull and the meninges (Sunderland). Between the dura mater and the arachnoid membrane is the subdural space; the subarachnoid space lies beneath the arachnoid membrane (Sunderland) (see Figure 5-2).

Malignant spinal cord compression most commonly is caused by metastatic disease rather than from a primary tumor of the spinal cord or spinal canal (Flounders & Ott, 2003). Three different types of spinal cord metastases exist: intramedullary, leptomeningeal, and epidural, referring to the location of metastatic disease (Flaherty, 2000). Metastasis to the epidural space is the most common type of spinal cord metastatic disease (Flaherty). Metastatic disease is rare in the intramedullary and leptomeningeal sites. Most metastatic disease (70%) occurs in the thoracic area of the spinal column (Grandt, 2000). Metastatic spread to the epidural space occurs through three mechanisms: "hematogenous spread; direct tumor extension; and direct metastatic deposits of tumor cells" (Bucholtz, 1999, p. 152). Hematogenous spread to vertebrae accounts for 85% of all cases of spinal cord compression (Bucholtz). In this case, metastatic growth of tumor within the vertebra leads to subsequent destruction of bone. Direct tumor extension usually occurs in patients with non-Hodgkin's lymphoma; direct metastatic deposits of tumor cells are seen in patients with leukemia (Bucholtz).

Neurologic abnormalities result from interruption of the vascular supply to the spinal cord by tumor or bone destruction, direct compression of the spinal cord, vertebral collapse secondary to pathologic bone destruction, and dislocation of vertebral bodies (Flounders & Ott, 2003). Cellular injury to nerve tissue occurs from pressure on the spinal cord exerted by the tumor (Flounders & Ott). Cellular injury is mediated by the following mechanisms: vasogenic edema; cytokines, including prostaglandin, interleukin-1, and interleukin-6, which cause demyelination and nerve tissue injury; serotonin and glutamide, which cause tissue damage; and cytotoxic edema, which causes irreversible paraplegia (Bucholtz, 1999).

Signs and Symptoms

Signs and symptoms of spinal cord compression depend on the site of vertebral metastases and the amount of tumor invasion. Back pain is the initial presenting symptom in nearly all patients (95%) and may precede neurologic signs and symptoms by days to months (Bucholtz, 1999). Pain is either localized or radicular in nature. Local pain occurs at or near the site of the tumor and characteristically tends to be constant, dull, and aching (Flounders & Ott, 2003). Radicular pain results from irritation of the nerve root by compression from tumor. It is shooting and burning in nature and can be exacerbated by coughing or movement. Constrictive-band-like pain is caused by compression of thoracic vertebrae, whereas involvement of cervical or lumbosacral vertebrae tends to cause pain in a limb (Flaherty, 2000). The pain associated with compression of thoracic vertebrae usually is bilateral, whereas pain associated with compression of cervical or a lumbosacral vertebra is usually unilateral (Flaherty). Pain radiating to the buttocks indicates compression at the sacral level (Weinstein, 2001).

The highest incidence of lung cancer is in the elderly. In this group, back pain is a common problem and may be caused by degenerative or disc disease. Consequently, these patients often minimize back pain, attributing it to arthritis or injury. Characteristically, pain from spinal cord compression is worse on lying down, whereas pain from degenerative disease usually is relieved by this measure. Therefore, any patient who reports worsening of pain when lying down should be evaluated for spinal cord compression (Manzullo, Rhines, & Forman, 2002). In patients with epidural spinal cord compression, neurologic symptoms tend to progress from pain to motor weakness, sensory loss, motor loss, and autonomic dysfunction (Flounders & Ott, 2003). Motor weakness often is described as heaviness or stiffness in the limbs, which may cause difficulty in walking. Sensory loss is characterized by numbness, tingling, and the inability to determine temperature. Sensory changes are detected in nearly half of patients at presentation (Weinstein, 2001). Late manifestations of motor and sensory loss include autonomic dysfunction, such as loss of sphincter control, loss of coordination, and ataxia (Flounders & Ott).

Some patients may have significant epidural compression with no neurologic signs or symptoms (Weinstein, 2001).

Figure 5-2. Cross-Section of the Spinal Cord

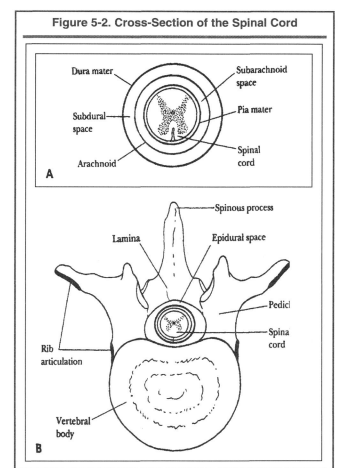

Note. From "Spinal Cord Compression" (p. 888) by A.M. Flaherty in C.H. Yarbro, M.H. Frogge, M. Goodman, and S.L. Groenwald (Eds.), *Cancer Nursing: Principles and Practice* (5th ed.), 2000, Sudbury, MA: Jones and Bartlett. Copyright 2000 by Jones and Bartlett. Reprinted with permission.

Physical exam in a patient with suspected epidural spinal cord compression may not be revealing. The exam should focus on the neurologic and musculoskeletal systems (Bucholtz, 1999). It should include gentle percussion and palpation over the spine, which may reveal tenderness at the level of tumor involvement. Findings on neurologic exam will depend on the degree of spinal cord compromise. Neurologic exam may reveal sensory deficits below the level of disease. Motor deficits include weakness and hyperreflexia. Autonomic dysfunction should be suspected in those with decreased rectal tone or a distended bladder.

Assessment and Diagnosis

Radiographic assessment may include plain x-rays of the spine, bone scan, myelogram CT scan, and MRI. Plain films are often the first exam to be performed and may demonstrate a mass or a lytic or blastic lesion within the vertebrae. For this to be evident on plain film, significant bone change from tumor must occur; therefore, a normal exam does not rule out epidural metastases (Peterson-Rivera & Watters, 1997; Weinstein, 2001). Additionally, the spinal cord and nerve roots are not visualized on plain films; therefore, CT, MRI, or myelogram must be performed (Novelline, 1997). When plain films are negative, a bone scan can be performed to detect possible bone disease. Bone scan has several disadvantages, however. It does not differentiate degenerative disease from metastatic disease, and it does not offer visualization of the spinal cord and nerve roots. When available, contrast-enhanced MRI is probably the best test to diagnose epidural spinal cord compression (Sitton, 1998). This test is safe and noninvasive, and the entire spine can be imaged easily. The spinal cord and nerve roots are visualized on MRI. Additionally, paraspinal masses are visible (Sitton) and MRI can distinguish between vertebral, extradural, intradural, extramedullary, and intramedullary lesions (Peterson-Rivera & Watters). Leptomeningeal disease also can be detected on MRI (Flaherty, 2000). If MRI is not available or the test is contraindicated (e.g., presence of pacemaker, claustrophobia), CT myelogram should be performed. An advantage to myelogram is that a sample of cerebral spinal fluid can be obtained for analysis. CT myelography also allows the neural elements to be visualized. CT myelography is an invasive test that requires a lumbar puncture and injection of a contrast agent (Novelline; Peterson-Rivera & Watters).

Treatment

For the majority of patients with lung cancer, epidural spinal cord compression is managed medically, and treatment is palliative in nature. The goals of treatment are preservation or restoration of neurologic function, pain control, and control of the tumor. Prompt intervention is required to prevent continued deterioration of the patient's functional status. The majority of patients who were ambulatory before treatment remain so, but only about 10% of patients who were paraplegic before treatment will regain some function with treatment (Peterson-Rivera & Watters, 1997)

Surgical intervention is reserved for those with spinal instability, compression from bone fragments in the canal, radioresistant primary (worsening disease on or after radiotherapy), and significant pain (Flaherty, 2000; Sullivan, 1996). In patients with lung cancer, surgical intervention should be considered on a case-by-case basis in patients with a good performance status and in whom the benefits outweigh the risks. Morbidity from surgical intervention has been estimated to be as high as 48% (Flaherty).

Medical management includes the use of corticosteroids, pain control, and radiation therapy. Corticosteroids often are the first intervention and are used regardless of the choice of definitive treatment (Sitton, 1998). They are used to decrease edema and inflammation and to help with pain control (Flounders & Ott, 2003). Additionally, neurologic deficits may improve with the use of corticosteroids. The best dose or schedule of administration has not been documented (Sullivan, 1996). However, many believe that high-dose corticosteroids, such as dexamethasone bolus IV followed by 96 mg/day, given orally, tapered quickly over a few weeks, are superior to the lower-dose regimens (Manzullo et al., 2002; Weinstein, 2001). Other studies have shown that lower-dose regimens are as effective and cause fewer steroid-related side effects (Heimdal, Hirschberg, Slettebo, Watne, & Nome, 1992; Vecht et al., 1989).

Radiation therapy is the treatment of choice for spinal cord compression, and response rates have ranged from 40%–80% (Bucholtz, 1999; Sullivan, 1996). Because the success of radiation therapy depends on the radiosensitivity of the tumor, it has varying effects in NSCLC, which is not considered particularly radiosensitive (Sullivan). Radiation therapy is believed to be more effective in patients with SCLC because SCLC is believed to be more radiosensitive; however, this has not been proven (Sullivan). The optimum fractionation schedule for the treatment of malignant spinal cord compression has not yet been determined (Rades et al., 2002). The most common dosage range of radiation is 30–40 Gy given over two to four weeks (Bucholtz; Flaherty, 2000; Peterson-Rivera & Watters, 1997). However, most courses are given in 10 fractions over 2.5 weeks (Bucholtz). The radiation field usually covers the area of spinal cord compression as well as one to two vertebral bodies above and below the area of compression (Flounders & Ott, 2003). Normal tissue is spared from the radiation as much as possible. Response to radiation therapy is measured as decrease in tumor mass, pain control, and preservation of function. In general, radiation therapy is well tolerated. The most common side effects include fatigue and skin changes.

Conclusions

Malignant epidural spinal cord compression is a true oncologic emergency that is seen in patients with lung cancer. For some patients, spinal cord compression may be the initial presentation of lung cancer. Outcome, including preservation of neurologic function, depends on prompt recognition and treatment. Early intervention, using corticosteroids when spinal cord compression is suspected or diagnosed followed by radiation therapy, most commonly is used in this group of patients.

References

Ahmann, F.R. (1984). A reassessment of the clinical implications of the superior vena cava syndrome. *Journal of Clinical Oncology, 2,* 961–969.

Baciewicz, F.A. (2000). Malignant pleural effusion. In H.I. Pass, J.B. Mitchell, D.H. Johnson, A.T. Turrisi, & J.D. Minna (Eds.), *Lung cancer: Principles and practice* (2nd ed., pp. 1027–1037). Philadelphia: Lippincott Williams & Wilkins.

Beauchamp, K.A. (1998). Pericardial tamponade: An oncologic emergency. *Clinical Journal of Oncology Nursing, 2,* 85–95.

Bern, M.M., Lokich, J.J., Wallach, S.R., Bothe, A., Benotti, P.N., Arkin, D.F., et al. (1990). Very low dose of warfarin can prevent thrombosis in central venous catheters. *Annals of Internal Medicine, 112,* 423–428.

Brubacher, S., & Gobel, B.H. (2003). Use of the Pleurex® catheter for the management of malignant pleural effusions. *Clinical Journal of Oncology Nursing, 7,* 35–38.

Bucholtz, J.D. (1999). Metastatic epidural spinal cord compression. *Seminars in Oncology Nursing, 15,* 150–159.

Camp-Sorrell, D. (1997). Cardiac tamponade. In R.A. Gates & R.M. Fink (Eds.), *Oncology nursing secrets* (pp. 329–331). Philadelphia: Hanley & Belfus, Inc.

Chiu, J., Atar, S., & Siegel, R.J. (2001). Comparison of serous and bloody pericardial effusion as an ominous prognostic sign. *Chest, 87,* 924–926.

Erasmus, J.J., Goodman, P.C., & Patz, E.F. (2000). Management of malignant pleural effusions and pneumothorax. *Radiology Clinics of North America, 38,* 375–383.

Ewer, M.S., Durand, J.B., Swafford, J., & Yusuf, S.W. (2002). Emergency cardiac problems. In S.-C.J. Yeung & C.P. Escalante (Eds.), *Holland-Frei oncologic emergencies* (pp. 304–314). Hamilton, ON: BC Decker.

Flaherty, A.M. (2000). Spinal cord compression. In C.H. Yarbro, M.H. Frogge, M. Goodman, & S.L. Groenwald (Eds.), *Cancer nursing: Principles and practice* (5th ed., pp. 887–899). Sudbury, MA: Jones and Bartlett.

Flounders, J.A., & Ott, B.B. (2003). Oncology emergency modules: Spinal cord compression. *Oncology Nursing Forum, 30,* E17–E21. Retrieved January 15, 2003, from http://www.ons.org/xp6/ONS/Library.xml/ONS_Publications.xml/ONF.xml/ONF2003/FebJan03/Members_Only/Flounders_article.xml

Fuller, B.G., Heiss, J.D., & Oldfield, E.H. (2001). Spinal cord compression. In V.T. De Vita, S. Hellman, & S.A. Rosenberg (Eds.), *Cancer: Principles and practice of oncology* (6th ed., pp. 2617–2632). Philadelphia: Lippincott Williams & Wilkins.

Girardi, L.N., Ginsberg, R.J., & Burt, M.E. (1997). Pericardiocentesis and intrapericardial sclerosis: Effective therapy for malignant pericardial effusions. *Annals of Thoracic Surgery, 64,* 1422–1428.

Grandt, C. (2000). Spinal cord compression. In D. Camp-Sorrell & R.A. Hawkins (Eds.), *Clinical manual for the oncology advanced practice nurse* (pp. 799–804). Pittsburgh, PA: Oncology Nursing Society.

Haapoja, I.S., & Blendowski, C. (1999). Superior vena cava syndrome. *Seminars in Oncology Nursing, 15,* 183–189.

Hayes, D.D. (2001). Stemming the tide of pleural effusions. *Nursing 2001, 31,* 49–52.

Heimdal, K., Hirschberg, H., Slettebo, H., Watne, K., & Nome, O. (1992). High incidence of serious side effects of high-dose dexamethasone treatment in patients with epidural spinal cord compression. *Journal of Neuro-Oncology, 12,* 141–144.

Kaplow, R. (2000). Cardiac tamponade. In C.H. Yarbro, M.H. Frogge, M. Goodman, & S.L. Groenwald (Eds.), *Cancer nursing: Principles and practice* (5th ed., pp. 857–868). Sudbury, MA: Jones and Bartlett.

Knoop, T., & Willenberg, K. (1999). Cardiac tamponade. *Seminars in Oncology Nursing, 15,* 168–173.

Labovich, T.M. (1994). Selected complications in the patient with cancer: Spinal cord compression, malignant bowel obstruction, malignant ascites, and gastrointestinal bleeding. *Seminars in Oncology Nursing, 10,* 189–197.

Mack, K.C. (1997). Superior vena cava syndrome. In R.A. Gates & R.M. Fink (Eds.), *Oncology nursing secrets* (pp. 356–362). Philadelphia: Hanley & Belfus, Inc.

Maher, E.A., Shephard, F.A., & Todd, T.J. (1996). Pericardial sclerosis as the primary management of pericardial effusion and cardiac tamponade. *Journal of Thoracic and Cardiovascular Surgery, 112,* 637–643.

Manzullo, E.F., Rhines, L.D., & Forman, A.D. (2002). Neurologic emergencies. In S.-C.J. Yeung & C.P. Escalante (Eds.), *Holland-Frei oncologic emergencies* (pp. 270–279). Hamilton, ON: BC Decker.

Mayo, D.J. (1999). Malignant pleural effusion. *Clinical Journal of Oncology Nursing, 3,* 36–38.

Moores, D.W.O., Allen, K.B., Faber, L.P., Dziuban, S.W., Gillman, D.J., Warren, W.H., et al. (1995). Subxiphoid pericardial drainage for pericardial tamponade. *Journal of Thoracic and Cardiovascular Surgery, 109,* 546–551.

Novelline, R.A. (1997). The central nervous system. In R.A. Novelline (Ed.), *Squires fundamentals of radiology* (pp. 506–547). Cambridge: Harvard University Press.

Peterson-Rivera, L., & Watters, M.R. (1997). Spinal cord compression. In R.A. Gates & R.M. Fink (Eds.), *Oncology nursing secrets* (pp. 329–331). Philadelphia: Hanley & Belfus.

Pinover, W.H., & Coia, L.R. (1998). Palliative radiation therapy. In A.M. Berger, R.K. Portenoy, & D.E. Weissman (Eds.), *Principles and practice of supportive oncology* (pp. 411–425). Philadelphia: Lippincott-Raven.

Rades, D., Karstens, J.H., & Alberti, W. (2002). Role of radiotherapy in the treatment of motor dysfunction due to metastatic spinal cord compression: Comparison of three different fractionation schedules. *International Journal of Radiation Oncology, Biology, Physics, 54,* 1160–1164.

Schindler, N., & Vogelzang, R.L. (1999). Endovascular and minimally invasive vascular surgery. *Surgical Clinics of North America, 79,* 683–694.

Schrump, D.S., & Nguyen, D.M. (2001). Malignant pleural and pericardial effusions. In V.T. De Vita, S. Hellman, & S.A. Rosenberg (Eds.), *Cancer: Principles and practice of oncology* (6th ed., pp. 2729–2744). Philadelphia: Lippincott Williams & Wilkins.

Shelton, B.K. (2000). Pericarditis/pericardial effusion/cardiac tamponade. In D. Camp-Sorrell & R.A. Hawkins (Eds.), *Clinical manual for the oncology advanced practice nurse* (pp. 307–316). Pittsburgh, PA: Oncology Nursing Society.

Sitton, E. (1998). Central nervous system metastases. *Seminars in Oncology Nursing, 14,* 210–219.

Sitton, E. (2000). Superior vena cava syndrome. In C.H. Yarbro, M.H. Frogge, M. Goodman, & S.L. Groenwald (Eds.), *Cancer nursing: Principles and practice* (5th ed., pp. 900–912). Sudbury, MA: Jones and Bartlett.

Stewart, I.E. (1996). Superior vena cava syndrome: An oncologic complication. *Seminars in Oncology Nursing, 12,* 321–317.

Stretton, F., Edmonds, P., & Marrinan, M. (1999). Malignant pleural effusions. *European Journal of Palliative Care, 6,* 5–9.

Sullivan, F. (1996). Palliative radiotherapy for lung cancer. In H.L. Pass, J.B. Mitchell, D.H. Johnson, & A.T. Turrisi (Eds.), *Lung cancer: Principles and practice* (pp. 775–789). Philadelphia: Lippincott Williams & Wilkins.

Sunderland, P.M. (1994). Structure and function of the nervous system. In K.L. McCance & S.E. Huether (Eds.), *Pathophysiology: The biologic basis for disease in adults and children* (pp. 397–436). St. Louis, MO: Mosby.

Taubert, J. (2001). Management of malignant pleural effusion. *Nursing Clinics of North America, 36,* 665–683.

Vecht, C.J., Haaxma-Reiche, H., van Putten, W.L., deVisser, M., Vries, E.P., & Twijnstra, A. (1989). Initial bolus of conventional versus high-dose dexamethasone in metastatic spinal cord compression. *Neurology, 39,* 1255–1257.

Wang, P.C., Yang, K.Y., Chao, J.Y., Liu, J.M., Perng, R.P., & Yen, S.H. (2000). Prognostic role of pericardial fluid cytology in cardiac tamponade associated with non-small cell lung cancer. *Chest, 118,* 744–749.

Weinstein, S.M. (2001). Spinal cord compression. In A.M. Berger, R.K. Portenoy, & D.E. Weissman (Eds.), *Principles and practice of supportive oncology: Updates 4* (pp. 1–16). Philadelphia: Lippincott Williams & Wilkins.

Works, C., & Maxwell, M.B. (2000). Malignant effusions and edemas. In C.H. Yarbro, M.H. Frogge, M. Goodman, & S.L. Groenwald (Eds.), *Cancer nursing: Principles and practice* (5th ed., pp. 813–830). Sudbury, MA: Jones and Bartlett.

Yahalom, J. (2001). Superior vena cava syndrome. In V.T. De Vita, S. Hellman, & S.A. Rosenberg (Eds.), *Cancer: Principles and practice of oncology* (6th ed.). Philadelphia: Lippincott Williams & Wilkins. Retrieved July 1, 2002, from http://lwwoncology.com/dynaweb/resources/devita/682573@Generic_Book TextView/6

Zwischenberger, J.B., & Bradford, D.W. (1996). In H.I. Pass, J.B. Mithcell, D.H. Johnson, & A.T. Turrisi (Eds.), *Lung cancer: Principles and practice* (pp. 655–662). Philadelphia: Lippincott Williams & Wilkins.

CHAPTER 6

Paraneoplastic Syndromes

Leslie B. Tyson, MS, ANP-C, OCN®

Introduction

Paraneoplastic syndromes are the result of remote clinical effects of cancer and are not directly related to the primary tumor or metastatic deposits. They are considered to have three interactive components: tumor, mediator, and target tissue (Nathanson & Hall, 1997). Overall, paraneoplastic syndromes are rare, occurring in 10% of patients with lung cancer, and are the result of substances (e.g., hormones, growth factors, cytokines, antibodies) secreted by the primary tumor or its metastases (Busick, Fretz, Galvin, & Peterson, 2003; Haapoja, 2000a). These substances have an effect on multiple systems of the body, including endocrine, neurologic, hematologic, and musculoskeletal systems (Haapoja, 2000a).

Seven criteria are used to distinguish a paraneoplastic syndrome from other clinical abnormalities in the patient with cancer (Nathanson & Hall, 1997, p. 265).

1. "Association of the syndrome with the presence of actively growing tumor.
2. "Identification of excess amounts of a factor in circulation, which decline with tumor removal.
3. "Identification of excess of amounts of a factor within tumor cells.
4. "An arteriovenous gradient of the factor across the tumor vascular bed.
5. "Production of the factor by tumor cells in vitro.
6. "Identification of mRNA in tumor cells specific for factor synthesis using reverse transcriptase polymerase chain reaction or similar techniques.
7. "Cloning of the gene for factor synthesis or proof of some other mechanism (e.g., neurological, immunologic) of paraneoplastic causation."

Paraneoplastic syndromes can occur with any cancer, but they occur more frequently in patients with lung carcinoma, particularly small cell lung cancer (SCLC) (Adams, 2002; Haapoja, 2000a). They may precede a lung cancer diagnosis and often lead clinicians to suspect and look for an undiagnosed cancer. This section will review the most common paraneoplastic syndromes seen in patients with lung cancer. They will be reviewed according to the systems that are affected. Anemia of malignancy and the anorexia-cachexia syndrome will not be covered.

Endocrine Paraneoplastic Syndromes

The most common and best understood of the paraneoplastic syndromes are those of the endocrine system. These syndromes are caused by hormones, steroids, or cytokines, with the most common cause being cancer production of hormones or hormone precursors (ectopic hormone production) (Odell, 1997). Classically, a hormone differs from a cytokine in that hormones affect tissue at distant sites, whereas cytokines affect local tissue. In patients with malignancy, hormones can be produced in such large quantities that they affect local tissues, and cytokines can be produced in such large quantities that they affect distant tissues (Adams, 2002; Odell). The most common endocrine paraneoplastic syndromes seen in patients with lung cancer are humoral hypercalcemia of malignancy, ectopic adrenocorticotropic hormone (ACTH) syndrome (Cushing's syndrome), and syndrome of inappropriate antidiuretic hormone (SIADH).

Humoral Hypercalcemia of Malignancy

Hypercalcemia is defined as an abnormal elevation in serum calcium. The normal range of serum calcium is 9–11 mg/dl. In adults, hypercalcemia is present when the serum calcium level exceeds 11 mg/dl. Hypercalcemia is a common medical problem and the most common metabolic complication in patients with cancer. In the general population, the primary cause of hypercalcemia is hyperparathyroidism. These patients are usually asymptomatic, and the diagnosis is made with an elevated serum parathyroid hormone level. Patients with hypercalcemia caused by a malignant process are usually symptomatic and have low serum parathyroid hormone levels (Bilezekian, 1992).

In patients with malignant disease, hypercalcemia most commonly is found with breast, lung, and genitourinary (kidney) cancers; multiple myeloma; and lymphomas. Overall, hypercalcemia is estimated to occur in 10%–40% of those with cancer (Wickham, 2000). In patients with lung cancer, it most often is seen in those with squamous cell histology (Barnett, 1999; Shuey, 1994) and occurs in up to 35% of those with squamous cell lung cancer (Wickham). Hypercalcemia is rare in patients with colon cancer, prostate cancer, or SCLC (Wickham). Most patients have skeletal metastases; however, hypercalcemia can occur in those who do not have bone metastases. Untreated, hypercalcemia will result in 50% mortality rate from renal failure, cardiac arrest, or coma (Jensen, 1997). The median survival of patients with untreated hypercalcemia is usually less than three months from time of diagnosis (Barnett). The control of hypercalcemia usually depends on control of the malignant process. New insights into the pathophysiology and new developments in the treatment of hypercalcemia have occurred in the last decade that may improve the prognosis of those with this disorder.

Calcium is the major cation involved in the structure of bone and teeth. Calcium's other functions include the maintenance of normal clotting functions, muscle contractility, transmission of nerve impulses, and maintenance of normal cellular membrane permeability (Smith, 2000). Most calcium (99%) is found in bone as hydroxyapatite, where it is responsible for bone rigidity (Huether, 1994). The remaining 1% is found in the extracellular fluid, where half is bound to plasma protein (albumin) (Smith) and half is in the ionized free form and is responsible for maintaining the most important of the calcium physiologic functions (Huether).

Maintenance of normal calcium levels occurs through bone remodeling, renal calcium reabsorption, and gastrointestinal absorption. Hormonal factors also play a role in calcium regulation. The three hormones responsible for extracellular calcium regulation are parathyroid hormone (PTH), calcitonin, and vitamin D.

Pathogenesis

Hypercalcemia occurs because of an imbalance of either osteoclastic bone resorption or osteoblastic bone formation (Morton & Ritch, 1998). An imbalance in either activity can lead to an increase in calcium in the extracellular fluid, which must be excreted by the kidneys. In severe hypercalcemia, bone resorption is accelerated by activation of osteoclasts (Bilezekian, 1992).

Hypercalcemia in malignancy is felt to be mediated by two independent mechanisms, humoral factors (humoral hypercalcemia of malignancy) and local osteolytic activity (local osteolytic hypercalcemia) (Barnett, 1999). They act to disrupt calcium balance by producing hormones, growth factors, or cytokines that interfere with normal calcium regulation. Humoral hypercalcemia accounts for approximately 80% of all hypercalcemia (Wickham, 2000). Local osteolytic hypercalcemia is seen in 20%–30% of patients with cancer (Wickham). The cause of local osteolytic hypercalcemia is tumor invasion of bone, which results in the release of large amounts of calcium from destroyed areas of bone. Humoral hypercalcemia is the result of tumor production of parathyroid hormone–related protein (PTHrP), which mimics PTH (Morton & Ritch, 1998). This causes increased renal tubular absorption and increased osteoclastic activity throughout the skeleton (Morton & Ritch). An increase in production of 1, 25 dihydroxyvitamin D in those with hematologic malignancies and immobility from weakness and fatigue further contributes to increases in bone resorption (Jensen, 1997).

Signs and Symptoms

Signs and symptoms of malignancy-generated hypercalcemia are seen in Table 6-1. The frequency and degree of symptoms are related to the rate at which hypercalcemia develops. Hypercalcemia that develops slowly has fewer symptoms than when serum calcium levels rise acutely. Acute rises in serum calcium may cause dramatic changes in mental status. Other symptoms are vague and include nausea, vomiting, anorexia, constipation, and fatigue. Many patients become dehydrated from the nausea, vomiting, and anorexia. Additionally, increased calcium in the extracellular fluid results in interference of the kidney's ability to resorb sodium (Jensen, 1997). This leads to sodium and water loss from polyuria (Jensen), which further exacerbates dehydration.

Diagnosis

The corrected serum calcium is the measurement most often used to diagnose hypercalcemia. This is done by obtaining serum calcium and albumin levels. The corrected serum calcium is calculated by adjusting the calcium level for every gram of albumin (see Figure 6-1) (Jensen, 1997).

If the corrected calcium levels are between 10.5–12.0 mg/dl, mild hypercalcemia exists. If they are between 12.0–13.5 mg/dl, moderate hypercalcemia exists. Hypercalcemia is considered severe when levels exceed 13.5 mg/dl (Boyle, 2001). Other important blood tests include assessment of renal function and measurement of parathyroid hormone to rule out hyperparathyroidism.

Assessment of patient history and symptoms, medication history, and physical examination also are important considerations in the patient with hypercalcemia. History should focus on the type and extent of cancer as well as treatment and response to treatment. Most cases of hypercalcemia are seen in patients with advanced cancer that is not responding to treatment. Assessment of symptoms (as seen in Table 6-1) and their duration will give clues about the onset of hypercalcemia. Medication history is important, as some medi-

Table 6-1. Signs and Symptoms of Hypercalcemia of Malignancy

System	Signs and Symptoms
Mental status and vision	Fatigue Weakness Hyporeflexia Visual disturbances Confusion Depression Lethargy Apathy Restlessness Somnolence Stupor Coma
Cardiovascular	Hypertension Bradycardia Electrocardiographic abnormalities Digitalis sensitivity Hypotension Heart block Cardiac arrest
Gastrointestinal tract	Anorexia Nausea and vomiting Pain and distension Constipation Adynamic ileus
Skeletal	Bone pain Pathologic fractures
Kidneys	Polyuria and nocturia Polydipsia Dehydration Azotemia and proteinuria Nephrocalcinosis Nephrolithiasis Renal failure
Systemic symptoms	Ectopic calcification Pruritus Metabolic alkalosis Hypercoagulopathy

Note. Based on information from Jensen, 1997.

Treatment

Treatment is aimed at the underlying disease and immediate management of the hypercalcemia. Immediate measures include rehydration and use of bisphosphonates. Ultimately, long-term control of hypercalcemia depends on control of the cancer. The degree of hypercalcemia determines whether patients can be managed in an ambulatory setting or must be admitted to the hospital.

IV fluids with isotonic saline usually are given initially to restore hydration and promote urinary excretion of calcium. Loop diuretics, such as furosemide, may be used to enhance calcium excretion, but these have a limited effect (Flombaum, 2000). Monitoring of renal function and electrolytes is important during rehydration.

These measures alone do little to control significant hypercalcemia; therefore, many patients also are treated with bisphosphonates, such as etidronate and pamidronate, which are used most often in the United States (Flombaum, 2000). Studies have shown that pamidronate is more effective and induces longer periods of response (Flombaum). Pamidronate usually is given in doses of 60 mg or 90 mg over 2, 4, or 24 hours. Research is being conducted to investigate shorter infusion times (less than two hours) of pamidronate (Body, 2001). The 90-mg dose of pamidronate has been shown to be more effective in reducing calcium levels (Flombaum). On average, the duration of effect is short (15 days on average, but may be as long as 28 days) and, therefore, pamidronate must be infused every 2–3 weeks (Flombaum). Side effects of pamidronate include flu-like symptoms, which are seen in 25%–33% of patients. Symptoms are more common after the first infusion and lessen with subsequent infusions (Body). Pamidronate is safe in patients with compromised renal function.

Zoledronic acid, a heterocyclic nitrogen-containing bisphosphonate, was approved for use in 2002 and has been shown to be effective in the treatment of moderate to severe hypercalcemia (Berenson et al., 2001). Double-blind, phase-III studies have shown that zoledronic acid is more effective than pamidronate (Berenson et al.). Zoledronic acid is given intravenously over 15 minutes, making it more convenient than pamidronate. The dose is 4 mg. Side effects are similar to those seen with pamidronate. Additionally, renal

cations (e.g., thiazide diuretics, lithium) can exacerbate hypercalcemia. Additionally, assessment of mental status and gastrointestinal symptoms is more difficult in patients using narcotics for pain control.

Physical examination should be thorough and focus on changes in mental status, extent of dehydration, bowel motility, muscle strength and tone, deep tendon reflexes (delayed in hypercalcemia), and heart rate and rhythm (bradycardia and dysrhythmias in hypercalcemia).

Figure 6-1. Formula for Determining Corrected Serum Calcium

1. Subtract the albumin level from 4.0.
2. Multiply the difference by 0.8.
3. If the result is a negative number, subtract it from the serum calcium; if it is positive, add it to the calcium.

Note. Based on information from Jensen, 1997.

function should be monitored. Other agents that may be used to treat hypercalcemia include calcitonin, plicamycin, and glucocorticoids, but these are used less often.

Conclusions

Hypercalcemia is the most common metabolic disorder in patients with cancer and is seen in moderate frequency in patients with squamous cell lung cancer. Healthcare providers must be aware of patients who are at greatest risk for hypercalcemia and the most common signs and symptoms of hypercalcemia so that therapy can be initiated early. Treatment response of the underlying malignancy will provide the longest period of normocalcemia. Bisphosphonates can provide symptom relief and prevent hypercalcemia from worsening. Additionally, they can be administered in the outpatient setting.

Ectopic Adrenocorticotropic Hormone Syndrome

Incidence and Pathogenesis

Ectopic ACTH syndrome (Cushing's syndrome) is most common in patients with SCLC. Cushing's syndrome from bronchogenic cancer represents 60%–70% of all cases of ectopic production of ACTH, and SCLC represents the predominant histology (Adams, 2002; Haapoja, 2000a). Cushing's syndrome also is seen in patients with benign pituitary tumors or hyperplasia. Cushing's syndrome results when the cancer produces large amounts of biologically active ACTH. The ACTH then stimulates the adrenal glands to produce excessive amounts of corticosteroids, which leads to the development of Cushing's disease (Haapoja, 2000a). The difference between benign and malignant Cushing's syndrome is that patients with the paraneoplastic syndrome have higher levels of precursor ACTH and higher concentrations of cortisol in the blood and urine (Adams). Additionally, hypokalemia is more prevalent in patients with ectopic production of ACTH (Odell, 1997).

Signs and Symptoms

The symptoms of patients with paraneoplastic ACTH syndrome include proximal muscle weakness, hypokalemia, metabolic alkalosis, glucose intolerance, and hypertension. Hypokalemic alkalosis is present in 70% of patients with the syndrome (Agarwala, 1996). Bilateral adrenal hyperplasia also can be seen in these patients (Agarwala). The more commonly associated signs and symptoms of increased ACTH production, such as moon face, buffalo hump, and hyperpigmentation of the skin, do not develop because, in general, the patients do not live long enough to develop these signs (Haapoja, 2000a).

Diagnosis

Diagnosis is based on the aforementioned findings above and through the use of laboratory studies. The cortisol suppression test involves giving an oral dose of dexamethasone at bedtime, followed by serum measurement of cortisol levels in the morning. In patients with ectopic production of ACTH, cortisol levels will not be suppressed by dexamethasone (Agarwala, 1996; Fischbach, 1996; Odell, 1997). However, the dexamethasone suppression test will suppress ACTH in patients with pituitary tumors (Midthun & Jett, 1996). A 24-hour urine collection for free cortisol will demonstrate elevated urinary-free cortisol levels. Levels in excess of 100 mcg/day in conjunction with elevated serum ACTH levels are diagnostic of the syndrome (Agarwala; Midthun & Jett).

Treatment

For patients with ectopic production of ACTH, treatment is aimed at management of the primary tumor. Control of the tumor should lead to control of this paraneoplastic syndrome. Often, one of the first signs of tumor recurrence is reemergence of this syndrome. Drug therapy often is used in the treatment of Cushing's syndrome. The most commonly used agent is ketoconazole. Ketoconazole has a rapid onset of action and inhibits corticosteroid production (Haapoja, 2000a). Common doses range from 400–1,200 mg per day. Ketoconazole can be used in conjunction with combination chemotherapy in those with SCLC (Midthun & Jett, 1996). Liver enzymes must be monitored closely, and patients must be evaluated for significant adrenal suppression that can occur from ketoconazole (Haapoja, 2000a). Other medications used in the treatment of ectopic ACTH production include metyrapone, aminoglutethimide, mitotane, and octreotide. The latter most often is used in management of ACTH secreting bronchial carcinoid tumors (Haapoja, 2000a). In patients diagnosed with SCLC and concurrent ectopic ACTH, the overall prognosis is poor. Cushing's syndrome has been found to be an adverse prognostic indicator if present at the time of diagnosis (Haapoja, 2000a). Quality-of-life issues must be considered when treating these patients.

Syndrome of Inappropriate Antidiuretic Hormone

Incidence and Pathogenesis

SIADH is a paraneoplastic syndrome characterized by abnormal production of antidiuretic hormone (ADH) (arginine vasopressin), which results in hyponatremia. Ectopic production of ADH is the most common cause of increased ADH levels. This most often occurs in patients with cancer, but it also can be seen in patients with infections, such as pneumonia or tuberculosis, and with central nervous system disorders (e.g., trauma, infection, cerebral vascular accident), as well as those taking drugs that potentiate ADH (e.g., diuretics, vincristine, cyclophosphamide) (Ezzone, 2000). SCLC is the cause of SIADH in 75% of cases (Keenan, 1999). This syndrome can be seen in as many as 40% of patients who are diagnosed with SCLC (Odell, 1997; Zumsteg & Casperson, 1998).

Classically, patients with SIADH from malignancy experience fluid excess (with expanded plasma volume), which leads to dilutional hyponatremia, serum hypo-osmolality, and urine hyperosmolality (inappropriate urine concentration) (Keenan, 1999). This is caused by an abnormal production and secretion of ADH and high serum levels of vasopressin. ADH acts on the tubular portion of the collecting duct system by increasing water permeability of the collecting duct system. Water then is reabsorbed, and only a small volume of concentrated urine is excreted (Keenan). Additionally, euvolemia is present in SIADH, along with normal thyroid, adrenal, and renal function (Kraut & Wozniak, 2000). Elevated serum levels of ADH usually are present but are not necessary to make the diagnosis.

Signs and Symptoms

Hyponatremia exists when serum sodium levels are below 135 mEq/l. Signs and symptoms result from water excess and depend on the degree of hyponatremia and the rate at which it occurs. Generally, hyponatremia is graded as mild, moderate, or severe. Patients with mild hyponatremia may be asymptomatic or have vague symptoms that include tiredness, headache, weakness, muscle cramps, or decreased appetite. Those with moderate hyponatremia may experience confusion or personality changes; gastrointestinal symptoms of nausea, vomiting, or diarrhea; decreased urine output; increased thirst; lethargy; or loss of deep-tendon reflexes. Although not common, severe symptoms include seizure activity and coma when serum sodium levels are between 100–115 mEq/l (Ezzone, 2000; Keenan, 1999). Patients with SIADH do not have edema, but weight gain is seen because of the excess water. This usually only occurs when levels drop acutely. In patients with chronic low serum sodium levels, clinical manifestations are less common.

Diagnosis

Diagnostic criteria are well established and include both laboratory and physical findings. An absolute diagnosis of SIADH is based on five criteria, which are shown in Figure 6-2. Other laboratory findings include low to normal BUN, serum creatinine, uric acid, and phosphate levels. Additionally, serum ADH levels may be increased (Ezzone, 2000). Findings on physical examination reveal the absence of edema, weight gain, loss or decreases in deep tendon reflexes, and changes in levels of consciousness.

Treatment

In patients with cancer-induced SIADH, treatment is aimed at correcting hyponatremia and reducing symptoms. For patients with SCLC, systemic chemotherapy, fluid restriction, and medications often are needed. SCLC usually is responsive to combination chemotherapy and will result in correction of the hyponatremia. Often, the first sign of progression of disease is a recurrence of SIADH. In patients with mild hyponatremia who are asymptomatic or have few symptoms, systemic chemotherapy and subsequent control of the tumor may lead to resolution of symptoms. Patients may or may not require restriction of fluid to 500–1,000 ml per day. In those with moderate hyponatremia, IV fluid administration with diuretics and electrolyte replacement may be required. Isotonic saline (0.9%) usually is used in these cases (Ezzone, 2000). Hypertonic saline (0.3%) is reserved for patients with severe hyponatremia. Guidelines direct the amount of sodium replacement needed to prevent serious neurologic problems; in general, sodium replacement should not exceed 1–2 mEq/l per hour until normalization or near normalization of sodium levels and resolution of symptoms occur (Ezzone). This is followed by additional sodium replacement of 12–15 mEq/l in 24 hours (Ezzone; Keenan, 1999). Overly rapid correction of sodium can lead to osmotic demyelination syndrome (central pontine myelinosis); this is characterized by progressive extremity weakness and other neurologic symptoms (Ezzone; Keenan). Drug therapy consists of the use of loop diuretics and demeclocycline. Furosemide commonly is used with IV fluid administration and also is helpful in the management of fluid overload. In patients with chronic hyponatremia or in those who have difficulty maintaining water restriction, demeclocycline often is used. Demeclocycline is a tetracycline derivative that inhibits the kidney's response to antidiuretic hormone, thus leading to diuresis (Ezzone; Haapoja, 2000b). Dosages usually range from 60–1,200 mg per day (Kozisek, 2000). Renal function should be monitored carefully, as demeclocycline is nephrotoxic, and pa-

---

Figure 6-2. Five Criteria for Diagnosis of Syndrome of Inappropriate Antidiuretic Hormone

- Serum sodium less than 135 mEq/l (hyponatremia)
- Plasma osmolality less than 275 mOsm/l (hypoosmolality)
- Urine osmolality greater than 300 mOsm/l
- Euvolemia
- Normal thyroid, renal, and adrenal function

Note. Based on information from Ezzone, 2000; Keenan, 1999.

tients need to be aware of photosensitivity and nausea (Kozisek). In summary, SIADH is a common paraneoplastic syndrome in patients with SCLC. Most often, the hyponatremia normalizes with systemic treatment of the tumor. For most patients, the hyponatremia is chronic in nature and rarely presents as an emergency.

Neurologic Paraneoplastic Syndromes

Neurologic paraneoplastic syndromes are rare and can involve any portion of the nervous system (Posner & Dalmau, 1997). Overall, 1% or less of patients with cancer are affected by neurologic paraneoplastic syndromes (Dalmau & Posner, 1997). Most of these paraneoplastic neurologic syndromes are associated with SCLC (Kraut & Wozniak, 2000). In many cases, they are present for months to years before the cancer is diagnosed and can even direct the oncology workup. For example, in patients found to have certain auto antibodies (anti-Hu indicates SCLC), the likelihood that the patient has a specific cancer is high (Dalmau & Posner). Although these paraneoplastic neurologic disorders often are present before a cancer diagnosis is made, they can occur at any time during the course of the malignancy (Zumsteg & Casperson, 1998).

In contrast to other paraneoplastic syndromes, neurologic disorders are believed to be the result of autoimmune dysfunction, whereby proteins ectopically produced by the tumor are recognized as foreign by the immune system, resulting in an autoimmune reaction (Dalmau & Posner, 1997; Haapoja, 2000a). In some instances, the presence of a paraneoplastic neurologic syndrome slows tumor growth or is associated with spontaneous tumor regressions, suggesting that the immune system also can attack the tumor (Dalmau & Posner).

The most common neurologic syndromes associated with SCLC are Lambert-Eaton myasthenic syndrome (LEMS) and syndromes associated with the anti-Hu antibody.

Lambert-Eaton Myasthenic Syndrome

Incidence and Pathogenesis
LEMS most commonly is seen in patients with SCLC, although it occurs in 3% or less of all patients with this diagnosis (Dalmau & Posner, 1997). This syndrome may be present for 2–5 years before an SCLC diagnosis is made, and 60% of patients with the syndrome will be diagnosed with SCLC (Newsom-Davis, 1998). Although it has been seen in patients with breast, prostate, and ovarian tumors, this paraneoplastic syndrome is rare in other cancers (Struthers, 1994). LEMS also may be seen in patients without an underlying malignancy in which the cause is not known, or it may be associated with autoimmune disorders such as rheumatoid arthritis, thyroid disease, or multiple sclerosis (Struthers).

LEMS is a paraneoplastic disease that affects the transmission of nerve impulses at the neuromuscular junction. In healthy individuals, transmission of a nerve impulse at the neuromuscular junction occurs with the release of a presynaptic neurotransmitter across the synaptic cleft and then binding of the neurotransmitter at the postsynaptic receptors on the muscle cell (Boss, Sunderland, & Heath, 1994). For a nerve impulse to be transmitted from one cell to another, several processes need to occur. First, the nerve impulse stimulates calcium to enter the axon from the extracellular fluid. Once in the axon, calcium stimulates the release of acetylcholine. Acetylcholine is a neurotransmitter that is released by voltage-gated calcium channels (VGCCs), which are located in the presynaptic nerve terminal. Acetylcholine then crosses the synaptic cleft and binds with the postsynaptic receptors on the muscle cell, as described earlier, and a muscle contraction occurs (Struthers, 1994). Anything that interferes with this process will cause muscular weakness.

The pathogenesis of LEMS is the result of antibodies directed against VGCCs (Dalmau & Posner, 1997; Lennon et al., 1994). Studies have found that in patients with LEMS, the tumor produces IgG antibodies against the calcium channels and the auto antibodies block the VGCCs in the presynaptic terminal, thus preventing or decreasing the amount of acetylcholine release (Haapoja, 2000a). The result is muscular weakness. The specific type of calcium-channel antibody is the P/Q-type; this type was found to be the most potent inhibitor of calcium influx and, in one study, was found in the serum of all patients diagnosed with LEMS and concurrent cancer (Lennon et al.).

Of all the paraneoplastic neurologic syndromes, LEMS provides the best evidence to support an autoimmune hypothesis for neurologic paraneoplastic disorders (Dalmau & Posner, 1997). This has been demonstrated by the transfer of serum IgG from patients with the disease to animals, which reproduces the disorder; this meets the criteria for antibody mediated autoimmune disease (Posner & Dalmau, 1997; Struthers, 1994). Symptoms also have improved in patients in whom VGCC antibodies are removed from the serum (Posner & Dalmau).

Signs and Symptoms
The hallmark symptoms in patients with LEMS are proximal muscle weakness and muscle fatigue with exercise. Most often, the patient will complain of difficulty arising from a chair. The muscle weakness often is more pronounced at the end of the day. Usually the lower extremities and pelvic girdle are first affected, with upper extremity weakness occurring later in the course of the disease in some (Zumsteg & Casperson, 1998). Additionally, patients report muscle stiffness and myalgias (Dalmau & Posner, 1997). Autonomic symptoms also may be present and include dry mouth, constipation, impotence, and postural hypotension (Zumsteg & Casperson).

On physical examination, patients will exhibit signs of proximal muscle weakness and loss or decrease in deep-tendon reflexes. An increase in muscle strength and a return of deep-tendon reflexes following maximal muscle contraction is a classic finding in LEMS (Dalmau & Posner, 1997). Additionally, cranial nerves may be involved. This condition is generally mild and includes symptoms of ptosis, diplopia, and dysarthria (Dalmau & Posner).

Diagnosis

The diagnosis of LEMS is accomplished largely by ruling out a similar neurologic disorder, myasthenia gravis (Haapoja, 2000a). The diagnosis is supported by blood studies, the patient's response to edrophonium chloride (Tensilon® [Valeant Pharmaceuticals International, Costa Mesa, CA]), and electromyography (EMG) studies (Boss et al., 1994). The serum of patients with LEMS does not contain anti-acetylcholine receptor antibodies, whereas the presence of these antibodies is diagnostic in patients with myasthenia gravis. Additionally, 90% of patients with LEMS have demonstrated the presence of serum anti-P/Q-type VGCC antibodies (Newsom-Davis, 1998). IV administration of edrophonium chloride will result in temporary improvement in muscle strength in those with myasthenia gravis; however, no improvement is noted in those with LEMS. Finally, EMG studies with repeated nerve stimulation demonstrate a decrease in muscle response in myasthenia gravis, whereas those with LEMS demonstrate a temporary increase in strength (Struthers, 1994).

Treatment

Treatment is twofold; it is aimed at treating the underlying tumor and suppressing the immune system. The use of chemotherapy for the treatment of SCLC has resulted in an improvement of LEMS symptoms in those whose cancers respond to treatment (Chalk, Murray, Newsom-Davis, O'Neill, & Spiro, 1990). However, irreversible nerve damage may limit improvement in others (Zumsteg & Casperson, 1998). If symptoms do not respond with the treatment of the tumor, other measures may be helpful. This can involve suppression of the immune response with medications, such as corticosteroids and azathioprine or a combination of both. Other agents that promote release of acetylcholine from the nerve terminal are sometimes useful, but their side effects may outweigh their benefits (Struthers, 1994). The agents in use are guanidine hydrochloride and 3,4-diaminopyridine (DAP). Generally, 3,4-DAP is beneficial for most patients. Side effects include perioral and distal paresthesias. Central excitation and seizures can occur with overdosage and sometimes are seen with recommended doses (Newsom-Davis, 1998). Usually, 3,4-DAP is the first choice for treatment because it is considered safer than guanidine. Guanidine should be considered if 3,4-DAP is unavailable because it can be very effective in reducing symptoms associated with LEMS. However, it should be used with caution because side effects can be serious and can include bone marrow suppression, renal failure, and atrial fibrillation (Newsom-Davis). In patients who do not respond to either

guanidine or 3,4-DAP, prednisolone with or without azathioprine is usually helpful (Newsom-Davis). Additionally, plasma exchange or treatment with IV immune globulin also may be effective (Dalmau & Posner, 1997).

Conclusions

LEMS is a neurologic paraneoplastic syndrome often seen in patients with SCLC. Symptoms often precede the diagnosis of cancer by months to sometimes years. A diagnosis of LEMS should prompt a search for cancer. In patients who have a prolonged period from the diagnosis of LEMS and SCLC, anti-VGCC antibodies are believed to play a role in controlling tumor growth or these patients may have a slower growing, well-differentiated cancer, rather than a poorly differentiated SCLC, which usually is a highly malignant, rapidly growing tumor (Newsom-Davis, 1998).

Anti-Hu Antibody-Associated Paraneoplastic Cerebellar Degeneration

The anti-Hu antibody and other autoantibodies (e.g., anti-Yo, anti-Ri, anti-Ma, and anti-Ta) are associated with several underlying cancers and neurologic syndromes (Dalmau & Posner, 1997). The cancers that these antibodies are associated with include SCLC and testicular, breast, and gynecologic cancers (Dalmau & Posner). The neurologic syndromes are paraneoplastic cerebellar degeneration (PCD), encephalomyelitis, sensory neuropathy, autonomic neuropathy, limbic encephalitis, and opsoclonus/myoclonus (Kraut & Wozniak, 2000). These syndromes are rare, even in patients with SCLC.

One of the most common of these neurologic syndromes is PCD, which is seen in patients with and without the anti-Hu antibody. Other antibodies (anti-Yo and anti-Ri) also are known to cause this condition (Haapoja, 2000a). As seen in patients with LEMS, PCD often predates the cancer diagnosis. Although this condition can occur in patients without the anti-Hu antibody, this discussion will be limited to PCD and the anti-Hu antibody.

Incidence and Pathogenesis

Overall, neurologic paraneoplastic syndromes are seen in 1% or less of all patients with cancer (Dalmau & Posner, 1997). One source indicates that only 300 incidents of PCD have been reported in the literature (Haapoja, 2000a). In patients with a neurologic disorder and the presence of the anti-Hu antibody, more than 90% will be diagnosed with SCLC (Dalmau & Posner). PCD was first described by Brain and Wilkinson in 1965 and was classified as "a clinico-pathologic concept characterized by the subacute onset of cerebellar dysfunction (gait difficulty and limb ataxia), sometimes associated with dysarthria, dysphagia, nystagmus, mental changes, and muscular and sensory deficits" (Mason et al., 1997, p. 1280). The most common pathologic finding is the absence of cerebellar Purkinje cells (Mason et al.). Additionally, some patients have inflammatory infiltrates within the cerebellum and other areas of the neurologic system (Mason et al.). The cerebellum is responsible for the coordinated action of skeletal muscles and voluntary muscular movement. With loss or dysfunction of cerebellar Purkinje cells, patients may have signs of ataxia, dysarthria, nystagmus, or loss of reflexes (Haapoja, 2000a).

Signs and Symptoms

As with patients with LEMS, signs and symptoms of PCD often predate the diagnosis of SCLC; however, this syndrome can occur at any time during the illness. The symptoms may appear acutely over a few days or over a longer period of time (Zumsteg & Casperson, 1998). Often, patients appear to be very ill and have severe ataxia, dysarthria, dysphagia, and difficulty speaking (Zumsteg & Casperson). Diplopia and sensory neuropathy also may be seen in patients with PCD (Mason et al., 1997).

In a study examining the serum of 57 patients with SCLC and presenting symptoms of PCD, Mason et al. (1997) found high anti-Hu antibody titers in 25 (44%) patients. Compared with those who had low anti-Hu antibody titers or those who were anti-Hu antibody negative, those who had high titers tended to be women, have multifocal neurologic disease, and be severely disabled (Mason et al.).

Diagnosis and Treatment

Cerebellar dysfunction is more likely to be the result of metastatic disease (intracranial or leptomeningeal metastases) or other neurologic problems (e.g., Wernicke's encephalopathy) rather than PCD (Zumsteg & Casperson, 1998). These disorders must be considered as part of the differential diagnosis. History, physical examination, and tests, such as magnetic resonance imaging (MRI), can help to rule out other neurologic problems or metastatic disease. Treatment is twofold, with the goals of controlling tumor and improving or stabilizing neurologic deficits with immune therapy. Spontaneous remissions have been reported, but are rare (Dalmau & Posner, 1997). Although improvement in neurologic symptoms has been noted in some patients with treatment of the tumor, in general, the course of PCD is independent of the tumor (Dalmau & Posner). Often, irreversible neurologic damage results, and this will not improve with treatment. Unlike patients with LEMS, immune suppression with corticosteroids, plasma exchange, and IV immune globulin have been helpful in individual patients, but studies have not shown them to be helpful for most (Dalmau & Posner; Mason et al., 1997). PCD is a rare and often devastating paraneoplastic syndrome. It is seen most often in patients with SCLC and is occasionally seen in patients with other tumors. Successful treatment of the tumor usually does not result in improvement in neurologic symptoms. Several authors report that PCD is especially difficult to treat when associated with SCLC or the presence of the anti-Hu antibody (Graus et al., 1992; Uchuya, Graus, Vega, Rene, & Delattre, 1996). Additionally, despite

successful treatment of the tumor, these patients are likely to die from neurologic disease (Dalmau & Posner).

Hematologic Paraneoplastic Syndromes

Trousseau's Syndrome

Trousseau's syndrome is one of several paraneoplastic conditions of the hematopoietic system. It is the earliest paraneoplastic syndrome described, and it demonstrates the association of thrombosis with malignancy (Staszewski, 1997). Other hematologic paraneoplastic syndromes may involve any of the corpuscular elements of the blood or hemostatic system (Staszewski). These syndromes include disorders of the platelets (thrombocytopenia, thrombocytosis), leukocytes (leukocytosis, neutropenia), and erythrocytes (erythrocytosis, anemia of malignancy); thrombosis (Trousseau's syndrome); and hemorrhage (disseminated intravascular coagulation [DIC]) (Staszewski). Anemia of malignancy is considered to be the most common of the hematologic paraneoplastic syndromes. Information regarding this syndrome is available elsewhere (Frenkel, Bick, & Rutherford, 1996; Haapoja, 2000a; Kraut & Wozniak, 2000). This section will focus on Trousseau's syndrome, which can be problematic in patients with lung cancer, causing deep vein thrombosis (DVT) and pulmonary emboli.

Incidence and Pathogenesis

Trousseau's syndrome often is the first manifestation of cancer. The initial description of Trousseau's syndrome was in patients with gastrointestinal tumors whose diagnosis was preceded by thrombophlebitis (Shannon & Ng, 2002). Currently, it is described as a hypercoagulable state with migratory thrombophlebitis (Zumsteg & Casperson, 1998). It is seen in patients with mucin-producing tumors, such as adenocarcinoma of the lung or gastrointestinal tract, and can occur in 40%–50% of patients with solid tumors (Staszewski, 1997; Zumsteg & Casperson). Other authors note that the highest incidence is in patients with adenocarcinoma of the lung (Shannon & Ng). Migratory thrombophlebitis also is seen in patients with SCLC, and, less often, in patients with breast, prostate, or ovarian cancer (Haapoja, 2000a). Post-mortem studies have documented multiple emboli in patients with advanced cancer (Naschitz, Yeshurun, & Lev, 1993). The hypercoagulable state in patients with cancer is well known; however, the pathogenesis is poorly understood. Multiple risk factors contribute to the development of thromboembolic disease (see Table 6-2).

Virchow's triad still provides the basis for the pathogenesis of thromboembolic disease. Virchow's triad describes a process of endothelial injury, venous stasis or alterations in normal blood flow, and alterations in coagulability (hypercoagulability) (Robbins, Cotran, & Kumar, 1995; Shannon & Ng, 2002). Patients with cancer and thromboembolic disease develop an alteration in the clotting pathway, caused either

Table 6-2. Pathogenesis of Thromboembolism in Patients With Cancer

Condition	Pathogenesis
Venous stasis	Venous obstruction by tumor Decreased mobility Increased blood viscosity Increased venous pressure
Vessel wall injury	Direct tumor injury to endothelium Chemotherapy-induced (e.g., carmustine, bleomycin vincristine, doxorubicin, taxanes?)
Hypercoagulability	Direct and indirect tumor-cell activation of clotting factors Overexpression of other procoagulants? Chemotherapy-induced reductions in protein C and protein S (e.g., cyclophosphamide, methotrexate, 5-fluorouracil) Antithrombin III reductions caused by surgery, chemotherapeutic agents (taxanes, L-asparaginase) and heparin
Platelet abnormalities	Reactive thrombocytosis (carcinomas of breast, lung, stomach, ovary, and colon) Spontaneous platelet aggregation Increased thrombopoietin

Note. From "Noninfectious Pulmonary Emergencies" (p. 193) by V.R. Shannon and A. Ng in S.-C.J. Yeung and C.P. Escalante (Eds.), *Holland, Frei Oncologic Emergencies,* 2002, Hamilton, ON: BC Decker Inc. Copyright 2002 by BC Decker Inc. Reprinted with permission.

directly or indirectly by the tumor cells (Haapoja, 2000a). Some of the alterations in the clotting pathway include overexpression of fibrin and clotting factors as well as alterations in protein C and S levels and antithrombin III (Shannon & Ng). Additionally, inflammatory cytokines may be generated from an interaction between cancer cells and leukocytes, also leading to the hypercoagulable state (Silverstein & Nachman, 1992). These alterations can then initiate the clotting cascade, causing the formation of thromboses.

Another theory comes from the tumor's ability to grow, metastasize, and activate the clotting cascade. To grow and metastasize, tumors must have proteolytic and adhesive qualities, which are necessary for invasion, implantation, and angiogenesis (Silverstein & Nachman, 1992). To do this, tumors are believed to form a fibrin gel (Haapoja, 2000a). Studies in animals support this theory by showing that antiplatelet and anticoagulant medicines have antineoplastic activity (Rickles, Hancock, Edwards, & Zacharski, 1988).

Other comorbid conditions and treatments that coexist in the patient with cancer play a role in the development of thromboembolic disease. A history of cardiac disease may predispose a patient for thromboses because of venous stasis. Immobility from pain or fatigue or following surgery contributes to the problem. Indwelling venous access devices are known to increase the risk of upper extremity venous thromboses (Blinder & Behl, 2002). Additionally, treatment with chemotherapy, hormonal therapy, and radiation therapy may increase the risk for venous thromboses (Blinder & Behl).

Signs and Symptoms

Symptoms of DVT include pain and swelling of the affected extremity. In extremity DVT, the swelling is usually unilateral. Edema from other causes is usually symmetrical. Early in the course, mild pain may occur in the affected area without swelling or the patient may be asymptomatic. Redness usually is seen in patients with superficial thrombophlebitis. With thrombosis associated with venous access devices, the swelling and pain usually are on the side of the implanted device. A thrombus in the superior vena cava (SVC) can cause swelling of the face and neck (SVC syndrome). Pulmonary embolus classically causes acute-onset shortness of breath and chest pain. Early on, chest pain may resemble angina, but, later in the course, this evolves to pleuritic chest pain. Pleuritic chest pain and dyspnea are the most common symptoms (Feied, 1998). In patients with pulmonary embolism documented on angiogram, dyspnea was present in 70%–90% (Shannon & Ng, 2002). Cough is present in approximately 50% of patients (Feied). Massive pulmonary embolus may result in death.

Budd-Chiari syndrome is a clot in the portal vein, and patients may present with acute-onset abdominal pain (Staszewski, 1997.) This syndrome primarily is seen in patients with gastrointestinal tumors. Signs on physical examination usually are indicative of the location of the thrombus. Patients with a lower-extremity DVT often will have swelling in the calf, ankle, or foot. Palpation of the calf may reveal a cord, and pain may be identified. Dorsiflexion of the foot with subsequent pain in the calf is known as Homan's sign. This test results in a high incidence of false-positives, and it is positive in less than 50% of patients with DVT (Story, 2000). In those with an upper-extremity DVT or SVC clot, swelling in the face, neck, or affected arm may be present. Additionally, examination may reveal the presence of prominent superficial vessels on the arm or chest wall.

In patients with a pulmonary embolus, physical examination can be unremarkable or it may reveal tachypnea (the most common sign of pulmonary embolism); crackles or wheezing may be heard on auscultation of the lungs (Goldhaber, 1998). Dyspnea, syncope, and cyanosis usually are indicative of a massive pulmonary embolus (Goldhaber). Oxygen saturation (via pulse oximeter) may be abnormal. Up to 40% of patients will have a low-grade fever (Henke, 2000). On cardiac examination, a gallop may be heard, or the pulmonary component of the second heart sound may be more prominent. In those with a pulmonary embolus, clinicians must look for signs and symptoms of a lower-extremity DVT. Lower-extremity thrombophlebitis is present in about a third of patients with pulmonary embolus (Feied, 1998).

Diagnosis

A DVT diagnosis is made based on clinical predictors and radiographic studies. Laboratory studies are not always used but may be helpful. Figure 6-3 outlines clinical predictors for diagnosis of DVT (Wells et al., 1995). Clinical predictors are based on patient history and physical examination.

Radiographic diagnosis of DVT is made by Doppler ultrasound, impedance plethysmography, contrast venography, or radionuclide scintigraphy. Doppler ultrasound is a noninvasive test that uses ultrasound to measure venous patency by showing the movement of red blood cells through a vein (Story, 2000). The accuracy of this test's results depend on the operator, but with a skilled technician, sensitivity and specificity are 95% (Story). Often, this is the test of choice because it is noninvasive and inexpensive. Impedance plethysmography also is a noninvasive test that monitors changes in venous volume of the leg and detects impaired venous emptying (Story). Contrast venogram involves the injection of contrast material into a vessel; for examination of a lower extremity, a vein in the dorsum of the foot is used. Following injection of contrast material, the deep venous system becomes opacified on conventional x-rays or electronically with digital subtraction (Novelline, 1997). This test is considered to be the gold standard for detection of DVT. Disadvantages include the cost and invasiveness. Additionally, it may be difficult to perform in patients who are critically ill, are obese, or have edema or local infection (Story).

Radionuclide scintigraphy testing uses radiolabeled agents that are injected to detect DVT. Imaging is performed at a delayed time period. These tests are expensive. They may be useful in patients with an equivocal Doppler study (Story, 2000).

Diagnostic exams for pulmonary embolism include chest radiograph, radioisotope perfusion and ventilation lung (V/Q) scan, spiral computed tomography (CT), MRI, and angiogram. Echocardiogram also may be used to rule out a clot, but it primarily is used to exclude other diagnoses (Shannon & Ng, 2002). Chest x-ray may be normal, or it may reveal atelectasis, focal infiltrates, and elevation of the hemidiaphragm on the same side as the pulmonary embolus. Again, its chief use is to rule out other pathology. Findings on chest x-ray are not diagnostic of pulmonary embolus (Shannon & Ng).

A V/Q scan usually is the next step in screening for a pulmonary embolus. This test contains two parts, as the abbreviation implies. The first part is a perfusion lung scan. Patients are given an IV injection of a radioisotope (technetium-99m tagged), and then the lungs are scanned using a gamma camera (Novelline, 1997). A normal scan (i.e., no pulmonary embolus) will result in images of two black homogeneous lungs. If an artery is blocked from pulmonary embolus, the scan will demonstrate a nonperfused (or nonblackened) area (Novelline). If the perfusion scan is normal, no further testing is needed, because a normal scan is considered to be similar to results of pulmonary angiography (Shannon & Ng, 2002). If the perfusion scan is abnormal, a ventilation scan is performed, which is the second part of the test. In this part, patients inhale a radioactive gas, usually xenon-133 (Novelline), which allows the degree of ventilation of the lungs to be im-

---

Figure 6-3. Clinical Model for Predicting Pretest Probability for Deep Vein Thrombosis

Checklist
- Major points
  - Active cancer (ongoing, within previous six months, or palliative treatment)
  - Paralysis, paresis, or recent plaster immobilization of the lower extremities
  - Recently bedridden for more than three days or major surgery within four weeks
  - Localized tenderness along the distribution of the deep venous system
  - Thigh and calf swollen (should be measured)
  - Calf swelling more than 3 cm on symptomless side (measured 10 cm below tibial tuberosity)
  - Strong family history of deep vein thrombosis (two or more first-degree relatives with history of deep vein thrombosis
- Minor points
  - History of recent trauma (60 days or fewer) to the symptomatic leg
  - Pitting edema, symptomatic leg only
  - Dilated superficial veins (non-varicose) in symptomatic leg only
  - Hospitalization within previous six months
  - Erythema

Clinical Probability
- High
  - Three or more major points and no alternative diagnosis
  - Two or more major points, two or more minor points, and no alternative diagnosis
- Low
  - One major point, two or more minor points, and an alternative diagnosis
  - One major point, one or more minor point, and no alternative diagnosis
  - No major points, three or more minor points, and an alternative diagnosis
  - No major points, two or more minor points, and no alternative diagnosis
- Moderate
  - All other combinations

Active cancer did not include non-melanomatous skin cancer; deep-vein tenderness had to be elicited either in the calf or thigh in the anatomical distribution of the deep venous system.

Note. From "Accuracy of Clinical Assessment of Deep Vein Thrombosis," by P.S. Wells, J. Hirsh, D.R. Anderson, A.W. Lensing, G. Foster, C. Kearon et al., 1995, *Lancet, 345*(8961), p. 1330. Copyright 1995 by Elsevier. Adapted with permission.

aged. Pulmonary embolus should not cause a ventilation defect, and the scan should appear normal. Other lung problems (e.g., pneumonia, emphysema, tumor) can cause an abnormal ventilation scan. Thus, a patient with a perfusion scan (Q) that shows a defect and a normal ventilation scan (V) is termed a V/Q mismatch; the probability of a pulmonary embolus is high, and anticoagulant treatment is initiated (Novelline).

Results of the majority of V/Q scans are deemed indeterminate and do not rule out pulmonary embolus (Shannon & Ng, 2002). This is not uncommon in patients with lung cancer, who may have other abnormalities in addition to a tumor in the lung. At this point, additional testing must be performed. Pulmonary angiography, although considered the gold standard for diag-

nosis, is invasive and expensive. If Doppler ultrasound reveals DVT and the patient is symptomatic for pulmonary embolus, the diagnosis of pulmonary embolus is supported and angiogram is not needed (Shannon & Ng).

Both spiral CT and magnetic resonance angiography (MRA) are used in the diagnosis of pulmonary embolus. Sensitivity and specificity for these tests are 80% and 90%, respectively (Shannon & Ng, 2002). In addition to confirming a diagnosis of pulmonary embolus, they may reveal other sources of pathology that are responsible for the symptoms. In one study, MRA was compared with pulmonary angiography, and the results demonstrated that MRA had high sensitivity and specificity for the diagnosis of pulmonary embolus (Meaney et al., 1997).

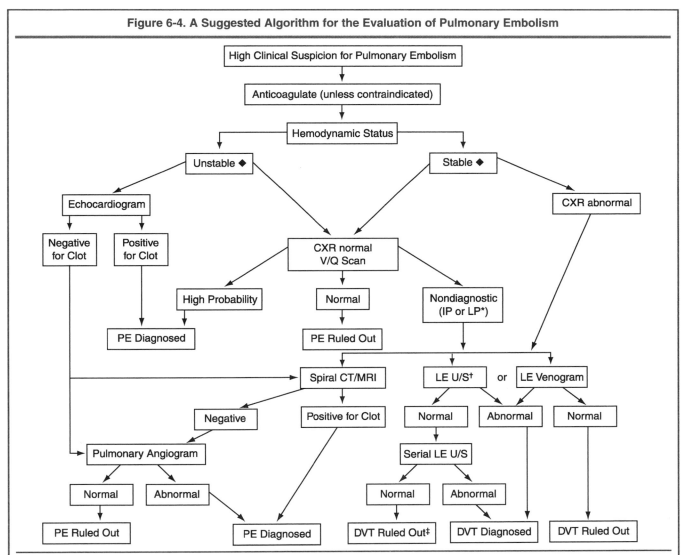

Figure 6-4. A Suggested Algorithm for the Evaluation of Pulmonary Embolism

*IP = Intermediate Probability; LP = Low Probability; †LE U/S = Lower extremity ultrasound; ‡May proceed to Spiral CT/MRI or pulmonary angiogram if clinical suspicion remains high. ◆Spiral CT may replace V/Q scan or echocardiogram as initial study in some patients.

Note. From "Noninfectious Pulmonary Emergencies" (p. 194) by V.R. Shannon and A. Ng in S.-C.J. Yeung and C.P. Escalante (Eds.), *Holland, Frei Oncologic Emergencies*, 2002, Hamilton, ON: BC Decker Inc. Copyright 2002 by BC Decker Inc. Reprinted with permission.

Additionally, MRA is less invasive than angiography because it does not expose the patient to ionizing radiation or iodinated contrast material. Others have shown that spiral CT may be a better test than MRA, and results using spiral CT have been shown to compare favorably with angiography. However, MRA is more invasive and requires contrast material (Shannon & Ng). Figure 6-4 outlines a suggested algorithm for the evaluation of pulmonary embolism (Shannon & Ng).

Laboratory studies are not diagnostic of thromboses, but they may be helpful in certain circumstances. Antithrombin III, protein S and C, and antiphospholipid antibodies may be obtained in patients with recurrent disease and in those without other risk factors (Story, 2000). Elevated D-dimer levels (> 500 ng/ml) usually are seen with acute thrombosis. However, elevated D-dimer levels are nonspecific. They may be elevated in other disorders such as sepsis, trauma, pneumonia, and malignancy (Shannon & Ng, 2002).

Treatment

Management will focus on treatment of DVT and patients with pulmonary embolus who are stable. Treatment of massive pulmonary embolus, the unstable patient with pulmonary embolus, and use of thrombolytic therapy is beyond the scope of this chapter, and information is available elsewhere (Shannon & Ng, 2002). Treatment of DVT or pulmonary embolus traditionally begins with anticoagulation with IV continuous-infusion unfractionated heparin. Clinicians have been using subcutaneous doses of low molecular weight heparin (LMWH). LMWHs (e.g., enoxaparin, tinzaparin) are approved by the U.S. Food and Drug Administration for outpatient management of patients with DVT and for inpatient treatment of patients with pulmonary embolus. The doses of LMWHs are based on the patient's body weight. They have been found to have better bioavailability, a longer half-life, and more predictable anticoagulant activity, and they do not require laboratory monitoring (Koopman et al., 1996). Studies have documented the efficacy and safety of LMWH administered subcutaneously when compared with continuous-infusion heparin for treatment of venous thromboses in hospitalized patients (Lensing, Prins, Davidson, & Hirsh, 1995; Prandoni et al., 1992). Koopman et al. randomly assigned patients with proximal DVT to receive either standard IV heparin in the hospital or subcutaneous fixed-dose LMWH on an outpatient basis. Results of the study demonstrated that subcutaneous LMWH was as safe and effective as standard heparin and 75% of patients treated with LMWH were able to be treated on an outpatient basis (Koopman et al.). Quality-of-life assessments also were made in this study, and results showed that patients treated with LMWH had less impairment of physical activity and social functioning (Koopman et al.). If oral anticoagulation is used to accomplish long-term anticoagulation, patients also are started on warfarin on the first day. Simultaneous administration is required because development of adequate anticoagulation takes several days on warfarin alone. Measurement of the international normalized ratio (INR) pro-

vides laboratory monitoring of warfarin. Administration of LMWH is recommended for at least five days in addition to warfarin. Once the patient is therapeutic on warfarin (INR 2.0–3.0), the LMWH is stopped. Guidelines for initiation and adjustment of warfarin therapy are seen in Table 6-4. In patients with lung cancer (or any cancer) and DVT or PE, continued anticoagulation is recommended for 12 months to lifetime or until the cancer is resolved (Story, 2000). Close, regular monitoring of warfarin is required to maintain therapeutic anticoagulation, as many different foods and medicines can affect the activity of warfarin. In patients in whom anticoagulation is contraindicated, a filter may be placed in the inferior vena cava. In patients with a proximal DVT, the risk for pulmonary embolus is increased. A filter in the inferior vena cava may prevent migration of thrombus to the pulmonary vasculature. Placement of a filter in a patient with cancer and a hypercoagulable state may prevent pulmonary emboli, but it does not prevent other incidents of thrombotic events.

Musculoskeletal Paraneoplastic Syndromes

Clubbing and Hypertrophic Pulmonary Osteoarthropathy

Clubbing and hypertrophic pulmonary osteoarthropy (HPOA) are considered to be paraneoplastic syndromes of the musculoskeletal system. These conditions often coexist, but they can occur separately (Fraser, Paré, Fraser, & Paré, 1994). They involve changes in the hands, toes, and long bones. Both are frequently associated with thoracic malignancies. Clubbing also is associated with other medical problems, such as chronic obstructive pulmonary disease, inflammatory bowel disease, heart disease, and cystic fibrosis (Stauffer, 1996). Some nonmalignant conditions can cause HPOA, but the most common cause is lung cancer (Kraut & Wozniak, 2000).

Incidence and Pathogenesis

Clubbing occurs in the fingers or toes or both. It is not a common manifestation, occurring in 2%–21% of patients with non-small cell lung cancer (NSCLC) (Busick et al., 2003). It was first described by Hippocrates more than 2,000 years ago. A prospective study by Sridhar, Lobo, and Altman (1998) demonstrated that clubbing was more frequent in patients with NSCLC than SCLC and more common in women. HPOA, an inflammation of the long bones of the limbs (osteitis), occurs in less than 5% of patients with NSCLC (Beckles, Spiro, Colice, & Rudd, 2003). The paraneoplastic syndrome of HPOA usually consists of clubbing and rheumatologic manifestations of arthralgias, synovitis, and periostitis (Burstein, Janicek, & Skarin 1997). The pathogenesis of clubbing and HPOA is unknown, but it is believed to be the result of vasodilator substances or increased blood flow to the digits (clubbing); others believe that humoral mediators (growth factors and inflammatory cytokines)

Table 6-4. Initiation and Dose Adjustment of Warfarin in Deep Vein Thrombosis

- Start warfarin and heparin on the same day, if possible.
- Obtain baseline prothrombin time (PT)/international normalized ratio (INR).
- Start with 5 mg by mouth, four times per day.
- Repeat PT/INR the next day.
- Repeat warfarin dose if PT/INR is unchanged.
- Obtain daily PT/INR until value is in therapeutic range.
- Reduce warfarin dose when PT/INR starts to rise.
- Overlap heparin with warfarin until at least two consecutive PT/INR values are in the therapeutic range.

Adjust total weekly warfarin dose using the following guidelines.

INR	Adjustment
1.1–1.4	Day 1: Add 10%–20% of total weekly dose (TWD) of warfarin Weekly: Increase TWD by 10%–20% Return: One week for PT/INR
1.5–1.9	Day 1: Add 5%–10% of TWD Weekly: Increase TWD by 5%–10% Return: Two weeks for PT/INR
2.0–3.0	No change Return: Four weeks for PT/INR
3.1–3.9	Day 1: Subtract 5%–10% of TWD Weekly: Reduce TWD by 5%–10% Return: Two weeks for PT/INR
4.0–5.0	Day 1: No warfarin Weekly: Reduce TWD by 10%–20% Return: One week for PT/INR
> 5.0	Stop warfarin; monitor INR until 3.0 is reached Weekly: Reduce TWD by 20%–50% Return: Daily for PT/INR
Recommended INR levels 1.2–1.5	For indwelling devices
2.0–3.0	To prevent thrombus in high-risk situations (e.g., high-risk surgery, chronic recurrent deep vein thrombosis, atrial fibrillation)
2.5–3.5	To prevent recurrent thrombus in patients with mechanical valves

Note. From *Disorders of Hemostasis and Thrombosis: A Clinical Guide* (p. 497), by W.E. Hathaway and S.H. Goodnight, Jr., 1993, New York: McGraw-Hill, Copyright 1993 by McGraw-Hill. Adapted with permission; "Oral Anticoagulation Therapy: Practical Aspects of Management," by M.L. Bridgen, 1996, *Postgraduate Medicine, 99*(6), pp. 84 and 87. Copyright 1996 by Postgraduate Medicine. Adapted with permission.

play a role (Burstein et al.; Fraser et al., 1994). HPOA leads to formation of new subperiosteal cancellous bone occurring most often in the long bones, specifically the distal ends of the radius, ulna (wrist), tibia, and fibula (ankles) (Busick et al.).

Signs and Symptoms

The early stages of clubbing may be difficult to detect, as the signs are subtle; later stages are easier to recognize. Clubbing cannot be verified by imaging modalities. Its diagnosis rests on the physical examination (Myers & Farquhar, 2001). Pain is not associated with clubbing. Clubbing most often is symmetrical and generally is graded according to five criteria on physical examination (see Figure 6-5) (Altman & Tenenbaum, 1997).

- Fluctuation and softening of the nail bed (feels spongy to touch)
- Loss of the normal 15-degree angle between the nail and the cuticle

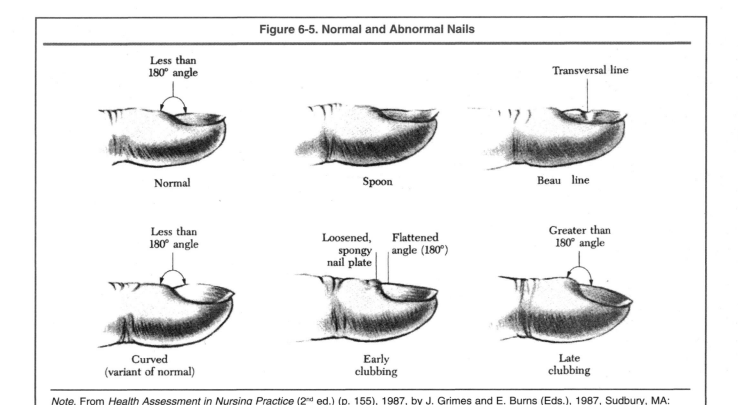

Figure 6-5. Normal and Abnormal Nails

Less than 180° angle — Normal

Spoon

Transversal line — Beau line

Less than 180° angle — Curved (variant of normal)

Loosened, spongy nail plate — Flattened angle (180°) — Early clubbing

Greater than 180° angle — Late clubbing

Note. From *Health Assessment in Nursing Practice* (2nd ed.) (p. 155), 1987, by J. Grimes and E. Burns (Eds.), 1987, Sudbury, MA: Jones and Bartlett. Copyright 1987 by Jones and Bartlett. Reprinted with permission.

- Accentuated convexity of the nail
- Development of a clubbed appearance at the fingertips
- Development of a shiny or glossy change with longitudinal striations of the nail

Patients with HPOA experience significant, usually symmetrical, pain in the wrists, ankles, feet, knees, and lower legs (Beckles et al., 2003). Joint effusions also may develop. Additionally, swelling and erythema often are seen in the affected joints (Busick et al., 2003). Pain can occur on palpation of the affected bone. Very often, these symptoms predate the diagnosis of cancer and often are initially mistaken for rheumatoid arthritis. Approximately 10% of patients have gynecomastia (Johnson, Spiller, & Faull, 1997).

Diagnosis

Clubbing is diagnosed by findings on physical examination. There are no imaging studies that demonstrate the abnormalities associated with clubbing. HPOA is diagnosed by signs and symptoms and presence of a cancer diagnosis. Without a cancer diagnosis, it often is mistaken for rheumatologic disease. Additionally, bone scan will demonstrate increased metabolic activity, and radiographs of the long bones will demonstrate new subperiosteal bone formation, which appears as linear calcification outside the cortex of the affected areas (Busick et al., 2003; Penson & Rudd, 1997).

Treatment

Treatment is aimed at control of symptoms and management of the cancer. Clubbing usually is asymptomatic and may resolve over many months with control of the tumor. For many with HPOA, the symptoms will abate with control of the lung tumor with chemotherapy or radiotherapy. Symptoms also have been known to resolve following resection of NSCLC (Burstein et al., 1997). Nonsteroidal anti-inflammatory agents, corticosteroids, and analgesics are used either alone or in combination to treat the arthralgias associated with HPOA. Low-dose colchicine also has been used (Penson & Rudd, 1997). One case report demonstrated significant relief of pain with subcutaneous octreotide in a patient with HPOA who had failed other conventional pain modalities (Johnson et al., 1997). Continued evaluation of octreotide is needed before it can be recommended in patients with HPOA.

Conclusions

HPOA is a paraneoplastic syndrome of the musculoskeletal system that often predates a cancer diagnosis. It is characterized by a constellation of signs and symptoms that include clubbing of the fingers and toes, pain in the distal long bones and associated joints, and periostitis, which can be demonstrated radiographically. The pain associated with

HPOA can be debilitating. Control of the tumor with radiotherapy, chemotherapy, or surgery usually results in improvement or resolution of symptoms. Symptomatic improvement also can be obtained with conventional pain control methods.

References

Adams, L. (2002). Paraneoplastic syndromes. *Radiation Therapist, 11,* 23–33.

Agarwala, S.S. (1996). Paraneoplastic syndromes. *Medical Clinics of North America, 80,* 173–184.

Altman, R.D., & Tenenbaum, J. (1997). Hypertrophic osteoarthropathy. In W.N. Kelly & E.D. Harris (Eds.), *Textbook of rheumatology* (5th ed., pp. 1514–1520). Philadelphia: W.B. Saunders.

Barnett, M.L. (1999). Hypercalcemia. *Seminars in Oncology Nursing, 15,* 190–201.

Beckles, M.A., Spiro, S.G., Colice, G.L., & Rudd, R.M. (2003). Initial evaluation fo the patient with vlung cancer. *Chest, 123* (Suppl. 1), 97S–104S.

Berenson, J.R., Rosen, L.S., Howell, A., Porter, L., Coleman, R.E., Morley, W., et al. (2001). Zoledronic acid reduces skeletal-related events in patients with osteolytic metastases. *Cancer, 91,* 1191–1200.

Bilezekian, J. (1992). Management of acute hypercalcemia. *New England Journal of Medicine, 326,* 1196–1203.

Blinder, M.A., & Behl, R. (2002). Coagulation disorders in cancer. In R. Govinday & M.A. Arquette (Eds.), *The Washington manual of oncology* (pp. 441–447). Philadelphia: Lippincott Williams & Wilkins.

Body, J.J. (2001). Dosing regimens and main adverse events of bisphosphonates. *Seminars in Oncology, 4,* 49–53.

Boss, B.J., Sunderland, P.M., & Heath, J. (1994). Alterations of neurologic function. In K.L. McCance & S.E. Huether (Eds.), *Pathophysiology: The biologic basis for disease in adults and children* (pp. 527–586). St. Louis, MO: Mosby.

Boyle, D. (2001). Oncologic emergency: Case 4. In E.M. Lin (Ed.), *Advanced practice in oncology nursing* (pp. 320–327). Philadelphia: W.B. Saunders.

Brain, W.R., & Wilkinson, M. (1965). Subacute cerebellar degeneration associated with neoplasms. *Brain, 88,* 465–478.

Burstein, H.J., Janicek, M.J., & Skarin, A.T. (1997). Hypertrophic osteoarthropathy. *Journal of Clinical Oncology, 15,* 2759–2760.

Busick, N.P., Fretz, P.C., Galvin, J.R., & Peterson, M.W. (2003). Neoplastic and paraneoplastic syndromes. *Virtual Hospital at the University of Iowa Web Site.* Retrieved January 20, 2003, from http://www.vh.org/adult/provider/radiology/LungTumors/ParaneoplasticProcesses/Text/ParaneoplasticProcesses.html

Chalk, C.H., Murray, N.M., Newsom-Davis, J., O'Neill, J.H., & Spiro, S.G. (1990). Response of the Lambert-Eaton myasthenic syndrome to treatment of associated small-cell lung carcinoma. *Neurology, 40,* 1552–1556.

Dalmau, J.O., & Posner, J.B. (1997). Paraneoplastic syndromes affecting the nervous system. *Seminars in Oncology, 24,* 318–328.

Ezzone, S.A. (2000). Syndrome of inappropriate antidiuretic hormone. In D. Camp-Sorrell & R.A. Hawkins (Eds.), *Clinical manual for the oncology advanced practice nurse* (pp. 571–575). Pittsburgh, PA: Oncology Nursing Society.

Feied, C. (1998). Pulmonary embolism. In P. Rosen & R. Barkin (Eds.), *Emergency medicine concepts and clinical practice* (pp. 1770–1805). St. Louis, MO: Mosby.

Fischbach, F. (1996). Chemistry studies. In F. Fischbach (Ed.), *A manual of laboratory and diagnostic tests* (pp. 302–440). New York: Lippincott Williams & Wilkins.

Flombaum, C.D. (2000). Metabolic emergencies in the cancer patient. *Seminars in Oncology, 27,* 322–334.

Fraser, R.S., Paré, J.A.P., Fraser, R.G., & Paré. P.D. (1994). Methods of clinical, laboratory, and functional investigation. In R.S. Fraser, J.A.P. Paré, R.G. Fraser, & P.D. Paré (Eds.), *Synopsis of diseases of the chest* (pp. 141–164). Philadelphia: W.B. Saunders.

Frenkel, E.P., Bick, R.L., & Rutherford, C.J. (1996). Anemia of malignancy. *Hematology-Oncology Clinics of North America, 10,* 861–871.

Goldhaber, S.Z. (1998). Pulmonary embolism. *New England Journal of Medicine, 339,* 93–104.

Graus, F., Vega, F., Delattre, J.Y., Bonaventura, I., Rene, R., & Arbaiza, D. (1992). Plasmapheresis and antineoplastic treatment in CNC paraneoplastic syndromes with antineuronal autoantibodies. *Neurology, 42,* 536–540.

Haapoja, I.S. (2000a). Paraneoplastic syndromes. In C.H. Yarbro, M.H. Frogge, M. Goodman, & S.L. Groenwald (Eds.), *Cancer nursing: Principles and practice* (5th ed., pp. 792–812). Sudbury, MA: Jones and Bartlett.

Haapoja, I.S. (2000b). Syndrome of inappropriate antidiuretic hormone. In C.H. Yarbro, M.H. Frogge, M. Goodman, & S.L. Groenwald (Eds.), *Cancer nursing: Principles and practice* (5th ed., pp. 913–919). Sudbury, MA: Jones and Bartlett.

Henke, S.C. (2000). Pulmonary embolism. In D. Camp-Sorrell & R.A. Hawkins (Eds.), *Clinical manual for the oncology advanced practice nurse* (pp. 183–188). Pittsburgh, PA: Oncology Nursing Society.

Huether, S.E. (1994). The cellular environment: Fluids and electrolytes, acids and bases. In K.L. McCance & S.E. Huether (Eds.), *Pathophysiology: The biologic basis for disease in adults and children* (pp. 91–123). St. Louis, MO: Mosby.

Jensen, G. (1997). Hypercalcemia of malignancy. In R.A. Gates & R.M. Fink (Eds.), *Oncology nursing secrets* (pp. 336–341). Philadelphia: Hanley & Belfus, Inc.

Johnson, S.A., Spiller, P.A., & Faull, C.M. (1997). Treatment of resistant pain in hypertrophic pulmonary osteoarthropathy with subcutaneous octreotide. *Thorax, 52,* 298–299.

Keenan, A.M. (1999). Syndrome of inappropriate secretion of antidiuretic hormone in malignancy. *Seminars in Oncology Nursing, 15,* 160–167.

Koopman, M.W., Prandoni, P., Piovella, F., Ockelford, P.A., Brandjes, D.P.M., van der Meer, J., et al. (1996). Treatment of venous thrombosis with intravenous unfractionated heparin administered in the hospital as compared with subcutaneous low-molecular-weight heparin administered at home. *New England Journal of Medicine, 334,* 682–687.

Kozisek, P. (2000). Hyponatremia. In M.R. Dambro (Ed.), *Griffith's 5-minute clinical consult* (pp. 546–547). Philadelphia: Lippincott Williams & Wilkins.

Kraut, M., & Wozniak, A. (2000). Clinical presentation. In H.L. Pass, J.B. Mitchell, D.H. Johnson, A.T. Turissi, & J.D. Minna (Eds.), *Lung cancer: Principles and practice* (2nd ed., pp. 521–534). Philadelphia: Lippincott Williams & Wilkins.

Lennon, V.A., Kryzer, T.J., Griesmann, M.S., O'Suilleabhain, P.E., Windebank, A.J., Whoppmann, A., et al. (1994). Calcium-channel antibodies in the Lambert-Eaton syndrome and other paraneoplastic syndromes. *New England Journal of Medicine, 332,* 1467–1474.

Lensing, A.W.A., Prins, M.H., Davidson, B.L., & Hirsh, J. (1995). Treatment of deep venous thrombosis with low-molecular-weight-heparins: A meta analysis. *Archives of Internal Medicine, 155,* 601–607.

Mason, W.P., Graus, F., Lang, B., Honnorat, J., Delattre, J.Y., Valldeoriola, F., et al. (1997). Small-cell lung cancer, paraneoplastic cerebellar degeneration and the Lambert-Eaton myasthenic syndrome. *Brain, 120,* 1279–1300.

Meaney, J.F.M., Weg, J.G., Chenevert, T.L., Stafford-Johnson, D., Hamilton, B.H., & Prince, M.R. (1997). Diagnosis of pulmonary embolism with magnetic resonance angiography. *New England Journal of Medicine, 336,* 1422–1427.

Midthun, D.E., & Jett, J.R. (1996). Clinical presentation of lung cancer. In H.L. Pass, J.B. Mitchell, D.H. Johnson, & A.T. Turissi (Eds.), *Lung cancer: Principles and practice* (pp. 775–789). Philadelphia: Lippincott Williams & Wilkins.

Morton, A.R., & Ritch, P.S. (1998). Hypercalcemia. In A.M. Berger, R.K. Portenoy, & D.E. Weissman (Eds.), *Principles and practice of supportive oncology* (pp. 411–425). Philadelphia: Lippincott-Williams & Wilkins.

Myers, K.A., & Farquhar, D.R.E. (2001). Does this patient have clubbing? *JAMA, 286,* 341–347.

Naschitz, J.E., Yeshurun, D., & Lev, L.M. (1993). Thromboembolism in cancer. *Cancer, 71,* 1384–1390.

Nathanson, L., & Hall, T.C. (1997). Introduction: Paraneoplastic syndromes. *Seminars in Oncology, 24,* 265–268.

Newsom-Davis, J. (1998). A treatment algorithm for Lambert-Eaton myasthenic syndrome. *Annals of the New York Academy of Sciences, 841,* 817–822.

Novelline, R.A. (1997). The diaphragm, the pleural space, and pulmonary embolism. In R.A. Novelline (Ed.), *Squires fundamentals of radiology* (pp. 126–139). Cambridge, MA: Harvard University Press.

Odell, W.D. (1997). Endocrine/metabolic syndromes of cancer. *Seminars in Oncology, 24,* 299–317.

Penson, R.T., & Rudd, R.M. (1997). Commentary: Octreotide and hypertrophic pulmonary osteoarthropathy. *Thorax, 52,* 297–298.

Posner, J.B., & Dalmau, J.O. (1997). Paraneoplastic syndromes affecting the central nervous system. *Annual Reviews of Medicine, 48,* 157–166.

Prandoni, P., Lensing, A.W.A., Buller, H.R., Carta, M., Cogo, A., Vigo, M., et al. (1992). Comparison of subcutaneous low-molecular-weight-heparin with intravenous standard heparin in proximal deep-vein thrombosis. *Lancet, 339*(8791), 441–445.

Rickles, F.R., Hancock, W.W., Edwards, R.L., & Zacharski, L.R. (1988). Antimetastatic agents. I. Role of cellular procoagulants in the pathogenesis of fibrin deposition in cancer and the use of anticoagulants and/or antiplatelet drugs in cancer treatment. *Seminars in Thrombosis and Hemostasis, 14,* 88–94.

Robbins, S.L., Cotran, R.S., & Kumar, V. (Eds.). (1995). *Pocket companion to Robbins pathologic basis of disease* (2nd ed.). Philadelphia: W.B. Saunders.

Shannon, V.R., & Ng, A. (2002). Noninfectious pulmonary emergencies. In S.-C.J. Yeung & C.P. Escalante (Eds.), *Holland, Frei oncologic emergencies* (pp. 191–248). Hamilton, ON: BC Decker.

Shuey, K.M. (1994). Heart, lung, and endocrine complications of solid tumors. *Seminars in Oncology Nursing, 10,* 177–188.

Silverstein, R.L., & Nachman, R.L. (1992). Cancer and clotting-Trousseau's warning. *New England Journal of Medicine, 327,* 1163–1164.

Smith, W.J. (2000). Hypocalcemia/hypercalcemia. In D. Camp-Sorrell & R.A. Hawkins (Eds.), *Clinical manual for the oncology advanced practice nurse* (pp. 849–858). Pittsburgh, PA: Oncology Nursing Society.

Sridhar, K.S., Lobo, C.F., & Altman, R.D. (1998). Digital clubbing and lung cancer. *Chest, 114,* 1535–1537.

Staszewski, H. (1997). Hematological paraneoplastic syndromes. *Seminars in Oncology, 24,* 329–333.

Stauffer, J.L. (1996). Lung. In L.M. Tierney, S.J. McPhee, & M.A. Papadakis (Eds.), *Current medical diagnosis and treatment* (pp. 215–294). Stamford, CT: Appleton & Lange.

Story, K.T. (2000). Deep vein thrombosis. In D. Camp-Sorrell & R.A. Hawkins (Eds.), *Clinical manual for the oncology advanced practice nurse* (pp. 235–243). Pittsburgh, PA: Oncology Nursing Society.

Struthers, C.S. (1994). Lambert-Eaton myasthenic syndrome in small cell lung cancer: Nursing implications. *Oncology Nursing Forum, 21,* 677–683.

Uchuya, M., Graus, F., Vega, F., Rene, R., & Delattre, J.Y. (1996). Intravenous immunoglobulin treatment in paraneoplastic neurological syndromes with antineuronal autoantibodies. *Journal of Neurology, Neurosurgery, Psychiatry, 60,* 388–392.

Wells, P.S., Hirsh, J., Anderson, D.R., Lensing, A.W., Foster, G., Kearon, C., et al. (1995). Accuracy of clinical assessment of deep vein thrombosis. *Lancet, 345*(8961), 1326–1330.

Wickham, R.S. (2000). Hypercalcemia. In C.H. Yarbro, M.H. Frogge, M. Goodman, & S.L. Groenwald (Eds.), *Cancer nursing: Principles and practice* (5th ed., pp. 776–791). Sudbury, MA: Jones and Bartlett.

Zumsteg, M.M., & Casperson, D.S. (1998). Paraneoplastic syndromes in metastatic disease. *Seminars in Oncology Nursing, 14,* 220–229.

CHAPTER 7

Small Cell Lung Cancer

Margaret Joyce, MSN, RN, AOCN®

Introduction

Small cell lung cancer (SCLC) has unique biological characteristics that distinguish it from the other major forms of lung cancer, which are collectively categorized as non-small cell lung cancer (NSCLC). These unique properties of SCLC include rapid cell growth, a tendency to be widely disseminated at the time of diagnosis, and prominent sensitivity to chemotherapy and radiotherapy (RT). If untreated, small cell carcinoma has the most aggressive clinical course of any type of pulmonary tumor, with a median survival from diagnosis of two to four months (Cancer.gov, 2003). Although current therapy has a significant impact on the natural history of SCLC, long-term disease-free survival is rare. Most studies cite median duration of survival at 8–20 months, depending on clinical stage at diagnosis (National Comprehensive Cancer Network [NCCN], 2002). Only about 10% of the total population of patients with SCLC remain free of disease two years from the start of therapy (Cancer.gov).

Prevalence and Presentation

In the United States, about 18% of all patients diagnosed with lung cancer annually have a histological diagnosis of small cell carcinoma (Murren, Glatstein, & Pass, 2001). Most SCLC tumors are centrally located, presenting in the main stem or lobar bronchi, and tend to disseminate early and widely into hilar and mediastinal nodes, often forming very bulky masses. SCLCs often show areas of necrosis, grossly, although they are not as prone to cavitation as are squamous cell carcinomas (Fraire, 1996). Superior vena cava (SVC) syndrome is not uncommon; it usually is caused by invasion of the vena cava or extrinsic compression by the tumor with or without intraluminal thrombosis. SCLC predominates as the cause of SVC syndrome, followed by squamous cell carcinoma of the lung (Vaporciyan et al., 2000).

SCLC accounts for about 75% of tumors associated with ectopic production of antidiuretic hormone (ADH). Although 50%–75% of patients with SCLC have elevated ADH levels, only 1%–5% of patients develop symptoms attributed to syndrome of inappropriate antidiuretic hormone release (Patel & Jett, 1996). Successful treatment of the tumor effectively controls the endocrine symptoms.

Small cell carcinoma also is the most common type of lung cancer associated with paraneoplastic autoimmune neurologic syndromes. Neurologic symptoms often precede the diagnosis of cancer and do not improve with successful antineoplastic therapy. Lambert-Eaton myasthenic syndrome (LEMS) is a neurologic impairment characterized by proximal muscle weakness that improves after repetitive movement or exertion. Approximately 50% of patients with LEMS have malignancy, with SCLC being the most common (Patel & Jett, 1996).

Relationship to Smoking

A strong relationship exists between SCLC and cigarette smoking (Cancer.gov, 2003; Murren et al., 2001). SCLC incidence parallels trends in cigarette smoking; a 20–50-year lag period or interval has been found between the initiation of smoking and the diagnosis of cancer (Murren et al.). Because of past smoking patterns, SCLC initially was more predominant among men. However, as the prevalence of smoking among women increased, so did the incidence of SCLC in women. As groups of individuals most heavily exposed to tobacco grow older, the median age at diagnosis for SCLC also will increase. Over the next few decades, the overall incidence of lung cancer should continue to decline in the United States. However, if the current increase in popularity of cigarette smoking among adolescents does not change, that decline in incidence of lung cancer will halt and eventually reverse.

Over the last decade, the incidence of the subhistologies of lung cancer has shifted in the United States; the frequency of small cell carcinoma has declined, and adenocarcinoma is now the most frequently diagnosed subform. Whether this reflects an industry change to filtered cigarettes, causing smokers to modify their smoking behavior by inhaling more deeply or blocking filter vents to increase nicotine yield, is speculative (Koh, Kannler, & Geller, 2001). These factors, along with changing demographics of the smoking population, will define who develops SCLC in future decades.

Cell Type

In 1988, the Pathology Committee of the International Association for the Study of Lung Cancer revised the classification of SCLC to include (a) small cell carcinoma, (b) mixed small and large cell carcinoma, and (c) combined small cell carcinoma (typical SCLC elements mixed with neoplastic squamous or adenocarcinoma) (Hirsch et al., 1988). More than 90% of untreated SCLCs fall into the pure small cell carcinoma category (Murren et al., 2001).

Although the diagnosis of small cell carcinoma rests primarily on morphologic assessment, immunocytochemistry plays a role. Virtually all SCLCs are immunoreactive for keratin and epithelial membrane antigen; negative staining for neuroendocrine markers can occur in 25% of cases and should not deter the diagnosis of SCLC (Guinee, Fishback, Koss, Abbondanzo, & Travis, 1994).

Whether the presence of a mixed cell or a combined histology confers a different prognosis or response to treatment than pure small cell carcinoma is not clear. Published reports have identified survival that is inferior to, superior to, or comparable to pure small cell (Murren et al., 2001). In a review of 429 patients, nine (2%) with combined small cell and nonsmall cell histologies were identified. Two of the nine patients were long-term survivors and underwent surgical resection in addition to chemotherapy. Although this circumstance is rare, surgery may play a role in the management of residual tumor in patients with combined histology (Mangum, Greco, Hainsworth, Hande, & Johnson, 1989).

Neuroendocrine Classification

SCLC is considered a neuroendocrine carcinoma, which represents a spectrum of disease that arises from basal neuroendocrine cells. SCLC, which has a poor prognosis, is at one end of the spectrum. At the other extreme end of the spectrum is bronchial carcinoid, which has an excellent prognosis after surgical excision. Between these extremes is well-differentiated neuroendocrine carcinoma of the lung. Like SCLC, it occurs primarily in cigarette smokers; however, it metastasizes less frequently and has a more favorable prognosis (Cancer.gov, 2003).

Molecular and Genetic Characteristics

Carcinogenesis occurs over time in a multistep process of initiation, promotion, and progression. Initiation refers to

genetic damage caused by carcinogens. If DNA damage is not repaired and the cell divides, the daughter cells inherit the abnormal DNA and are called initiated cells. Tumor promotion occurs with excessive proliferation of the initiated cell. Cigarette smoke contains chemicals that are both initiators and promoters. Progression is the final step of tumor invasion and metastasis.

Each stage of carcinogenesis may involve various oncogenes, tumor suppressor genes (TSGs), growth factors, and growth factor receptors (Works & Gallucci, 1996). Identification of specific abnormal cell targets may lead to development of directed therapies. The technology of molecular biology has allowed for the identification of gene families implicated in lung carcinogenesis, including proto-oncogenes and TSGs. A proto-oncogene is a gene in a normal cell that influences the control of cellular proliferation and differentiation. Mutations or amplifications of proto-oncogenes cause them to act as oncogenes. Oncogenes are capable of inducing one or more characteristics of cancer cells. TSGs normally inhibit cellular proliferation. When mutated or deleted, TSGs promote the development of cancer (Works & Gallucci). Many of the proto-oncogene and TSG changes are present in both major lung cancer subtypes (SCLC and NSCLC), although certain mutations have small cell specificity (see Table 7-1).

Tumor Initiation

Deletion of the short arm of chromosome *3p* occurs in virtually 100% of SCLCs and up to 80% of lung adenocarcinomas. Chromosome *3p* is believed to contain a TSG that, when lost as a result of damage from tobacco smoke, allows malignant transformation to occur. Other TSGs involved in lung cancer include *p53* and the retinoblastoma (*Rb*) gene. The *Rb* gene encodes a nuclear regulatory protein, which acts as a "brake" on cell proliferation. Point mutations or deletions of this gene lead to uncontrolled cell division. The *Rb* product is inactivated in more than 90% of SCLCs (Works & Gallucci, 1996).

Tumor Promotion

Gastrin-releasing peptide (GRP) or bombesin is a growth factor for normal bronchial epithelium. Chronic proliferation of bronchial epithelium from prolonged exposure to cigarette smoke produces excessive GRP. SCLC cells synthesize and secrete GRP. GRP serves as an autocrine growth factor that stimulates their proliferation. Small cell carcinoma cell lines express a high-affinity, saturable-binding receptor for bombesin or GRP (Vaporciyan et al., 2000).

The *p53* gene normally prevents genetically damaged cells from replicating. If cell damage repair is unsuccessful in the G1 phase of replication, *p53* triggers apoptosis, or cell death. Cells with inactivated *p53* (through deletion or point mutation) contribute to cancer promotion by replicating damaged DNA and passing the abnormality on to many more cells.

Table 7-1. Oncogenes and Tumor Suppressor Genes in Small Cell Lung Cancer

Oncogenes	Mutation	Frequency	Stage of Carcinogenesis	Clinical Applications
Myc family	Amplification	20%	Progression	Prognostic indicator
Tumor-suppressor genes				
3p	Deletion	100%	Initiation	Early detection marker
p53	Point mutation	80%	Promotion or initiation	Gene therapy
Rb	Deletion or point mutation	90%	Initiation or promotion	Early detection marker

Note. From "Biology of Lung Cancer," by C.R. Works and B.G. Gallucci, 1996, *Seminars in Oncology Nursing, 12,* p. 281. Copyright 1996 by Elsevier, Inc. Adapted with permission.

Mutation or deletion of the *p53* gene is the most common genetic abnormality in human cancer. Fifty percent of lung cancers have *p53* gene deletion, and mutations have been found in 80% of SCLCs and 45% of NSCLCs (Works & Gallucci, 1996).

Tumor Progression

The Myc family of oncogenes may be involved in lung cancer progression. Amplified *Myc* genes overexpress nuclear regulatory proteins, which stimulate other growth regulatory genes. The cell divides continually, becoming immortal. *Myc* gene amplification occurs in 20% of SCLCs and 8% of NSCLCs.

In summary, considerable information exists about the molecular abnormalities involved in the pathogenesis of SCLC. Both common and distinct genetic pathways exist in the major subtypes of lung cancer (SCLC and NSCLC) that are consistent with markedly biological and clinical features. New strategies for detection, prevention, and treatment are being developed based on an understanding of the basic underlying molecular genetic abnormalities.

Staging

Accurate clinical staging is important to determine prognosis and define therapy. It also is critical for entry into clinical trials that evaluate outcomes based on comparable patient populations. The usual tumor, node, metastasis (TNM) staging classification is not used for SCLC because most patients (90%) with SCLC have locally advanced or systemic metastases at the time of diagnosis. Pathologic nodal assessment is not required because surgery is not a primary approach in SCLC management. Patients commonly have radiologic evidence of hilar or mediastinal node involvement at initial presentation. For this reason, the Veterans Administration Lung Cancer Study Group developed a simple two-stage system. This system classifies patients with limited disease (LD) when the tumor is confined to one hemithorax and its regional lymph nodes, including the ipsilateral mediastinal, ipsilateral supraclavicular, and contralateral hilar nodes (Feld, Sagman, & LeBlanc, 1996). In essence, LD SCLC is localized disease that easily can be encompassed within an acceptable or tolerable RT port. Extensive disease (ED) means that the tumor is too widespread to be included within the definition of limited-stage disease.

Pericardial involvement or bilateral parenchyma involvement are considered signs of ED because the RT portal required to encompass this bulk of tumor would be too large and associated with significant risk of unacceptable toxicity. Any evidence of distant disease or disease outside of the thorax is considered ED. Common distant sites of metastasis are the adrenals, bone, liver, bone marrow, and brain.

Chemotherapy is the mainstay of treatment for SCLC. Combination therapy (i.e., chemotherapy with concurrent RT) is employed in LD SCLC to augment primary control. Thus, accurate clinical staging (LD or ED) is important in SCLC to determine when adding RT to chemotherapy is necessary.

Areas of controversy remain within this simple LD/ED staging system. Patients with pleural effusion have been both included and excluded from the limited-stage group. Several large series have failed to identify a difference in survival between patients with an isolated ipsilateral pleural effusion compared with other patients with limited-stage SCLC (Murren et al., 2001). All patients with contralateral pleural effusions should be included in the ED category (Feld et al., 1996).

Staging Procedures

Staging procedures aim to determine whether patients with SCLC have LD or ED. Initial workup includes a complete history and physical, computed tomography (CT) of the thorax, and blood tests that include complete blood count and biochemistry, such as electrolytes, liver function enzymes, alkaline phosphatase, and lactate dehydrogenase (LDH). Several investigators have found LDH to be a useful prognostic factor (Murren et al., 2001). It is an independent prognostic variable, and serial measurement of LDH often mirrors clinical response (Feld et al., 1996).

Staging tests are applied to define extrathoracic sites of disease and include CT of upper abdomen (to evaluate the liver and adrenals), radionuclide bone scan, and CT or magnetic resonance imaging (MRI) of the brain. Demonstration of one extrathoracic site of involvement is sufficient to complete the staging evaluation; hence, bone marrow aspiration and biopsies now are performed infrequently.

The role of positron emission tomography (PET) in SCLC is evolving and may streamline the staging evaluation. Data from several small studies reveal PET to be a suitable imaging method in SCLC (Chin et al., 2002; Hauber et al., 2001; Shen, Shiau, Wang, Ho, & Kao, 2002). The efficacy of PET in the staging of patients with SCLC appears to be comparable to the initial staging of conventional modality findings. Whether PET will replace other, more established staging modalities remains to be determined by larger, prospective, randomized controlled trials.

Treatment

Historically, the therapeutic approach to SCLC has been based on poor results of surgical resection. Surgical reports from before the 1970s found only one or two patients alive at five years. This led the Medical Research Council of Great Britain to prospectively randomize patients to surgical resection or RT. The median survival of patients in the surgery and RT arms was 199 and 300 days, respectively. At five years, one and three patients were alive in the surgery and RT arms, respectively. At 10 years, there were no surgical survivors. Researchers concluded that RT was preferable to surgery but that neither of the treatment modalities was effective. The investigators suggested that other modalities, such as chemotherapy or various combination therapies, might be more successful (Shepherd, 1996).

Preoperative radiation was investigated next; again, it yielded no long-term survivors. Patients were dying of systemic metastases, which suggested that no treatment with local therapy would lead to long-term survival without primary systemic chemotherapy. In the 1970s, the Medical Research Council Lung Working Party (1979) compared low-dose cyclophosphamide and lomustine (CCNU) given adjuvantly with radiation in patients with LD to radiation alone in patients with LD. A modest prolongation of progression-free survival was seen for patients in the chemotherapy arm, although overall survival and long-term survival benefit were not seen. Earlier, starting in 1958, the Veterans Administra-

tion Lung Cancer Study Group conducted randomized studies testing alkylating agents in bronchiogenic carcinoma and found that three courses of cyclophosphamide more than doubled the median survival compared with a placebo-treated control group in disseminated SCLC (Green, Humphrey, Close, & Patno, 1969). This initiated the chemotherapy era for treatment of SCLC and, hence, the quest for the most efficacious chemotherapy agent or agents. Today, oncology practitioners acknowledge SCLC as a remarkably chemosensitive disease, and systemic chemotherapy is considered the cornerstone or primary treatment modality for both stages of SCLC.

Extensive-Stage Disease

Several single chemotherapy agents have documented activity in SCLC (see Figure 7-1). Despite many active agents, SCLC rarely is treated with single agents largely because complete remissions are relatively infrequent and remission durations tend to be brief with single agents (DeVore & Johnson, 1996). Response rates of 60%–80% (8%–30% complete remissions) have been achieved in ED with combination chemotherapy (NCCN, 2002). Duration of response, however, is very short, with median survivals of 7–14 months.

Figure 7-1. Chemotherapeutic Agents With Documented Activity Against Small Cell Lung Cancer

Group 1 (Activity known before 1980)
- Cyclophosphamide
- Mechlorethamine (nitrogen mustard)
- Doxorubicin
- Methotrexate
- Altretamine (hexamethylmelamine)
- Etoposide
- Vincristine

Group 2 (Activity documented after 1980)
- Carboplatin
- Teniposide
- Ifosfamide
- Cisplatin

Group 3 (Newer agents)
- Paclitaxel
- Docetaxel
- Irinotecan (CPT-11)
- Topotecan
- Gemcitabine
- Vinorelbine

Note. From "Small Cell Lung Cancer" (p. 920) by D.C. Ihde, H.I. Pass, and E. Glatstein, in V.T. DeVita, S. Hellman, and S.A. Rosenberg (Eds.), *Cancer: Principles and Practice of Oncology* (5th ed.), 1997, Philadelphia: Lippincott-Raven. Copyright 1997 by Lippincott-Raven. Adapted with permission.

Platinum-based chemotherapy is the established mainstay of therapy for extensive SCLC (Simon, Wagner, & American College of Chest Physicians, 2003). Etoposide combined with a platinum compound is an important consideration of the initial drug treatment regimen. Although several regimens yield approximately equivalent survival results, etoposide plus cisplatin has become the most frequently used combination for SCLC (NCCN, 2002). The combination of etoposide and cisplatin appears to have the best therapeutic index, with fewer episodes of life-threatening toxicities (Johnson, 1999).

In clinical practice, clinicians often substitute carboplatin for cisplatin in combination with etoposide. Brahmer and Ettinger (1998) concluded that the combination of carboplatin and etoposide resulted in comparable efficacy, had less non-hematologic toxicity, and was easier to administer than cisplatin plus etoposide. The Hellenic Oncology Group conducted a prospective trial comparing the two regimens (Kosmidis et al., 1994). The study included patients with both limited and extensive SCLC. The median survival time was comparable and not statistically different. The carboplatin plus etoposide regimen caused significantly less nausea, vomiting, nephrotoxicity, and neurotoxicity; however, increased myelosuppression can be expected with the carboplatin plus etoposide regimen.

A phase III trial conducted in Japan compared the cisplatin plus etoposide regimen to a combination of cisplatin plus irinotecan (Noda et al., 2002). A statistically significant benefit was found in the group of patients randomized to the cisplatin plus irinotecan arm compared with the group of patients randomized to the cisplatin plus etoposide arm (median survival time 12.8 months versus 9.4 months respectively, p = 0.002). Severe or life-threatening myelosuppression was more frequent in the etoposide plus cisplatin group. Severe or life-threatening diarrhea was more frequent in the irinotecan plus cisplatin group. Confirmatory trials are under way in Europe and the United States (Cancer.gov, 2003; Sandler, 2003).

Several general principles have evolved in pursuit of improved outcomes in SCLC therapy.

- Alternating blocks of chemotherapy combinations have not yielded superior results when compared to sustained treatment with one combination (Martin & Comis, 1996).
- Higher doses of chemotherapy, even chemotherapy of the intensity used in autologous bone marrow transplant regimens, has not been shown to improve survival in patients with SCLC (Cancer.gov, 2003).
- Adding a third drug (i.e., paclitaxel) to the standard two-drug regimen has not provided a survival advantage but has added toxicity (Simon et al., 2003).
- Maintenance therapy beyond induction chemotherapy offers no proven survival benefit. Furthermore, maintenance therapy may be associated with inferior quality of life. Four to six cycles of induction therapy appear to be optimal in the management of both limited and extensive SCLC (Murren et al., 2001).

In summary, although improvements have been made in the treatment of both stages of SCLC with chemotherapy, the overall outcome remains disappointing with only a small percentage of patients achieving long-term survival. Investigation of newer agents and combination agents continues. Given the strong association of SCLC and smoking, primary prevention through tobacco abstinence and cessation remains paramount.

Limited-Stage Disease

Limited-stage SCLC is disease confined to one hemithorax within a single radiation port. At the time of diagnosis, approximately 30% of patients with small cell carcinoma have LD (Cancer.gov, 2003). The addition of thoracic RT to chemotherapy has improved survival for patients with limited-stage disease, with median survivals of 14–18 months (NCCN, 2002).

Two meta-analyses of randomized trials compared chemotherapy alone with chemotherapy combined with thoracic RT to evaluate the hypothesis that thoracic RT contributes to a moderate increase in overall survival in LD SCLC. Warde and Payne (1992) showed a small but significant improvement in two-year survival and a major improvement in tumor control in the thorax in patients receiving thoracic radiation therapy. However, this was achieved at the cost of a small increase in treatment-related mortality. Pignon et al. (1992) reported a meta-analysis that collected individual data on patients enrolled in 13 randomized trials before December 1988. They found that the relative risk of death in the combined therapy group as compared with the chemotherapy group was 0.86, which corresponds to a 14% reduction in the risk of death with combined therapy. The benefit in terms of overall survival at three years (± SD) was 5.4% (±1.4%). A subgroup analysis showed a significant trend (p = 0.01) toward a larger proportional effect on survival in favor of the combined therapy group among younger patients (younger than 55) compared with older patients. Pignon et al. were unable to evaluate the nonlethal toxicity of treatment because information about toxicity was heterogeneous. These two meta-analyses shifted the debate from whether to employ thoracic RT to how to best integrate it with chemotherapy (Simon et al., 2003). Controversies in chest RT include the sequencing and timing of chemotherapy and RT (concurrent versus sequential and early versus late), volume of the radiation port (original tumor versus shrinking field as the tumor responds), and dose and fractionation of therapy. Descriptions of these individual RT issues follow.

Sequencing and Timing of Chemotherapy and Radiotherapy

The combination of etoposide and cisplatin has offered marked improvements in safety and efficacy of concurrent chemoradiation compared with earlier trials that used alkylating agents and doxorubicin. Concurrent combined modality therapy has demonstrated a survival advantage compared with a sequential plan, in which RT is administered after chemotherapy, or a "sandwich," in which chemotherapy is administered initially, is interrupted during radiation therapy, and is reinstated thereafter (Martin & Comis, 1996; NCCN, 2002; Simon et al., 2003).

Optimizing radiation in conjunction with chemotherapy is an important issue because small cell carcinoma is very radiosensitive. Murray et al. (1993) studied the timing of radiation in a randomized controlled trial with chemotherapy given concurrently with RT commencing early on week 3 or later on week 15. A statistically significant advantage was found in progression-free survival and overall survival for the earlier RT application. Early RT was associated with improved local and systemic control and a survival advantage. Patients in the late (week 15) RT arm had a higher risk of brain metastasis ($p = 0.0006$).

In one meta-analysis, the best results were seen with thoracic RT beginning 3–5 weeks from the start of chemotherapy (Murray & Coldman, 1995). As radiation was further delayed, the benefit decreased and survival approached that seen with chemotherapy alone (Simon et al., 2003). Delayed chemoradiation usually is associated with a long-term survival rate of approximately 10%, which differs little from the 9% rate of chemotherapy alone. Long-term survival for early concurrent platinum and etoposide plus thoracic radiation consistently exceeds 20% at five years. This should be considered the minimum standard at this time for limited-stage SCLC (Erridge & Murray, 2003).

Radiation Target Volumes

SCLC often presents with bulky mediastinal lymphadenopathy and with a mixture of tumor mass and atelectasis in the lung parenchyma. This requires a large area of tissue to be irradiated, which is known as the radiation target volume. The three main potential toxicities of thoracic RT are esophagitis, pneumonitis, and radiation myelopathy. For both the esophagus and the lungs, the risk of toxicity depends not only on dose, but also on the volume of tissue irradiated (Erridge & Murray, 2003); hence, oncologists have attempted to define the minimal appropriate target volume and dose. The idea of using either a shrinking volume technique or a very reduced volume, treating just gross disease, is appealing to minimize toxicity. These approaches have not been compared in a randomized trial to more "standard" therapy. One Southwest Oncology Group (SWOG) randomized clinical trial examined the issue of radiation volume (Kies et al., 1987). Patients in this study, who achieved a partial or stable response after four cycles of chemotherapy, were randomized to RT with one of two arms of tumor volume. One arm included treatment portals based on the tumor volume before induction chemo-

therapy, and the other arm was based on the reduced volume postinduction chemotherapy. No appreciable differences were detected in either overall survival or recurrence patterns between the two arms, suggesting that if RT is started after several cycles of chemotherapy, the post-chemotherapy target volume can be employed. The North American Intergroup trial studied the concept of using limited elective radiation with no intentional radiation to normal-appearing lymph nodes in the contralateral hilum or supraclavicular nodes, except with bulky adenopathy (Turrisi, Glover, & Mason, 1988). This trial produced the best five-year survival rate reported by a cooperative group (Simon et al., 2003).

Dose and Fractionation

Because SCLC is a rapidly proliferating tumor, researchers hypothesized that it may be more responsive to thoracic radiation given twice daily than once daily. The theory was that the use of multiple daily fractions may allow cells to redistribute to more sensitive phases of the cell cycle during the interval from the first to the second or subsequent dose of irradiation, thus enhancing cytotoxicity (Johnson, 1999). Giving two fractions per day, with a modest reduction in fraction size from the usual 1.8–2.0 Gy to 1.5 Gy, accelerates treatment. Two prospective trials compared this approach to conventional daily fractionation. Turrisi et al. (1999) showed a modest survival advantage in favor of twice daily radiation therapy given over 3 weeks, compared to once daily radiation given over 5 weeks (26% versus 16% at 5 years [$p = 0.04$]). Esophagitis was increased with twice daily treatment. Bonner et al. (1999) also compared twice daily to daily fractionation but with a different regimen. In both arms of this study, RT was administered with the fourth and fifth cycles of chemotherapy. The twice daily irradiation dose was 48 Gy in 32 fractionations with a 2.5-week break after the initial 24 Gy. The once daily thoracic radiation was 50.4 Gy in 28 fractions. This trial demonstrated no differences in local control or survival. A criticism of the trial was that, unlike the Turrisi et al. trial, the rest interval resulted in no overall acceleration of the radiation course (Simon et al., 2003). The NCCN (2002) guidelines recommend that for limited-stage disease, radiation should be delivered concurrently with chemotherapy at a dosage of 1.5 Gy twice daily to a total dose of 45 Gy or 1.8 Gy per day to at least 54 Gy.

Prophylactic Cranial Irradiation

Patients experience a high risk (50%–60%) of developing central nervous system (CNS) metastases within 2–3 years after induction treatment. Most chemotherapeutic agents do not readily cross the blood-brain barrier. CNS-only relapse occurs in 17%–28% of patients who achieve a complete response with improved systemic control (NCCN, 2002). Overt metastatic disease to the brain, although often responding temporarily to radiation, is rarely, if ever, cured. Prophylactic cranial irradiation evolves from the hypothesis that moderate doses of radiation given to patients without detectable CNS involvement might eradicate occult metastases, improve CNS control, and prolong survival.

The Prophylactic Cranial Irradiation (PCI) Overview Collaborative Group (Auperin et al., 1999) performed a meta-analysis on individual data from 987 patients with SCLC in complete remission from seven trials that compared cranial irradiation with no prophylactic cranial irradiation. The main end point was survival. The findings showed that PCI significantly decreased the cumulative incidence of brain metastases by about 50% and improved overall survival at three years (15.3% in the control group compared with 20.7% in the treated group). Higher RT doses (30–36 Gy using 2 Gy fractions) tended to have better results than 20 Gy doses, but this was not a randomized comparison, and the effect on survival did not differ significantly according to dose. Auperin et al. concluded that prophylactic cranial irradiation improves both overall survival and disease-free survival among patients with SCLC who achieve complete remission.

An earlier nonrandomized study of long-term survivors treated with PCI suggested that patients may have a higher incidence of CNS impairment. The small sample of patients reported common signs and symptoms of memory loss, gait abnormalities, and coordination defects (Johnson et al., 1990). However, recent data from prospective trials (Arriagada et al., 1995; Komaki et al., 1995) found cognitive dysfunction in more than 90% of patients with SCLC before they underwent PCI. This dysfunction did not appear to worsen in any patients on completion of therapy or at two-year follow-up. This baseline impairment may in fact be related to the underlying malignancy. Ahles et al. (1998) showed neurocognitive deterioration after PCI in which the PCI was administered concomitantly with chemotherapy. Brain irradiation is believed to disrupt the blood-brain barrier so that chemotherapy given concomitantly or following PCI seems to enhance the toxicity of irradiation (Vines, Le Pechoux, & Arriagada, 2003). A balanced discussion between the patient and his or her physician disclosing therapy benefit and potential adverse effects is necessary to make the decision to administer PCI.

In summary, evidence currently suggests that PCI is effective in decreasing the rate of brain metastasis in patients with limited SCLC who achieve a complete response to therapy. This translates into an overall survival advantage. No demonstrable neurologic functional impairment secondary to PCI has been found when neuropsychological evaluations are conducted prospectively. Data do not lend support to the idea that PCI is associated with significant neurotoxicity. Therefore, PCI is considered the standard of care for the aforementioned subgroup of patients with SCLC (Vines et al., 2003).

Role of Surgery in Limited-Stage Small Cell Lung Cancer

Surgery for SCLC was abandoned when the British Medical Research Council showed inferior results for resection in an early study that compared surgery with RT. With the introduction of multidrug chemotherapy and combination therapies in limited-stage SCLC, many considered surgical treatment in this disease inappropriate. However, a most favorable subset of patients with T1 N0 tumors identified either at the time of surgery or on postoperative pathologic examination showed long-term survival. This very limited disease (VLD) is rare and diagnosed in fewer than 10% of patients (NCCN, 2002). Surgical resection of patients with VLD should only be attempted after very careful staging, and all VLD patients should undergo mediastinoscopy prior to resection. Surgery alone is not recommended, and postoperative platinum-based chemotherapy should be given to this group (NCCN; Simon et al., 2003). If nodal disease is found at surgery, postoperative RT also is recommended (Szczesny, Szczesna, Shepherd, & Ginsberg, 2003).

A large, prospective randomized trial failed to prove any added value for surgery after induction chemotherapy in the treatment of LD SCLC (Lad et al., 1994). All patients in this study received five cycles of induction chemotherapy (cyclophosphamide, doxorubicin [Adriamycin® (Pfizer, New York, NY)], and vincristine [CAV]). Patients who achieved a partial or complete response were randomized to surgery or no surgery. Both arms then received chest irradiation and prophylactic cranial irradiation. Median survival times for the nonsurgical and surgical arms were 18.6 and 15.4 months, respectively (p = 0.78). Thus, this study failed to demonstrate any survival advantage for the addition of surgery to standard chemotherapy and RT. This study is criticized because it included patients with LD SCLC but few patients with VLD. Szczesny et al. (2003) concluded that results of retrospective analyses and prospective nonrandomized trials suggest that in a highly select subgroup of patients with VLD SCLC, the addition of surgery to standard treatment results in cure for some patients.

Recurrent Disease

Although patients typically respond to first-line treatment with systemic chemotherapy, most patients inevitably relapse with a very poor prognosis. When previously treated patients relapse, their median survival is 4–5 months (NCCN, 2002). Two predictors of response to salvage or second-line therapy in SCLC patients are response to initial therapy and the duration of disease-free interval. Patients who relapse less than 3 months after first-line therapy commonly are called refractory. Patients who respond initially and relapse more than 3 months following treatment are called "sensitive" and are more likely to respond to additional chemotherapy. In patients with an initial complete response of 6 months or more of progression-free survival (a late relapse), retreatment with the original therapy can be considered. In the case of local or isolated recurrence, local treatment should be considered. Patients with symptomatic bone or CNS recurrences can benefit from RT if it has not been used previously.

A second-line regimen can be offered to early relapsers pending performance status, comorbidities, and sites of progression. In a multicenter randomized trial, von Pawel et al. (1999) evaluated second-line treatment in SCLC with either CAV or topotecan. No significant differences were found in response rates or survival (25 weeks for topotecan and 24.7 weeks for CAV) between the two arms, but palliation of four of eight common lung cancer symptoms (dyspnea, anorexia, hoarseness, and fatigue) was improved in the topotecan group. Further randomized studies compared the IV versus oral routes of administration of topotecan (von Pawel et al., 2001). Initial results suggested no difference in efficacy and less-severe neutropenia with the oral drug. A larger phase III trial comparing the two routes of administration is pending (Glisson, 2003).

At relapse, all salvage therapy is palliative. Topotecan reasonably can be recommended for "sensitive" relapsed SCLC in the absence of an appropriate clinical trial (Glisson, 2003). However, topotecan is associated with significant myelosuppressive toxicity and a logistically difficult administration schedule. The opportunity for inclusion in a phase I clinical trial certainly also represents a treatment of choice. The rationale for this approach includes the limited curability of SCLC with currently available therapy and the low probability of false negative results if the agent is truly active against SCLC. Alternatively, for some patients, symptom palliation and quality of life through supportive care are the more important factors in the design of a treatment plan than prolonged survival.

Older Patients

Lung cancer incidence increases with age. At least 25% of patients with SCLC are older than 70. Chronological age is meaningless, as documented by practitioner comments such as "a young 70 year old," indicating parameters of a person's organ function and functional status. Limited data are available from clinical trials about older patients. Performance status and comorbid health status usually guide decisions regarding therapy for SCLC. If both parameters are acceptable, the recommendation is to treat with full-dose platinum standard chemotherapy and RT if indicated. More myelosuppression can be expected in older patients, especially with etoposide, and greater ancillary support may be required (NCCN, 2002; Simon et al., 2003).

A comparison trial with oral etoposide monotherapy versus CAV as palliative therapy in patients with poor performance status was stopped early because the etoposide was found to be inferior to standard multidrug therapy with more grade 2 or worse hematologic toxicity (Girling, 1996). Souhami et al. (1997) also compared oral etoposide with IV alternating CAV and platinum/etoposide regimens in patients with extensive SCLC. Overall and progression-free survival were worse in the oral etoposide arm. With the exception of acute nausea and vomiting associated with the IV arm, all aspects of symptom control and quality of life were the same or worse in the oral etoposide group. Study closure was recommended, and it was concluded that oral etoposide should not be used as first-line therapy in SCLC. This "gentler chemotherapy" is inferior to optimal combination chemotherapy.

Patients with poor functional status or poor prognostic factors may benefit from either an abbreviated treatment plan (two cycles of CAV with thoracic irradiation) (Murray et al., 1998) or CAV and etoposide in reduced doses (Westeel et al., 1998). Both of these studies were associated with acceptable toxicity and have potential for useful palliation, but these treatments need to be investigated further.

Future Directions

Areas of active clinical evaluation in SCLC include new combinations, such as irinotecan plus cisplatin, and novel agents, such as targeted therapy. Advances in molecular biology since the mid-1980s have led to identification of specific molecular abnormalities that contribute to proliferation and progression of SCLC. Glisson (2003) reported three molecular targeted agents with potential in small cell carcinoma. A monoclonal antibody (2A11) is being tested in preclinical in vitro and in vivo models because it shows potential to inhibit proliferation of SCLC through interruption of GRP effect. Genasense (G3139) is an antisense peptide that can suppress intracellular levels of *bcl-2,* which is commonly overexpressed in SCLC. Although SCLC tumor cell lines do not commonly overexpress epidermal growth factor receptor (EGFR), the EGRF-tyrosine kinase inhibitor ZD1839 (Iressa™ [AstraZeneca, Wilmington, DE]) may have an impact even for cancer cells that express little of the EGFR alternatively acting via inhibition of a different signal in this setting. All of these represent new avenues for therapy with translational research.

Outcomes

Current treatment options have undoubtedly had an impact on survival in SCLC during the past three decades. However, SCLC remains a formidable clinical problem. Despite improvements, the majority (80%) of patients with this cancer will die from the disease. If a person is fortunate to be a long-term (greater than two years) survivor of SCLC, the risk for development of a second smoking-related malignancy, most notably NSCLC, is significant (Johnson et al., 1986). Prevention is paramount in this malignancy. An effective worldwide public health effort to stop smoking initiation in children and to promote smoking cessation in current smokers is a critical intervention. The elimination of cigarette smoking would virtually eliminate SCLC.

References

Ahles, T.A., Silberfarb, P.M., Herndon, J., Maurer, L.H., Kornblith, A.B., Aisner, J., et al. (1998). Psychologic and neuropsychologic functioning of patients with limited small cell lung cancer treated with chemotherapy and radiation therapy with or without warfarin: A study by the Cancer and Leukemia Group B. *Journal of Clinical Oncology, 16,* 1954–1960.

Arriagada, R., LeChevalier, T., Borie, F., Riviere, A., Chomy, P., Monnet, I., et al. (1995). Prophylactic cranial irradiation for patients with small cell lung cancer in remission. *Journal of National Cancer Institute, 87,* 183–190.

Auperin, A., Arriagada, R., Pignon, J., Le Pechoux, C., Gregor, A., Stephens, R.J., et al. (1999). Prophylactic cranial irradiation for patients with small cell lung cancer in complete remission. *New England Journal of Medicine, 341,* 476–484.

Bonner, J.A., Sloan, J.A., Shanahan, T.G., Brooks, B.J., Marks, R.S., Krook, J.E., et al. (1999). Phase III comparison of twice-daily split-course irradiation versus once-daily irradiation for patients with limited stage small cell lung cancer. *Journal of Clinical Oncology, 17,* 2681–2691.

Brahmer, J.A., & Ettinger, D.S. (1998). Carboplatin in the treatment of small cell lung cancer. *The Oncologist, 3,* 143–154.

Cancer.gov. (2003). *Small cell lung cancer (PDQ®): Treatment.* Retrieved February 12, 2003, from http://www.cancer.gov/cancerinfo/

Chin, R., McCain, T.W., Miller, A.A., Dunagan, D.P., Acostamadieo, J., Case, L.D., et al. (2002). Whole body FDG-PET for the evaluation and staging of small cell lung cancer: A preliminary study. *Lung Cancer, 37*(1), 7.

DeVore, III, R.F., & Johnson, D.H. (1996). Chemotherapy of small cell lung cancer. In H.L. Pass, J.B. Mitchell, D.H. Johnson, & A.T. Turrisi (Eds.), *Lung cancer: Principles and practice* (pp. 825–835). Philadelphia: Lippincott Williams & Wilkins.

Erridge, S.C., & Murray, N. (2003). Thoracic radiotherapy for limited-stage small cell lung cancer: Issues of timing, volumes, dose and fractionation. *Seminars in Oncology, 30,* 26–37.

Feld, R., Sagman, U., & LeBlanc, M. (1996). Staging and prognostic factors: Small cell lung cancer. In H.L. Pass, J.B. Mitchell, D.H. Johnson, & A.T. Turrisi (Eds.), *Lung cancer: Principles and practice* (pp. 495–509). Philadelphia: Lippincott Williams & Wilkins.

Fraire, A.E. (1996). Pathology of lung cancer. In J. Aisner, R. Arriagada, M.R. Green, N. Martini, & M.C. Perry (Eds.), *Comprehensive textbook of thoracic oncology* (pp. 245–275). Philadelphia: Lippincott Williams & Wilkins.

Girling, D.J. (1996). Comparison of oral etoposide and standard intravenous multidrug chemotherapy for small cell lung cancer: A stopped multicenter randomized trial. Medical Research Council Lung Cancer Working Party. *Lancet, 348*(9027), 563–566.

Glisson, B.S. (2003). Recurrent small cell lung cancer: Update. *Seminars in Oncology, 30,* 72–78.

Green, R.A., Humphrey, E., Close, H., & Patno, H.E. (1969). Alkylating agents in bronchogenic carcinoma. *American Journal of Medicine, 46,* 515–525.

Guinee, D.G., Fishback, N.F., Koss, M.N., Abbondanzo, S.L., & Travis, W.D. (1994). The spectrum of immunohistochemical staining of small cell lung carcinoma in specimens from transbronchial and open lung biopsies. *American Journal of Clinical Pathology, 102,* 406–414.

Hauber, H.P., Bohuslavizki, K.H., Lund, C.H., Fritscher-Ravens, A., Meyer, A., & Pforte, A. (2001). Positron emission tomography in the staging of small cell lung cancer: A preliminary study. *Chest, 119,* 950–954.

Hirsch, F.R., Matthews, M.J., Aisner, S., Campobasso, O., Elema, J.D., Gazdar, A.F., et al. (1988). Histopathologic classification of small cell lung cancer. Changing concepts and terminology. *Cancer, 62,* 973–977.

Johnson, B.E., Ihde, D.C., Matthews, M.J., Bunn, P.A., Zabell, A., Makuch, R.W., et al. (1986). Non-small cell lung cancer. Major cause of late mortality in patients with small cell lung cancer. *American Journal of Medicine, 80,* 1103–1110.

Johnson, B.E., Patronas, N., Hayes, W., Grayson, J., Becker, B., Gnepp, D., et al. (1990). Neurologic computed cranial tomographic and magnetic resonance imaging abnormalities in patients with small-cell lung cancer: Further follow-up of 6 to 13 year survivors. *Journal of Clinical Oncology, 8,* 48–56.

Johnson, D.H. (1999). Management of small cell lung cancer. Current state of the art. *Chest, 116*(Suppl. 6), 525S–530S.

Kies, M.S., Mira, J.G., Crowley, J.J., Chen, T.T., Pazdur, R., Grozea, P.N., et al. (1987). Multimodal therapy for limited small cell lung cancer: A randomized study of induction combination chemotherapy with or without thoracic radiation in complete responders; and with wide-field versus reduced-field radiation in partial responders: A Southwest Oncology Group study. *Journal of Clinical Oncology, 5,* 592–600.

Koh, H.K., Kannler, C., & Geller, A.C. (2001). Cancer prevention: Preventing tobacco-related cancers. In V.T. DeVita, S. Hellman, & S.A. Rosenberg (Eds.), *Cancer: Principles and practice of oncology* (6th ed., pp. 549–560). Philadelphia: Lippincott Williams & Wilkins.

Komaki, R., Meyers, C.A., Shin, D.M., Garden, A.S., Byrne, K., Nickens, J.A., et al. (1995). Evaluation of cognitive function in patients with limited small cell lung cancer prior to and shortly following prophylactic cranial irradiation. *International Journal of Radiation Oncology, Biology, Physics, 33*(1), 179–182.

Kosmidis, P.A., Samantas, E., Fountzilas, G., Pavlidis, N., Apostolopoulou, F., & Skarlos, D. (1994). Cisplatin/etoposide versus carboplatin/etoposide chemotherapy and irradiation in small cell lung cancer: A randomized phase III study. Hellenic Cooperative Oncology Group for Lung Cancer Trials. *Seminars in Oncology, 21*(3 Suppl. 6), 23–30.

Lad, T., Piantadosi, S., Thomas, P., Payne, D., Ruckdeschel, J., & Giaccone, G. (1994). A prospective randomized trial to determine the benefit of surgical resection of residual disease following response of small cell lung cancer to combination chemotherapy. *Chest, 106*(Suppl. 6), 320S–323S.

Mangum, M.D., Greco, F.A., Hainsworth J.D., Hande, K.R., & Johnson, D.H. (1989). Combined small-cell and non-small cell lung cancer. *Journal of Clinical Oncology, 7,* 607–612.

Martin, V.R., & Comis, R.L. (1996). Small cell carcinoma of the lung: An "updated" overview. *Seminars in Oncology Nursing, 12,* 295–303.

Medical Research Council Lung Working Party. (1979). Radiotherapy alone or with chemotherapy in the treatment of small cell carcinoma of the lung. *British Journal of Cancer, 40,* 1–10.

Murray, N., & Coldman, A. (1995). The relationship between thoracic irradiation timing and long term survival in combined modality therapy of limited stage small cell lung cancer (LSCLC)

[Abstract]. *Proceedings of the American Society of Clinical Oncology, 14,* 360.

Murray, N., Coy, P., Pater, J.L., Hodson, I., Arnold, A., Zee, B.C., et al. (1993). Importance of timing for thoracic irradiation in the combined modality treatment of limited-stage small cell lung cancer. The National Cancer Institute of Canada Clinical Trials Group. *Journal of Clinical Oncology, 11,* 336–344.

Murray, N., Grafton, C., Shah, A., Gelmon, K., Kostashuk, E., Brown, E., et al. (1998). Abbreviated treatment for elderly, infirm, or noncompliant patients with limited stage small cell lung cancer. *Journal of Clinical Oncology, 16,* 3323–3328.

Murren, J., Glatstein, E., & Pass, H.I. (2001). Small cell lung cancer. In V.T. DeVita, Jr., S. Hellman, & S.A. Rosenberg. (Eds.), *Cancer: Principles and practice of oncology* (6th ed., pp. 983–1018). Philadelphia: Lippincott Williams & Wilkins.

National Comprehensive Cancer Network. (2002). Small cell lung cancer. *Clinical Practice Guidelines in Oncology-v.1.2002.* Retrieved May 12, 2003, from http:// www.nccn.org/physicians-gls/f-guidelines.html

Noda, K., Nishiwaki, Y., Kawahara, M., Negoro, S., Sugiura, T., Yokoyama, A., et al. (2002). Irinotecan plus cisplatin compared with etoposide plus cisplatin for extensive small cell lung cancer. *New England Journal of Medicine, 346,* 85–91.

Patel, A.M., & Jett, J.R. (1996). Clinical presentation and staging of lung cancer. In J. Aisner, R. Arriagada, M.R. Green, N. Martini, & M.C. Perry (Eds.), *Comprehensive textbook of thoracic oncology* (pp. 293–318). Philadelphia: Lippincott Williams & Wilkins.

Pignon, J.P., Arriagada, R., Ihde, D.C., Johnson, D.H., Perry, M.C., Shouhami, R.L., et al. (1992). A meta-analysis of thoracic radiotherapy for small cell lung cancer. *New England Journal of Medicine, 327,* 1618–1624.

Sandler, A.B. (2003). Chemotherapy for small cell lung cancer. *Seminars in Oncology, 30*(1), 9–25.

Shen, Y.Y., Shiau, Y.C., Wang, J.J., Ho, S.T., & Kao, C.H. (2002). Whole-body 18F-2-deoxyglucose positron emission tomography in primary staging small cell lung cancer. *Anticancer Research, 22*(2B), 1257–1264.

Shepherd, F.A. (1996). Role of surgery in the management of small cell lung cancer. In J. Aisner, R. Arriagada, M.R. Green, N. Martini, & M.C. Perry (Eds.), *Comprehensive textbook of thoracic oncology* (pp. 439–455). Philadelphia: Lippincott Williams & Wilkins.

Simon, G.R., Wagner, H., & American College of Chest Physicians. (2003). Small cell lung cancer. *Chest, 123*(Suppl. 1), 259S–271S.

Souhami, R.L., Spiro, S.G., Rudd, R.M., Ruiz de Elvira, M.C., James, L.E., Goy, N.H., et al. (1997). Five-day oral etoposide treatment for advanced small cell lung cancer: Randomized comparison with intravenous chemotherapy. *Journal of the National Cancer Institute, 89,* 577–580.

Szczesny, T.J., Szczesna, A., Shepherd, F.A., & Ginsberg, R.J. (2003). Surgical treatment of small cell lung cancer. *Seminars in Oncology, 30,* 47–56.

Turrisi, A.T., Glover, D.J., & Mason, B.A. (1988). A preliminary report: Concurrent twice-daily radiotherapy plus platinum-etoposide chemotherapy for limited small cell lung cancer. *International Journal of Radiation Oncology, Biology, Physics, 15,* 183–187.

Turrisi, A.T., Kim, K., Blum, R., Sause, W.T., Livingston, R.B., Komaki, R., et al. (1999). Twice daily compared with once daily thoracic radiotherapy in limited small-cell lung cancer treated concurrently with cisplatin and etoposide. *New England Journal of Medicine, 340,* 265–271.

Vaporciyan, A.A., Nesbitt, J.C., Lee, J.S., Stevens, C., Komaki, R., & Roth, J.A. (2000). Cancer of the lung. In J.F. Holland & E. Frei III (Eds.), *Cancer medicine* (5th ed., pp. 1227–1292). Hamilton, ON: BC Decker.

Vines, E.F., Le Pechoux, C., & Arriagada, R. (2003). Prophylactic cranial radiation in small cell lung cancer. *Seminars in Oncology, 30,* 38–46.

von Pawel, J., Gatzemeier, U., Pujol, J., Moreau, L., Bildat, S., Ranson, M., et al. (2001). Phase II comparator study of oral versus intravenous topotecan in patients with sensitive small cell lung cancer. *Journal of Clinical Oncology, 19,* 1743–1749.

von Pawel, J., Schiller, J.H., Shepherd, F.A., Fields, S.Z., Kleisbauer, J.P., Chrysson, N.G., et al. (1999). Topotecan versus cyclophosphamide, doxorubicin, and vincristine for the treatment of recurrent small cell lung cancer. *Journal of Clinical Oncology, 17,* 658–667.

Warde, P., & Payne, D. (1992). Does thoracic irradiation improve survival and local control in limited-stage small cell carcinoma of the lung? A meta-analysis. *Journal of Clinical Oncology, 10,* 890–895.

Westeel, V., Murray, N., Gelmon, K., Shah, A., Sheehan, F., McKenzie, M., et al. (1998). New combination of the old drugs for elderly patients with small cell lung cancer: A phase II study of the PAVE regimen. *Journal of Clinical Oncology, 16,* 1940–1947.

Works, C.R., & Gallucci, B.G. (1996). Biology of lung cancer. *Seminars in Oncology Nursing, 12,* 276–284.

CHAPTER 8

Non-Small Cell Lung Cancer

Leslie B. Tyson, MS, ANP-C, OCN®

Introduction

An estimated one million men and women worldwide die of lung cancer each year (Carney, 2002). Approximately 80% of these patients have non-small cell lung cancer (NSCLC) (Beckles, Spiro, Colice, & Rudd, 2003). The median survival of untreated patients with metastatic NSCLC is estimated at 4–5 months, with one-year survival estimated at 10% (Schiller et al., 2002). Elimination of tobacco use, ultimately, will do the most to decrease incidence; however, elimination of tobacco-related lung disease is years away. Even if efforts to eliminate smoking today were successful, lung cancer would continue to kill people for decades, because more former smokers than active smokers are diagnosed (Alberts, 2003). We must rely on researchers and dedicated professionals for newer, more effective treatment modalities.

Presentation and Paraneoplastic Syndromes

Characteristic signs and symptoms of lung cancer have been discussed previously (see Chapter 5). Lung cancer is broadly classified into two groups: small cell and non-small cell. Prognosis, staging, and treatment of each type are different, thus making the determination of cell type of utmost importance. In general, small cell lung cancer (SCLC) differs from NSCLC in several respects (Ingle, 2000). SCLC usually is centrally located, is thought to be more aggressive and therefore is more likely to be metastatic at diagnosis, and more often is associated with paraneoplastic syndromes.

In contrast, NSCLC can present as a peripheral tumor, or it can be centrally located. NSCLC tumors can grow within the lung parenchyma or the bronchial wall. Tumors can grow in and around the bronchial lumen, at times causing complete obstruction of the bronchus. Progression of the tumor is by lymphatic invasion or direct extension to the chest wall or diaphragm (Ingle, 2000; Joyce & Houlihan, 2001). Other pulmonary structures can be involved and include lymphatic

channels, nerves, alveolar tissue, and pulmonary vasculature (Ingle). Metastatic disease results from progression of the tumor in the same way and most frequently involves bone, liver, adrenal glands, pericardium, and brain.

Overall, paraneoplastic syndromes occur in 10% of patients with lung cancer (Beckles, Spiro, Colice, & Rudd, 2003). Paraneoplastic syndromes most often seen in patients with NSCLC are humoral hypercalcemia of malignancy and hypertrophic pulmonary osteoarthropathy (HPOA) (Ingle, 2000). Approximately 15% of patients with squamous cell lung cancer, a subtype of NSCLC, develop hypercalcemia at some point in their illness (Haapoja, 2000). Eighty-eight percent of all patients diagnosed with HPOA have adenocarcinoma or large cell lung cancer, both of which are subtypes of NSCLC (Haapoja). The hypercoagulable state is seen in those with either type of lung cancer (Ingle). For more information on paraneoplastic syndromes in patients with lung cancer, see Chapter 6.

Studies have identified clinical, histopathologic, and molecular factors that affect prognosis in patients with NSCLC. Despite this, the tumor, node, metastasis (TNM) stage of disease at diagnosis remains the most important determinant of survival at this time (Lau, D'Amico, & Harpole, 2000). Those patients diagnosed with a lower stage (i.e., stage I) of disease at the outset have the best chance for cure (Ingle, 2000; Mountain, 1997; Smythe & American College of Chest Physicians [ACCP], 2003). Survival advantages for a specific histologic subtype of NSCLC (i.e., adenocarcinoma, squamous cell carcinoma, large cell carcinoma) have not been supported in the literature. Results of clinical studies examining the impact of specific subtypes have been mixed (Gail et al., 1984; Harpole, Herndon, Young, Wolfe, & Sabiston, 1995; Nesbitt, Putnam, Walsh, Roth, & Mountain, 1995; Padilla et al., 2002).

The current staging system does not take into account clinical symptoms or molecular markers. The presence of weight loss and poor performance status (PS) most often are correlated with poor survival in patients with NSCLC, despite the stage of disease at diagnosis (Harpole et al., 1995). In a study examining 289 patients with stage I NSCLC, 189 patients had no symptoms at diagnosis and 100 were symptomatic; the five-year survival rates were 74% and 41%, respectively (Harpole et al.). In particular, cough, hemoptysis, and chest pain were predictive of shorter survival (Harpole et al.). Other factors that confer poor prognosis include male gender, elevated serum lactate dehydrogenase (LDH), and bone or liver metastases (Ingle, 2000).

Since the early 1990s, investigators have discovered a great deal about the molecular biology of lung cancer (Bunn, Soriano, Johnson, & Heasley, 2000). Several investigators have been studying molecular markers of lung cancer to determine their effect on prognosis, tumor virulence, sites of metastatic disease, and early progression of disease (D'Amico et al., 2001; Lau, Moore, Brooks, D'Amico, & Harpole, 2002). Additionally, molecular markers may allow clinicians to diagnose NSCLC earlier than current testing methods allow (Lau et al., 2002).

Studies have found that biological and molecular markers have an impact on outcomes and that they influence the treatment of patients with NSCLC. These markers include, but are not limited to, the epidermal growth factor family and its receptors, markers of neuroendocrine differentiation, and mutations of the Ras family (Johnson, 1995). Patients who have tumors that test positive for epidermal growth factor receptors (EGFRs) face shortened survival times (Veale, Kerr, Gibson, Kelly, & Harris, 1993). Tumors that exhibit neuroendocrine differentiation show improvement in response to chemotherapy, but overall survival is not affected (Shaw et al., 1993). In addition, shortened survival has been documented in patients whose tumors test positive for K-ras (Rosell et al., 1993; Ross, 2003). Additionally, studies have found that patients with aneuploid tumors have decreased survival times compared with patients who have diploid tumors (Salgia & Skarin, 1998; Zimmerman, Bint, Hawson, & Parsons, 1987). More research is needed to determine the significance of biological markers, molecular markers, and ploidy.

Histologic Subtypes

Approximately 80% of all lung cancers are classified as NSCLCs (Haas, 2003). NSCLC has three major histologic subtypes: adenocarcinoma, squamous cell carcinoma, and large cell carcinoma. These cell types have multiple subclassifications, according to the World Health Organization (Travis, Colby, Corrin, Shimosato, & Brambilla, 1999). This section will discuss the three major subtypes as well as bronchoalveolar carcinoma (BAC), a subtype of adenocarcinoma.

Adenocarcinoma is the most common type of lung cancer, occurring in more than 30% of patients with NSCLC (Travis, Linder, & Mackay, 2000). Although it is seen in patients with histories of tobacco use, it also is the most common cell type seen in nonsmokers. The recent rise in the numbers of adenocarcinoma cases is attributed to improvements in histologic classification that distinguish adenocarcinoma

from undifferentiated large cell carcinoma (Ingle, 2000). In addition, the incidence of this disease is on the rise in women, a fact that also may be attributable to improvements in pathologic identification (Joyce & Houlihan, 2001).

Adenocarcinomas arise from alveolar surface epithelium or bronchial mucosal glands. Adenocarcinomas form glands and produce mucin. Patients with adenocarcinoma usually present with peripheral lesions, but adenocarcinomas also can present as multifocal disease. Adenocarcinomas may form in scars or fibrous tissue and sometimes are referred to as "scar tumors" (Ginsberg, Vokes, & Rosenzweig, 2001). The doubling time of these tumors is six months (Ingle, 2000). In nearly half of the patients, these tumors are unresectable at diagnosis because of metastatic disease (Ingle). K-ras mutations are present in about a third of tumors, and this is associated with shortened survival (Ingle).

BAC is an uncommon subtype of adenocarcinoma that occurs in about 3% of all patients with lung cancer (Travis et al., 2000). The incidence of this tumor is also on the rise, largely because of the increases seen in adenocarcinoma (Ebright et al., 2002). BAC typically presents in younger patients, women, and nonsmokers (Ebright et al.). It appears to arise from type 2 pneumocytes and grows along alveolar septa by lepidic ("scale-like") growth (Travis et al., 2000). This tumor is believed to be radioresistant and chemoresistant (Barkley & Green, 1996). However, compared to other NSCLCs, it has a decreased frequency of lymph node and extrathoracic metastases, and patients have a better prognosis when compared to those with non-BAC adenocarcinomas (Ebright et al.).

Approximately 30% of all lung cancers are squamous cell carcinomas. These carcinomas tend to occur more often in smokers and have a dose-response relationship with tobacco use. Two-thirds of these tumors present as central tumors, commonly arising in the proximal bronchi; the remaining are peripheral in location (Joyce & Houlihan, 2001; Travis et al., 2000). Cavitation most often is seen in patients with squamous cell carcinoma, compared with other types of lung cancer (Travis et al., 2000). Histologically, tumors are characterized by intercellular bridging, squamous pearl formation, and individual cell keratinization (Ingle, 2000). They may be well or poorly differentiated. They are slow-growing tumors; the doubling time is between 90–100 days (Ingle). The cells are shed easily, and, if expectorated, diagnosis can be made by sputum cytology. Squamous cell lung cancers are more likely to be associated with hypercalcemia (see Chapter 6).

Large cell carcinoma is the least common of the subtypes, occurring in 9%–15% of patients (Ingle, 2000; Travis et al., 2000). Large cell carcinoma is a diagnosis of exclusion; it is a poorly differentiated tumor that does not have features of either squamous cell or adenocarcinoma (Travis et al., 2000). Tumors may be central or peripheral in location, and they tend to be necrotic (Travis et al., 2000). These tumors tend to metastasize early and often spread to the gastrointestinal tract (Ingle).

The doubling time is about three months (Ingle). The prognosis with large cell tumors is similar to that of adenocarcinoma; large cell tumors with neuroendocrine features carry a poor prognosis (Joyce & Houlihan, 2001).

Staging

The importance of the International Staging System for Lung Cancer cannot be overemphasized; this system provides a common language worldwide for clinicians who care for patients with lung cancer. This system was revised in 1996, and the American Joint Committee on Cancer (AJCC) and the International Union Against Cancer adopted the revisions, which were published in 1997 (Mountain, 1997). Recommendations for revision of the system resulted from trends that emerged over time; heterogeneity was noted in the end results of TNM subsets of patients in stage I and stage IIIA, and different classification systems were used for staging regional lymph nodes (Mountain, Libshitz, & Hermes, 1999). The 1996 classification provided new rules for the stage grouping of the TNM subsets and new, consistent mapping of regional lymph nodes. As mentioned earlier,

accurate staging is essential in determining prognosis and making decisions regarding curative or palliative treatment. Data confirm the relationship between disease extent and prognosis (Mountain).

The TNM classification remains the same in the new system, except for revisions in the classification of multiple lung nodules. Ipsilateral satellite nodules associated with the primary tumor are now designated T4, and other separate nodules in the nonprimary tumor lobe are designated M1 (Mountain et al., 1999). See Table 8-1 for TNM descriptors. Because the majority of patients are not surgical candidates, most patients are clinically staged, designated cTNM. Those with surgical pathologic staging are designated pTNM. Note that the TNM descriptors do not change regardless of whether the patient is clinically or pathologically staged.

The new classification system has eight stage subsets instead of six. However, to be consistent with other solid tumor AJCC staging, four stage groupings of disease still exist (stage I–IV). Stages I and II now are divided into A and B, thus adding two new categories, and the definition for stage IIIA has been modified. Patients with stage T3 N0 M0, originally designated IIIA, have been moved to stage IIB. Analysis of more than 5,000 patients in a collected database

Table 8-1. TNM Descriptors	
Classification	**Description**
Primary tumor (T)	
TX	Primary tumor cannot be assessed or tumor proven by the presence of malignant cells in sputum or bronchial washings but not visualized by imaging or bronchoscopy
T0	No evidence of primary tumor
Tis	Carcinoma *in situ*
T1	Tumor $\leq$ 3 cm in greatest dimension, surrounded by lung or visceral pleura, without bronchoscopic evidence of invasion more proximal than the lobar bronchus[a] (i.e., not in the main bronchus)
T2	Tumor with any of the following features of size or extent • > 3 cm in greatest dimension • Involves main bronchus, $\geq$ 2 cm distal to the carina • Invades the visceral pleura • Associated with atelectasis or obstructive pneumonitis that extends to the hilar region but does not involve the entire lung
T3	Tumor of any size that directly invades any of the following: chest wall (including superior sulcus tumors), diaphragm, mediastinal pleura, or parietal pericardium; tumor in the main bronchus, 2 cm distal to the carina, but without involvement of the carina; or associated atelectasis or obstructive pneumonitis of the entire lung
T4	Tumor of any size that invades any of the following: mediastinum, heart, great vessels, trachea, esophagus, vertebral body, or carina; or tumor with a malignant pleural or pericardial effusion[b] or with satellite tumor nodule(s) within the ipsilateral primary tumor lobe of the lung
Regional lymph nodes (N)	
NX	Regional lymph nodes cannot be assessed.
N0	No regional lymph node metastasis
N1	Metastasis to ipsilateral peribronchial and/or ipsilateral hilar lymph nodes, and intrapulmonary nodes involved by direct extension of the primary tumor
N2	Metastasis to ipsilateral mediastinal and/or subcarinal lymph node(s)

(Continued on next page)

Table 8-1. TNM Descriptors *(Continued)*

Classification	Description
Regional lymph nodes (N) **(cont.)**	
N3	Metastasis to contralateral mediastinal, contralateral hilar, ipsilateral or contralateral scalene, or supra-clavicular lymph node(s)
Distant metastasis (M)	
MX	Presence of distant metastasis cannot be assessed.
M0	No distant metastasis
M1	Distant metastasis present [c]

[a] The uncommon superficial tumor of any size with its invasive component limited to the bronchial wall, which may extend proximal to the main bronchus, is also classified T1.

[b] Most pleural effusions associated with lung cancer are as a result of tumor. However, in a few patients, multiple cytopathologic examinations of pleural fluid show no tumor. In these cases, the fluid is nonbloody and is not an exudate. When these elements and clinical judgment dictate that the effusion is not related to the tumor, the effusion should be excluded as a staging element, and the patient's disease should be staged T1, T2, or T3. Pericardial effusion is classified according to the same rules.

[c] Separate metastatic tumor nodule(s) in the ipsilateral nonprimary-tumor lobe(s) of the lung also are classified M1.

Note. From "Revisions in the International System for Staging Lung Cancer," by C.F. Mountain, 1997, *Chest, 111,* p. 1711. Copyright 1997 by the American College of Chest Physicians. Reprinted with permission.

documented significant survival differences in patients with stage T3 N0 M0, compared with patients with T1–3 and nodal (N) disease (Mountain, 1997). Table 8-2 outlines stage grouping by TNM subsets. For graphic examples of stages IA through IIIB, see Figures 8-1, 8-2, 8-3, 8-4, 8-5, and 8-6. Stage IV patients have any T, any N, and M1 disease. Lymph node mapping and definitions are seen in Figure 8-7 and Table 8-3, respectively.

The five-year survival rate for patients with clinical stage IA is 61%; however, the five-year survival rate drops off significantly in patients with stage IB and more extensive stages. The five-year survival rate is less than 1% in patients with stage IV disease. These dismal statistics are driving research efforts, including molecular biology, early diagnosis, and all aspects of treatment in patients at risk for and with a diagnosis of lung cancer.

Treatment

Treatment decisions for patients with NSCLC are determined by disease stage, although these are not absolute indicators because other patient characteristics and the presence of comorbid disease must be considered as well. In general, treatment for lung cancer includes surgery, radiation therapy, and chemotherapy. Depending on the stage of disease, multimodality treatment with two or more combinations may be recommended. In January 2003, the ACCP published evidence-based guidelines on the diagnosis and management of lung cancer (Block, 2003). As research into treatments of the various stages of disease continues, recommendations will be revised.

Table 8-2. Stage Grouping—TNM Subsets[a]

Stage	TNM Subset
0	Carcinoma in situ
IA	T1 N0 M0
IB	T2 N0 M0
IIA	T1 N1 M0
IIB	T2 N1 M0
	T3 N0 M0
IIIA	T3 N1 M0
	T1 N2 M0
	T2 N2 M0
	T3 N2 M0
IIIB	T4 N0 M0
	T4 N1 M0
	T4 N2 M0
	T1 N3 M0
	T2 N3 M0
	T3 N3 M0
	T4 N3 M0
IV	Any T Any N M1

[a] Staging is not relevant for occult carcinoma, designated TX N0 M0.

Note. From "Revisions in the International System for Staging Lung Cancer," by C.F. Mountain, 1997, *Chest, 111,* p. 1712. Copyright 1997 by the American College of Chest Physicians. Reprinted with permission.

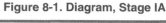

Figure 8-1. Diagram, Stage IA

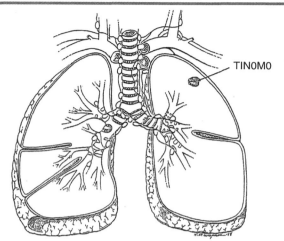

T1N0M0

Stage IA is reserved for classifying tumors 3 cm or less in greatest dimension, with no evidence of invasion proximal to a lobar bronchus and no evidence of metastasis, the T1 N0 M0 subset. The prognosis for these patients is significantly better than that for any other group.

Note. From *Lung Cancer. A Handbook for Staging, Imaging, and Lymph Node Classification* (p. 28), by C.F. Mountain, H.I. Libshitz, and K.E. Hermes, 1999, Houston, TX: Charles P. Young Company. Copyright 1999 by The Clifton F. Mountain Foundation. Reprinted with permission.

Surgery

Surgical intervention is considered to be the "gold standard" in treatment for patients with stage I and II disease, and complete resection is nearly always possible (Ginsberg & Port, 2000; Joyce & Houlihan, 2001). Five-year survival rates for patients with clinical stage IB, IIA, and IIB tumors are 38%, 34%, and 24%, respectively (Mountain, 1997). Stage IIIA (T3 N1) tumors are potentially operable, with a five-year survival rate of 22% (Mountain; Pisters et al., 2000). Following resection, the majority of these patients have recurrent disease and die of metastatic disease (Pisters et al.). Postoperative treatment (adjuvant treatment) with radiation therapy, chemotherapy, or a combination has shown no survival advantage over surgery alone (Ginsberg & Port; Pisters et al.). In contrast, clinical trials employing neoadjuvant or induction chemotherapy or chemoradiotherapy (before surgery) have shown improvements in survival rates (Martini et al., 1993; Pisters et al.; Rusch et al., 1993).

Approximately 20% of all patients with a lung cancer diagnosis present with stage I or II disease (Scott, Howington, Movsas, & ACCP, 2003; Smythe & ACCP, 2003). Significant five-year survival differences have been noted between stages IA and IB. In two retrospective series, the combined five-year survival rate for stage IA was 71.25%, whereas the

rate for stage IB was only 57% (Mountain, 1997; Naruke, Goya, Tsuchiya, & Suemasu, 1988). In patients who are able to tolerate surgery, the recommended procedure is lobectomy or pneumonectomy (Smythe & ACCP). In those who are unable to tolerate extensive procedures, lesser procedures, such as wedge or bronchopulmonary resections, are recommended (Smythe & ACCP). As noted, clinical trials are being conducted to investigate the use of adjuvant and neoadjuvant treatment in patients with stage IB disease. At this time, the routine use of adjuvant and neoadjuvant therapy is not recommended outside the clinical trial setting (Smythe & ACCP). However, patients who are found to have positive surgical margins should receive either surgical re-resection of margins or radiotherapy for local control (Smythe & ACCP).

Stage II disease is seen in only 5% of patients diagnosed with NSCLC overall and comprises the subsets seen in Table 8-2 (Scott et al., 2003). Stage II is divided into the subsets of IIA and IIB. As noted earlier, the five-year survival rates following resection are poor for both groups. Complete surgical resection is recommended in this group of patients, even in those with N1 disease (Scott et al.). Again, clinical trials using adjuvant radiotherapy have demonstrated mixed results in improving survival (Scott et al.). However, guidelines recommend radiation therapy for the improvement of local control (Scott et al.). Neoadjuvant and adjuvant chemotherapy are not recommended outside of a clinical trial setting for patients with stage II disease (Scott et al.). For patients with T3 disease and an incomplete resection, radiation therapy may improve survival (Scott et al.).

Figure 8-2. Diagram, Stage IB

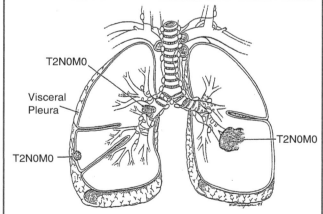

T2N0M0

Visceral Pleura

T2N0M0

T2N0M0

Patients with T2 primary tumors and no evidence of lymph node metastasis, the T2 N0 M0 subset, are assigned to stage IB.

Note. From *Lung Cancer. A Handbook for Staging, Imaging, and Lymph Node Classification* (p. 29), by C.F. Mountain, H.I. Libshitz, and K.E. Hermes, 1999, Houston, TX: Charles P. Young Company. Copyright 1999 by The Clifton F. Mountain Foundation. Reprinted with permission.

Stage III disease is divided into A and B subsets. In general, patients with stage IIIB are considered unresectable, as complete excision of all disease is not possible except in rare, carefully selected patients (Jett, Scott, Rivera, & Sause, 2003; Joyce & Houlihan, 2001). The standard of care for the majority of patients in this group is combined modality treatment with chemotherapy and radiotherapy (Jett et al.). Surgery for stage IIIA disease is deemed technically possible (except for those with unresectable bulky N2 disease), but five-year survival rates in this group of patients are poor with this modality alone. Stage IIIA patients represent a heterogeneous group (in terms of treatment and prognosis), and some advocate the use of four subsets when making treatment decisions (Robinson, Wagner, & Ruckdeschel, 2003).

The treatment of stage IIIA disease has been the subject of many clinical trials employing multimodality treatments. However, because of the variability of this stage, the optimal treatment strategies have not yet been defined (Robinson et al., 2003). Several trials have demonstrated five-year survival benefit with multimodal treatment compared to surgery or radiation therapy alone in patients with stage IIIA disease. These trials were reviewed in a meta-analysis published by the Non-Small Cell Lung Cancer Collaborative Group (1995). The recent ACCP guidelines recommended that selected pa-

Figure 8-4. Diagram, Stage IIB

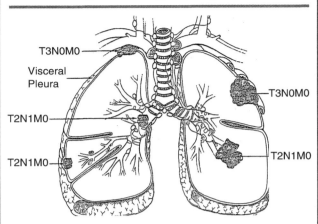

Two anatomic subsets that have nearly identical survival rates, T2 N1 M0 and T3 N0 M0 tumors, are designated stage IIB. T2 N1 M0 includes tumors of any size that invade the visceral pleura or the main bronchus more than 2 cm from the carina, or those more than 3 cm in greatest dimension with metastasis involving the intrapulmonary, including hilar, lymph nodes. T3 N0 M0 includes tumors with limited, circumscribed, extrapulmonary extension and no evidence of lymph node or other metastasis.

Note. From Lung Cancer. A Handbook for Staging, Imaging, and Lymph Node Classification (p. 33), by C.F. Mountain, H.I. Libshitz, and K.E. Hermes, 1999, Houston, TX: Charles P. Young Company. Copyright 1999 by The Clifton F. Mountain Foundation. Reprinted with permission.

Figure 8-3. Diagram, Stage IIA

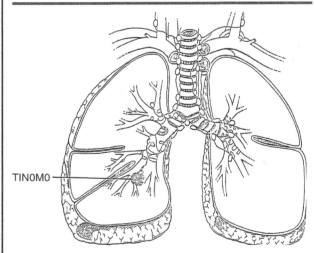

Patients with tumors classified as T1 N1 M0 are assigned to stage IIA. A clinical presentation of stage IIA disease is infrequent; however, stage migration based on surgical pathologic finding is common.

Note. From Lung Cancer. A Handbook for Staging, Imaging, and Lymph Node Classification (p. 31), by C.F. Mountain, H.I. Libshitz, and K.E. Hermes, 1999, Houston, TX: Charles P. Young Company. Copyright 1999 by The Clifton F. Mountain Foundation. Reprinted with permission.

tients with completely resected stage IIIA disease receive radiation therapy because it has been shown to reduce local recurrence (Robinson et al., 2003). Radiation therapy does not improve overall survival in this population (Robinson et al.). In patients with potentially resectable disease, multimodal therapy is better than surgery alone but, when possible, should be carried out in a clinical trial setting (Robinson et al.). Adjuvant and neoadjuvant trials of multimodal therapy are ongoing, and the future recommendations regarding stage IIIA may change (Robinson et al.).

Survival in the majority of patients with stage IV disease is not improved by surgery. In selected cases of patients with solitary brain, adrenal, or lung metastases and an otherwise resectable lung primary, surgery may be recommended for both the primary tumor and the metastatic site (Martini, 1993; Pearson, 1994). Improved survival and quality of life have been observed in these patients (Pearson). The recent ACCP guidelines support this approach (Detterbeck, Jones, Kernstine, Naunheim, & ACCP, 2003).

Preoperative Assessment

Following appropriate clinical staging procedures, patients with operable cancers must be evaluated to determine feasibility of the procedure. Thoracic surgery is associated with a high risk of complications, and patients must be carefully evaluated prior to surgery (Ingle, 2000). Many of these patients are either current or former smokers and, thus, may have tobacco-related pulmonary and cardiovascular disease or other comorbid conditions. Several guidelines have been published regarding the evaluation of patients for thoracic surgery. The British Thoracic Society (2001) and the American College of Cardiology and American Heart Association Task Force on Practice Guidelines (Eagle et al., 1996) have published guidelines for perioperative cardiovascular evaluation in patients undergoing noncardiac surgery. Cardiopulmonary status must be evaluated carefully prior to surgical intervention. Multidisciplinary decision making is essential, and physiologic assessment must include consideration of the perioperative risk from comorbid cardiovascular disease, the potential for long-term disability from pulmonary resection, and the lethal risk of untreated lung cancer (Beckles, Spiro, Colice, Rudd, & ACCP, 2003).

The most important causes of postoperative morbidity and mortality are significant cardiovascular disease, late tumor stage, and extent of resection (Ginsberg, 2002). Clinicians must take a careful cardiac history in patients undergoing resection for lung cancer. Remote myocardial infarction and angina increase risks to these patients. In addition, a history of recent infarction (within three months) markedly increases risk (Ginsberg). Pulmonary function testing, including

Figure 8-6. Diagram, Stage IIIB

Stage IIIB classifies extensive extrapulmonary tumor invasion of structures such as the trachea, esophagus, heart, and major vessels and metastasis to the contralateral mediastinal and hilar lymph nodes and the ipsilateral and contralateral supraclavicular/scalene lymph nodes—T4 Any N M0 and Any T N3 M0, stage IIIB disease.

Note. From *Lung Cancer. A Handbook for Staging, Imaging, and Lymph Node Classification* (p. 38), by C.F. Mountain, H.I. Libshitz, and K.E. Hermes, 1999, Houston, TX: Charles P. Young Company. Copyright 1999 by The Clifton F. Mountain Foundation. Reprinted with permission.

spirometry and estimation of carbon monoxide diffusing capacity (DLCO), should be performed in all patients prior to surgery. Most experts agree that the forced expiratory volume in one second (FEV1) is the major predictor of resectability and postoperative function (Ginsberg). Measurement of DLCO also can predict outcome in patients with thoracic resections. A recent study demonstrated that DLCO, not FEV1, was the better predictor of postoperative quality of life following lung cancer surgery (Handy et al., 2002). Adequate pulmonary function must be determined prior to surgery. In some instances, unplanned greater surgical resections are required, and this is not known until the time of surgery. Other factors that must be considered include history of diabetes or other chronic illness, weight loss of more than 10%, and age over 70 years. Older patients have increased morbidity and mortality following lung resection than younger patients (Quinn, 2003), a fact that may not be strictly related to age but, rather, increased comorbidities in older patients. In addition, a recent study examining outcomes of resection for lung cancer found lower mortality rates when board-certified thoracic surgeons perform resection rather than general surgeons (Silvestri, Handy, Lackland, Corley, & Reed, 1998), a fact that is echoed in the recent ACCP guidelines (Smythe & ACCP, 2003).

Figure 8-5. Diagram, Stage IIIA

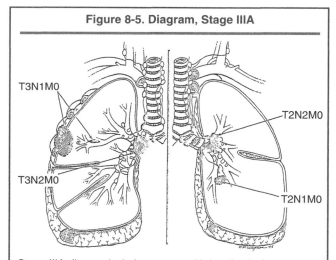

Stage IIIA disease includes tumors with localized, circumscribed extrapulmonary extension and ipsilateral intrapulmonary (including hilar) lymph node metastasis, the T3 N1 M0 subset, and T1, T2, and T3 tumors with metastasis limited to the ipsilateral mediastinal and subcarinal lymph nodes, the T1 N2 M0, T2 N2 M0, and T3 N2 M0 subsets.

Note. From *Lung Cancer. A Handbook for Staging, Imaging, and Lymph Node Classification* (p. 35), by C.F. Mountain, H.I. Libshitz, and K.E. Hermes, 1999, Houston, TX: Charles P. Young Company. Copyright 1999 by The Clifton F. Mountain Foundation. Reprinted with permission.

Figure 8-7. Regional Lymph Node Stations for Lung Cancer Staging

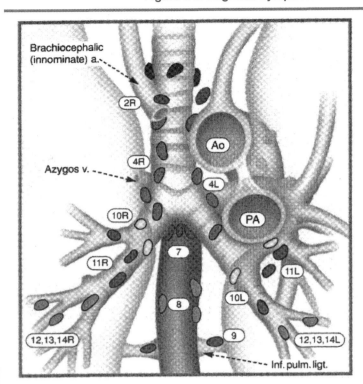

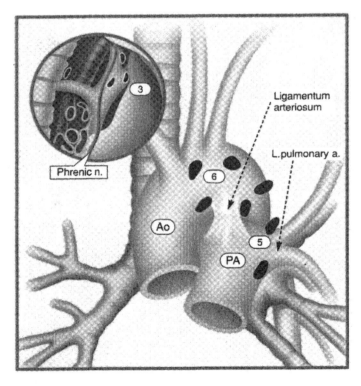

Superior Mediastinal Nodes

● **1** Highest Mediastinal

● **2** Upper Paratracheal

● **3** Pre-vascular and Retrotracheal

● **4** Lower Paratracheal
(including Azygos Nodes)

N_2 = single digit, ipsilateral
N_3 = single digit, contralateral or supraclavicular

Aortic Nodes

● **5** Subaortic (A-P window)

● **6** Para-aortic (ascending
aorta or phrenic)

Inferior Mediastinal Nodes

● **7** Subcarinal

● **8** Paraesophageal
(below carina)

● **9** Pulmonary Ligament

N₁ Nodes

○ **10** Hilar

● **11** Interlobar

● **12** Lobar

● **13** Segmental

● **14** Subsegmental

Note. From "Regional Lymph Node Classification for Lung Cancer Staging," by C.F. Mountain and C.M. Dresler, 1997, *Chest, 111,* p. 1719. Copyright 1997 by the American College of Chest Physicians. Reprinted with permission.

Table 8-3. Lymph Node Map Definitions

Nodal Station	Anatomic Landmarks
N2 nodes—All N2 nodes lie within the mediastinal pleural envelope.	
1 Highest mediastinal nodes	Nodes lying above a horizontal line at the upper rim of the brachiocephalic (left innominate) vein where it ascends to the left, crossing in front of the trachea at its midline
2 Upper paratracheal nodes	Nodes lying above a horizontal line drawn tangential to the upper margin of the aortic arch and below the inferior boundary of No. 1 nodes
3 Prevascular and retrotracheal nodes	Prevascular and retrotracheal nodes may be designated 3A and 3P; midline nodes are considered to be ipsilateral
4 Lower paratracheal nodes	The lower paratracheal nodes on the right lie to the right of the midline of the trachea between a horizontal line drawn tangential to the upper margin of the aortic arch and a line extending across the right main bronchus at the upper margin of the upper lobe bronchus, and contained within the mediastinal pleural envelope; the lower paratracheal nodes on the left lie to the left of the midline of the trachea between a horizontal line drawn tangential to the upper margin of the aortic arch and a line extending across the left main bronchus at the level of the upper margin of the left upper lobe bronchus, medial to the ligamentum arteriosum and contained within the mediastinal pleural envelope. Researchers may wish to designate the lower paratracheal nodes as No. 4s (superior) and No. 4i (inferior) subsets for study purposes; the No. 4s nodes may be defined by a horizontal line extending across the trachea and drawn tangential to the cephalic border of the azygos vein; the No. 4i nodes may be defined by the lower boundary of No. 4s and the lower boundary of No. 4, as described above.
5 Subaortic (aorto-pulmonary window)	Subaortic nodes are lateral to the ligamentum arteriosum or the aorta or left pulmonary artery and proximal to the first branch of the left pulmonary artery and lie within the mediastinal pleural envelope
6 Para-aortic nodes (ascending aorta or phrenic)	Nodes lying anterior and lateral to the ascending aorta and the aortic arch or the innominate artery, beneath a line tangential to the upper margin of the aortic arch
7 Subcarinal nodes	Nodes lying caudal to the carina of the trachea, but not associated with the lower lobe bronchi or arteries within the lung
8 Paraesophageal nodes (below carina)	Nodes lying adjacent to the wall of the esophagus and to the right or left of the midline, excluding subcarinal nodes
9 Pulmonary ligament nodes	Nodes lying within the pulmonary ligament, including those in the posterior wall and lower part of the inferior pulmonary vein
N1 nodes—All N1 nodes lie distal to the mediastinal pleural reflection and within the visceral pleura.	
10 Hilar nodes	The proximal lobar nodes, distal to the mediastinal pleural reflection and the nodes adjacent to the bronchus intermedius on the right; radiographically, the hilar shadow may be created by enlargement of both hilar and interlobar nodes
11 Interlobar nodes	Nodes lying between the lobar bronchi
12 Lobar nodes	Nodes adjacent to the distal lobar bronchi
13 Segmental nodes	Nodes adjacent to the segmental bronchi
14 Subsegmental nodes	Nodes around the subsegmental bronchi

Note. From "Regional Lymph Node Classification for Lung Cancer Staging," by C.F. Mountain and C.M. Dresler, 1997, *Chest, 111,* p. 1720. Copyright 1997 by the American College of Chest Physicians. Reprinted with permission.

Although no data exist from randomized trials to support the use of preoperative pulmonary rehabilitation, its use is advocated (Ginsberg, 2002; Martinez, Iannettoni, & Paine, 2000). The most common postoperative pulmonary complications following lung resection are atelectasis, bronchitis, bronchospasm, pneumonia, pulmonary thromboemboli, and respiratory failure (Martinez et al.). Many patients who present for resection for lung carcinoma have chronic obstructive pulmonary disease (COPD) from cigarette smoking. A strong relationship exists between COPD and the postoperative complications listed (Martinez et al.). Patients with COPD have increased respiratory secretions, which often can be colonized with bacteria; diminished air flow from obstructive lung disease results in ineffective cough and inability to clear secretions effectively (Martinez et al.). Postoperative morbidity and mortality may be reduced if pulmonary rehabilitation with antibiotics and bronchodilators and smoking cessation are employed. Additionally, patients can be taught to cough more effectively. For some patients in whom surgery initially is contraindicated, surgery may become an option if sufficient time is available for preoperative pulmonary rehabilitation (Ginsberg). For example, all patients at Memorial Sloan-Kettering Cancer Center in New York are given instructions for a preoperative exercise program because this has shown improved results (see Figure 8-8). One investigator found that patients who participated in a preoperative exercise program had "increased power" compared with patients who did not participate in the exercise program (Wall, 2000).

Surgical Procedures

As noted earlier, surgical resection is the treatment of choice for early-stage lung cancers. Surgical oncologists should follow several basic guidelines to optimize complete resection and TNM staging. These guidelines, which Ginsberg and Port (2000, p. 685) advocated, are as follows.

- "The tumor and its draining intrapulmonary lymphatic tributaries should be resected in their entirety whenever possible.
- "The tumor should be completely excised without spilling or traversing it.
- "The surgeon should resect *en bloc* any structure invaded by tumor in order to achieve negative margins.
- "A complete ipsilateral mediastinal lymph node dissection or sampling should be performed in all patients."

Pneumonectomy was first performed in 1933 in a patient with bronchogenic carcinoma. The procedure became the standard treatment for patients with resectable lung cancer in the 1940s (Waters, 2002). Pneumonectomy involves resection of the entire lung. Today, this procedure is limited to patients in whom a total resection (including negative margins) cannot be obtained with lobectomy (Ingle, 2000). This includes tumors that involve the proximal bronchus, several lobes of the lung, or the hilum (Ingle). This procedure is classified as simple or radical. Simple pneumonectomy involves removal of the lung with stapling of the bronchus. Radical pneumonectomy also includes removal of the mediastinal lymph nodes. To prevent mediastinal shift, the remaining pneumonectomy space is allowed to fill naturally with fluid. Mortality following pneumonectomy is twice that of lobectomy, estimated at 6% (Ingle; Quinn, 2003).

Lobectomy was first performed in 1912 but did not become routine until the 1950s, following a report of long-term survival in a patient with a peripheral tumor (Martini & Ginsberg, 2002). Lobectomy is the complete resection of a lobe of the lung. Lobectomy with lymph node sampling of hilar and mediastinal nodes is the procedure of choice in patients with stage I NSCLC, in whom the cancer is confined to a single lobe (Ginsberg & Port, 2000). One or two chest tubes are placed

---

Figure 8-8. Preoperative Exercise Program*

This program includes strengthening and flexibility exercises to improve muscle conditioning before surgery.

Arm exercises improve strength and flexibility.
1. Sitting or standing position
2. Place arms out at shoulder level; arms are straight, parallel to floor.
3. On breathing in: raise arms above head, touching both palms above head, hold for two seconds.
4. On breathing out: lower arms slowly, exhale through pursed lips; stop when arms are parallel to floor.

Leg exercises improve strength.
1. Sitting position
2. Lift leg off chair, tightening muscles on top of thigh, then extend leg straight, hold for three seconds.
3. Bend knee and lower slowly, relax then repeat.
Repeat 10 times; perform 10 times daily.

Sniff and blow—improve strength of diaphragm
1. Sitting position
2. Sniff twice; hold breath for two to three seconds.
3. Tighten stomach muscles and blow out slowly.
Repeat 10 times; perform 10 times daily.

Walk one mile, twice daily, in less than 20 minutes.
Climb two flights of stairs, quickly, four times daily.
Use incentive spirometer for 10 minutes, four times daily.

Mobilization—improve mobility and flexibility
1. Sitting position
2. Breathe in, raise arms above head, crossing wrists
3. Breathe out, pursed-lip breathing
   Bend forward touching chest to top of thigh (if possible).
   Lower arms to floor (try to touch fingers to floor).
4. Uncross arms.
   Breathe in.
   Raise upper body upright.
   Stretch arms above head.

Cough technique
1. Sitting position
2. Breathe in deeply five times, then
3. Hold breath for two seconds.
4. Contract abdominal muscles (bearing down).
5. Cough, while maintaining contraction of abdominal muscles.
6. Practice this four times daily.

---

* Developed by the Memorial Sloan-Kettering Cancer Center Thoracic Surgical Service in association with D. Wilson, RN, RT, and L. Wall, RN, and given to patients at their initial encounter.

Note. From "Preoperative Assessment of the Thoracic Surgical Patient: A Surgeon's Viewpoint" (p. 44), by R.J. Ginsberg, 2002, in F.G. Pearson, J.D. Cooper, J. Deslauriers, R.J. Ginsberg, C.A. Hiebert, G.A. Patterson, et al. (Eds.), *Thoracic Surgery*, 2002, New York: Churchill Livingstone. Copyright 2002 by Churchill Livingstone. Reprinted with permission.

following lobectomy; this practice varies from surgeon to surgeon (Martini & Ginsberg). The lobe is excised from the remaining lung, and, eventually, the remaining lung tissue expands to fill the space (Ingle, 2000). The mortality associated with lobectomy is approximately 3% (Ingle). Bilobectomy, a more extensive procedure, may need to be performed when the tumor crosses a major fissure or if more than one lobe is involved (Martini & Ginsberg). Empyema and bronchopleural fistula are more common in patients with bilobectomy involving the middle and lower lobes of the lung (Martini & Ginsberg).

Limited resections include segmentectomy and wedge resection. Segmental resection first was performed in 1939 and initially was performed for the surgical management of patients with tuberculosis and bronchiectasis (Fell & Kirby, 2002). It is defined as the excision of one or more bronchopulmonary segments of a lobe (Fell & Kirby). Because of the anatomy of segmental lymphatic drainage, most or all of the lymphatic drainage is resected during segmentectomy (Ginsberg & Port, 2000). Another procedure, the wedge resection, is a nonanatomic operation (Quinn, 2003). This procedure generally is reserved for patients who are unable to tolerate greater resections because of poor pulmonary reserve or comorbid conditions. It also is used for removal of small peripheral tumors. The 2003 ACCP guidelines recommend lobectomy over lesser resections, as clinical trials have demonstrated higher local recurrence rates in patients with wedge or segmental resections compared with those having greater resections (Smythe & ACCP, 2003).

The first true sleeve resection with broncoplastic reconstruction was performed in 1955 (Tsuchiya, 2002). Today, this procedure is performed when tumor is protruding from the main bronchus (Quinn, 2003). If tumor is confined to the bronchus, the involved area can be removed and the remaining bronchus can be reattached, thereby preserving unaffected lung tissue (Ingle, 2000). This procedure also can be performed in conjunction with lobectomy, often eliminating the need for pneumonectomy (Quinn).

At the time of surgery, lymph node sampling must be performed for adequate nodal staging. Accurate lymph node staging is especially important in early-stage lung cancers. Patients whose nodal status is determined by clinical methods have been shown to have decreased survival compared to those with pathologically staged lymph nodes (Haigentz & Keller, 2002). Controversy exists as to the most accurate way to sample lymph nodes to determine involvement by tumor (Ginsberg & Port, 2000). In general, lymph node sampling is performed in one of three ways: lymph node "sampling" refers to the removal of abnormal lymph nodes; "systematic sampling" refers to routine sampling of lymph nodes at different nodal stations; and "complete mediastinal lymph node dissection" refers to the removal of all lymph node tissue at levels specified by the surgeon (Haigentz & Keller). Two recent clinical trials have compared systematic sampling with complete mediastinal lymph node dissection (Keller, Adak, Wagner, & Johnson, 2000; Wu, Huang, Wang, Yang, & Ou, 2002). In

the first trial, Keller et al. demonstrated that complete mediastinal lymph node dissection identified significantly more N2 lymph nodes, and this group had improved survival. Wu et al. found that complete mediastinal lymph node dissection was associated with significant improvements in survival. The patients in the Wu et al. trial were followed for up to 10 years following surgery. Investigators are examining the technique of sentinel lymph node sampling in an effort to eliminate systematic dissection (Liptay et al., 2000; Little, DeHoyos, Kirgan, Arcomano, & Murray, 1999). More data need to be accumulated before this procedure can be recommended routinely.

Minimally invasive surgery, including video-assisted thoracoscopic surgery (VATS), may be used for lung resection in selected circumstances. VATS is used for both diagnostic and therapeutic purposes. Potential advantages of VATS over conventional surgery include decreased postoperative pain, better preservation of pulmonary function, and earlier return to normal activities (Yim, 2002). A distinct disadvantage for VATS is the inability to perform adequate mediastinal lymph node sampling (Yim). Very often, VATS is used in patients who are unable to tolerate a thoracotomy or who have poor pulmonary reserve. Before this technique can be widely recommended, more research must be conducted.

Nursing care of patients prior to and following lung resection is complex. Post-resection complications largely are determined by the physical status of the patient. The most common complications following lung resection are pain and atelectasis (Ingle, 2000). As noted earlier, most postoperative pulmonary complications are related directly to COPD. The focus of nursing care on the patient undergoing thoracic surgery should begin at the time the patient is being evaluated for resection and continue through the postoperative and ambulatory period.

Preoperative improvement in pulmonary function in patients with COPD may improve outcomes following resection. Patients with obstructive disease may benefit from a preoperative regimen using inhalers, antibiotics, and breathing exercises (e.g., incentive spirometer, cough and deep breathing exercises). Preoperative evaluation of all patients should include respiratory function and extremity range of motion so that appropriate instruction can occur. Instruction should include diaphragmatic breathing exercises and range of motion exercises, which can be performed in the initial postoperative period. The exercise program should be initiated prior to surgery (see Figure 8-8). In those who are current or recent smokers, the importance of smoking cessation cannot be overemphasized. Patients must be assessed carefully for smoking history and understand the importance of becoming tobacco free. The initial postoperative period presents many challenges, including, but not limited to, prevention of post-thoracotomy pain, promotion of pulmonary toilet, prevention of infection, and early recognition of cardiac arrhythmias. Adequate pain control must be assessed frequently, and medication should be adjusted as needed. With successful pain control, pulmonary exercises and coughing, as well as pulmonary toilet, will be easier to perform. Range of motion exercises and early ambulation are promoted to prevent venous stasis and decrease the risk of thromboembolic disease. Continuous assessment for incisional infection or other pulmonary infection should be performed. Early recognition of infection and judicious pulmonary toilet may prevent more serious complications.

Following hospital discharge, respiratory function and smoking status must be assessed. Patients must be aware that optimal respiratory function will not be immediate. Continuation of the exercise program may help to restore optimal respiratory function. If needed, patients may be referred to a pulmonary rehabilitation program. Smoking cessation efforts and encouraging patients to remain tobacco free are also important during this period.

Radiation Therapy

Radiation therapy for NSCLC has been used since the 1950s. Since the early days, much research has been done to determine the optimum dose and fractionation schedule, as well as the integration of radiation therapy into multimodality treatment. Radiation therapy kills both cancer cells and normal cells. The effect of radiation therapy on normal tissue surrounding the tumor determines the maximal dose of radiation and the resulting toxicities (Maher, 2000). This effect is termed the "therapeutic ratio" (Maher). One dose of ionizing radiation will have the greatest effect, or cell kill, on both normal cells and cancer cells. The therapeutic ratio is accomplished by dividing the total dose of radiation into equal fractions or doses and giving it over a specified time period (Maher). Fractionating radiation doses accomplishes the goal of destroying cancer cells and reducing the probability of any remaining viable cells while maintaining the integrity of normal cells (Weisenburger, 2002).

In recent years, several innovations have been developed in the field of radiation therapy. The goals of these innovations are to improve outcomes and decrease side effects. Hyperfractionation is when the total daily dose of radiation is given in two divided doses. This method allows for delivery of a slightly overall higher dose over the same time or a shorter period with fewer side effects, including a reduction in late side effects (Jett et al., 2003). Results of clinical trials comparing hyperfractionated radiotherapy with standard radiation have been mixed (Jett et al.). Because of the mixed results of trials, at this time hyperfractionated radiation therapy cannot be recommended over standard treatment in patients with stage IIIB disease (Jett et al.).

Continuous hyperfractionated accelerated radiotherapy (CHART) is delivered in three fractions per day over 12 days (Ingle, 2000). Again, the total dose delivered is greater than that for standard radiotherapy and with multiple smaller frac-

tions, normal cells receive less toxicity. Several studies have shown advantages for patients receiving CHART compared to standard radiation therapy (Belani, 1993; Hazuka & Turissi, 1993). As yet, CHART is not widely used in the United States in part because it requires radiotherapy to be given three times per day (Jett et al., 2003).

A study using proton-beam radiation therapy in early-stage lung cancer demonstrated safety with comparable local control and disease-free survival compared to conventional photon radiation therapy (Bush et al., 1999). Proton-beam therapy uses protons (as opposed to photons, which are used in standard radiotherapy) to kill cancer cells (Moore-Higgs, 2003). Because of the radiobiology of protons, radiation oncologists are able to deliver maximal doses of radiation to the tumor with significantly less toxicity to surrounding normal cells (Moore-Higgs). As a result, higher doses of proton-beam therapy may be delivered to the tumor, leading to better control with reduced side-effects (Bush et al.). Presently, proton-beam therapy is expensive and not widely available. More research is needed before recommendations can be made.

Three-dimensional conformational radiation therapy (3D-CRT) provides the prescribed dose of radiation to the configuration of the tumor but is able to deliver lower doses to the surrounding tissue. Treatment planning and dose delivery are based on computer-assisted programs. This type of treatment primarily has been used in patients with prostate cancer. Its use in lung cancer has been described, but, at this time, it is not widely used (Armstrong & McGibney, 2000; Martel, TenHaken, & Hazuda, 1999).

Brachytherapy is the placement of sealed radioactive sources in contact or close proximity to the target tissue. In patients with lung cancer, brachytherapy primarily is used in one of two ways: endobronchial or interstitial. Endobronchial brachytherapy is achieved by the bronchoscopic placement of a radioactive source beyond the distal margin of the tumor (Ingle, 2000). Endobronchial brachytherapy has been shown to be an excellent method for palliation of symptoms, such as dyspnea, cough, or hemoptysis, from endobronchial lesions (Ingle). Side effects are minimal, although bronchoesophageal fistula and hemoptysis have been reported (Ingle; Speiser & Kresl, 2000). Interstitial brachytherapy involves the placement of radioactive seeds by needle to the target tissue. It is best used for local control of tumor following surgical resection when the margins are close or positive (Speiser & Kresl). Interstitial brachytherapy is not used as commonly as external beam radiotherapy because of a lack of expertise with the technique (Speiser & Kresl). At this time, interstitial brachytherapy has no proven lung cancer treatment role, either alone or in combination with surgery, external beam radiation therapy, or chemotherapy (Speiser & Kresl). High dose rate brachytherapy has been used to palliate symptoms of obstructive lung cancer, such as dyspnea, cough, and hemoptysis (Ingle).

Radiation therapy is used as primary treatment for medically inoperable stage I and II NSCLC, in patients with early-stage unresectable disease (either alone or combined with chemotherapy), as prophylactic treatment (e.g., for impending superior vena cava syndrome), or for palliative treatment (e.g., for painful bone metastases). Additionally, radiation therapy is used in the adjuvant setting for patients with early-stage lung cancer and positive resection margins (Smythe & ACCP, 2003). In patients with NSCLC, standard treatment is delivered to the primary tumor as well as the regional lymphatics. The standard dose is considered to be 50–65 Gy over a five- to six-week period. Management of side effects, specifically radiation pneumonitis, fibrosis, and esophagitis, will be discussed in Chapter 9.

Studies examining the use of adjuvant or neoadjuvant radiation therapy in patients with early-stage lung cancer have not shown a survival benefit over surgery alone (Smythe & ACCP, 2003). A recent meta-analysis reported that postoperative radiotherapy had a significant adverse effect on survival in patients with completely resected lung cancer (PORT Meta-Analysis Trialists Group, 1998). These results may be affected by older treatment modalities; with newer approaches in radiation therapy, these data may change.

In patients with locally advanced disease (stage III), standard radiation therapy has not achieved long-term control of disease. Several trials have compared radiation therapy alone with combination chemotherapy and radiation therapy treatment in patients with nonoperable stage III disease. Both concurrent and sequential regimens have been used. Results of these trials have demonstrated improved survival and local control with the combination treatment (Curran, 2000; Johnson & Turrisi, 2000). Trials using cisplatin-based chemotherapy have shown an advantage (Sause et al., 2000). Combination radiation therapy and chemotherapy is the current standard for patients with unresectable stage III disease.

In a phase III trial involving patients with regional advanced, unresectable NSCLC, patients were randomized to one of three arms: standard radiation, induction chemotherapy (cisplatin-based) followed by standard radiation, and hyperfractionated radiation (Sause et al., 2000). The purpose of the trial was to demonstrate that either hyperfractionated radiation or the combination of chemotherapy and radiation would improve survival in patients with regionally advanced lung cancer. The study did not confirm the benefit of hyperfractionated radiation; however, patients who received combination therapy had superior survival over the other groups (Sause et al.).

Palliative radiation therapy plays an important role in patients with advanced incurable NSCLC. Palliative radiation can improve symptoms and, in some cases, survival. Several factors must be considered in patients receiving palliative radiation therapy. These include the natural history of the disease, resources for treatment, likelihood of achieving meaningful benefit, and patient condition. Radiation therapy for malignant spinal cord compression and superior vena cava syndrome is discussed in Chapter 5.

External beam whole brain radiation therapy (WBRT) is used most commonly in patients with NSCLC who have metastatic disease to the brain. Prompt treatment often is required to prevent or minimize progressive neurologic deterioration. The use of steroids in conjunction with WBRT reduces swelling from tumor and neurologic symptoms. The steroids are tapered slowly after completion of the WBRT.

Bone metastases occur in 20%–40% of patients with lung cancer. The most common sites of metastases are vertebrae, pelvis, and femora. The skull and extremities are involved less often. Often, bone metastases cause pain, immobility, and pathologic fractures. Radiation therapy can improve pain and mobility and prevent pathologic fractures in these patients. Additionally, it has been shown to stop osteolytic bone destruction and promote reossification (Greenberg et al., 1972).

Radiation therapy is an important treatment modality in the management of patients with nearly all stages of NSCLC. Clinical trials of newer methods such as 3-DCRT, intensity-modulated radiation therapy (an advanced form of 3-DCRT), and proton beam therapy continue to refine and improve outcomes. Management of patients with NSCLC will improve as newer radiation therapy strategies and combined modality treatments emerge.

Chemotherapy for Non-Small Cell Lung Cancer

Chemotherapy for NSCLC has been used widely for decades. Early treatments using alkylating agents, such as nitrogen mustard, were not very successful. Treatment outcomes improved with the second generation of platinum-based regimens. In the 1990s, researchers made greater progress with third-generation agents, including the taxanes (paclitaxel and docetaxel), vinorelbine, gemcitabine, and irinotecan.

Chemotherapy is used in several different approaches for NSCLC, including adjuvant and neoadjuvant treatment, multimodality treatment (most notably in the neoadjuvant setting), treatment for patients with unresectable stage III disease, and patients with stage IV disease. For patients with stage IV disease, chemotherapy is considered to be the primary treatment despite what have been only modest improvements in survival with modern regimens (Johnson, 2000; Non-Small Cell Lung Cancer Collaborative Group, 1995). Based on the less-than-satisfactory results of chemotherapy trials in this group, clinicians are recommending treatments aimed at new therapeutic targets currently in development (Bonomi et al., 2000; Carney, 2002).

Treatment of Advanced Non-Small Cell Lung Cancer

Advanced NSCLC includes patients with unresectable stage III disease and those with stage IV disease. The American Society of Clinical Oncology (ASCO) treatment guidelines and the more recent ACCP *Diagnosis and Management of Lung Cancer: Evidence-Based Guidelines* (Block, 2003) recommend platinum-based chemotherapy in patients with a good PS ("Clinical Practice Guidelines," 1997; Socinski, Morris, Masters, & Lilenbaum, 2003). These guidelines are based on the results of multiple clinical trials and meta-analyses.

Multiple trials published between 1988–1999 have compared best supportive care with platinum-based chemotherapy in patients with advanced lung cancer (Socinski et al., 2003). In all 10 trials, the median survival of the patients given chemotherapy was significantly superior to those receiving best supportive care. The median survival in patients receiving best supportive care was 3.6 months versus 6.5 months in the patients given chemotherapy. Additionally, a meta-analysis of 52 randomized clinical trials (representing 9,387 patients) demonstrated that chemotherapy improved survival in all stages of disease (Non-Small Cell Lung Cancer Collaborative Group, 1995). Results of this meta-analysis also demonstrated that cisplatin-based regimens were better than other chemotherapy regimens not containing cisplatin. Another randomized trial comparing best supportive care to a platinum-based regimen demonstrated reduced symptoms and improved quality of life for the patients given chemotherapy (Cullen et al., 1999). Despite this, no recommendation was given on the best cisplatin regimen or best dose for use in this population (Bengtson & Rigas, 1999). Given the results of the data presented, future randomized trials containing a best supportive care regimen are not likely (Thomas, 2003).

To date, cisplatin-based chemotherapy regimens have been referred to as first generation (e.g., cisplatin, mitomycin, ifosfamide), second generation (e.g., cisplatin, etoposide), or third generation (e.g., cisplatin, gemcitabine) (Schiller et al., 2002). Several trials have shown the benefits, including high response rates and improved one-year survival, of newer (i.e., third-generation) agents in combination with a platinum compound (Schiller et al.). However, no reports of a randomized trial were reported until 2002 (Schiller et al.). In this trial, patients were randomized to receive cisplatin and paclitaxel (referred to as the "reference regimen"), cisplatin and gemcitabine, cisplatin and docetaxel, or carboplatin and paclitaxel (Bonomi et al., 2000). This trial randomized 1,207 patients over nearly a three-year period. Patients were stratified according to PS, weight loss, stage of disease, and presence or absence of brain metastases. The trial concluded that no one regimen was clearly better than another in terms of response or survival. Additionally, survival was significantly improved in patients with a better PS. Based on the results of this trial and others, the current ACCP evidence-based guidelines recommend that patients with advanced NSCLC be treated with a platinum compound (carboplatin, cisplatin) and one of the newer agents as first-line chemotherapy (Socinski et al., 2003).

Other issues in patients with advanced NSCLC have included PS, duration of chemotherapy, and second-line chemotherapy in those with progressive disease following first-line treatment. Over the years, the most important prognostic factor in patients with NSCLC has been PS (Socinski et al., 2003). The two most common scales used to identify PS were developed by Karnofsky (Karnofsky & Burchenal, 1949) and the Eastern Cooperative Oncology Group (ECOG). Several trials have documented the impact of PS on survival; two of the largest are those by Schiller et al. (2002) and Finkelstein et al. (1986). The Schiller et al. trial was described previously. The Finkelstein et al. trial is considered to be the landmark study in answering this question (Socinski et al., 2003). In this study, which included nearly 900 patients, one-year survival for patients with PS level 0 was 36%, PS level 1 was 16%, and PS level 2 was 9%, a statistically significant difference (ECOG PS level 0 = normal, ECOG PS level 1 = fatigue without significant decrease in activity, ECOG PS level 2 = fatigue with significant impairment of daily activities or bed rest < 50% of waking hours). Based on these results and others, the ACCP guidelines recommend platinum-based chemotherapy for patients with advanced NSCLC and good PS (ECOG levels 0 or 1) (Socinski et al., 2003).

Multiple courses of varying regimens of chemotherapy frequently are used in the treatment of NSCLC. In many instances, first-line chemotherapy is continued until disease progression or intolerable chemotherapy-related toxicity. The 1997 ASCO treatment guidelines recommended no more than eight cycles of chemotherapy. This recommendation was based on the results of trials showing no survival advantage for patients receiving longer duration chemotherapy. (Buccheri, Ferrigno, Curcio, Vola, & Rosso, 1989; Smith et al., 2001; Socinski et al., 2002). Patients given the shorter duration of treatment had less toxicity and an improved quality of life. Socinski et al. (2002) randomized patients to receive four cycles of chemotherapy versus continuous treatment (until progression of disease). The median number of chemotherapy courses was four in the continuous-treatment arm. As a result of these trials, the ACCP guidelines recommend no more than three or four cycles of chemotherapy in patients with advanced NSCLC (Socinski et al., 2003).

Most patients with advanced NSCLC experience progression of disease following first-line treatment. Many of these patients remain well with good PS and choose to continue treatment with additional chemotherapy. Although many agents have been used, only one is approved for treatment in this setting. Docetaxel is approved by the U.S. Food and Drug Administration for second-line use in patients with advanced NSCLC. Data from two phase-three studies supported the use of docetaxel as second-line therapy in patients with advanced NSCLC (Fossella et al., 2000; Shepherd et al., 2000). Other agents such as gemcitabine, vinorelbine, and irinotecan have been tested in the second-line setting. At this time, no phase III trials have documented the advantage of one drug over the other (Socinski et al., 2003).

The results of these trials have made important contributions to the treatment of advanced NSCLC, but progress has been slow and increases in survival, although statistically significant in some cases, are small. To improve on the results of these data, investigators are looking for new treatments and combinations of treatments. Clinical trials comparing the best of the two drug combinations (doublets) versus modern chemotherapy regimens with three agents (triplets) have been and continue to be investigated (Kelly, 2000). Clinicians also are investigating the value of sequential single agents and sequential doublets. Additionally, trials are investigating newer, more active cytotoxic agents such as tirapazamine, multitargeted antifolates, oxaliplatin, and tegafur-uracil (Kelly). Trials with these agents continue.

In addition to response rates and survival, other important endpoints include quality of life and symptom management. Numerous tools have been specifically developed to measure quality of life in patients with lung cancer. Two such tools are the FACT-L, developed by Cella et al. (1995), and the Lung Cancer Symptom Scale (LCSS), developed by Hollen et al. (1994). Controlling chemotherapy and disease-related symptoms has been the subject of much research over the last 10–15 years, with entire textbooks devoted to the topic (Yarbro, Frogge, & Goodman, 2004).

Treatment Based on the Biology and Molecular Biology of Lung Cancer

Since the 1990s, researchers have developed a significant understanding of the biology and molecular biology of lung cancer. This new information includes the effect of the following on lung cancer: growth factors, oncogenes, tumor suppressor genes, signal transduction, and angiogenesis pathways (Bunn et al., 2000). As a result of this information, many new treatment strategies have been developed and tested in patients with NSCLC. Table 8-4 lists new agents that are in use for lung cancer prevention and treatment. Table 8-5 lists molecular targets for new lung cancer therapies.

To date, the best studied of this group are the EGFR inhibitors. The epidermal growth factor is believed to be involved in the growth of NSCLC. Overexpression of the EGFR is found in many solid tumors, including NSCLC. Interruption of signaling pathways with EGFR inhibitors in tumors that overexpress EGFR results in decreased cell proliferation, decreased angiogenesis, and promotion of apoptosis. The first of this class (gefitinib) is the best studied and was approved in May 2003 for the treatment of NSCLC.

Extensive studies have been conducted with gefitinib in patients with NSCLC. Two phase II studies assessing safety and efficacy were conducted in previously treated and symptomatic patients with NSCLC. These two studies tested gefitinib in more than 400 patients with advanced NSCLC. Results demonstrated mild toxicity and improvement in disease-related symptoms and quality of life (Fukuoka et al., 2002; Kris et al., 2002). In one study, two different daily oral doses were examined: 250 mg and 500 mg (Kris et al.). Response rates were 8.8% and 11.8%, respectively. Symptom response rates were 43% and 35%, respectively. The majority of patients experienced symptom improvement within two weeks of starting therapy. Side effects were mild and reversible and predominantly included an acne-like rash and diarrhea. In another trial, patients again were randomized to two different dose levels, 250 mg and 500 mg (Fukuoka et al.). Response rates were similar: 18.4% in those receiving the lower dose and 19% in the others. A favorable adverse event profile was seen and was similar to that of Kris et al.

Table 8-4. New Agents for Lung Cancer Prevention and Therapy Based on Biological Abnormalities

Agents	Types
Growth factor inhibitors	
Epidermal growth factor (EGF) inhibitors	EGF and EGF receptor antibodies, EGF fusion toxins, EGF receptor immunotoxins
Peptide hormone antagonists	Substance P derivatives, bradykinin antagonist dimmers
Matrix metalloproteinase inhibitors	Marimastat, batimastat Ag33340 Bay 12-9566
Antiangiogenesis agents	Endostatin, angiostatin Anti-VEGF antibodies, ribozymes Anti-VEGF-receptor antibodies, ribozymes Thalidomide
NSAIDs, cyclooxygenase, lipooxygenase inhibitors	Sulindac, sulindac sulfone (FGN-1)
Protein kinase C inhibitors	Bryostatin Dolostatin

Note. From "New Therapeutic Strategies for Lung Cancer: Biology and Molecular Biology Come of Age," by P.A. Bunn, A. Soriano, G. Johnson, and L. Heasley, 2000, *Chest, 117*, p. 164S. Copyright 2000 by the American College of Chest Physicians. Reprinted with permission.

Table 8-5. Molecular Targets for New Lung Cancer Therapies

Therapies	Targets
Tumor suppressor gene replacement	*p53* (SCLC and NSCLC) RB (SCLC) *p16* (NSCLC)
Dominant oncogene inhibition	Cyclin D1 antisense, phosmidosine *ras* antisense anf farnesylation inhibitors HER-2/*neu* antibodies and antisense *myc* antisense *bcl*-2 antisense

NSCLC = non-small cell lung cancer; SCLC = small cell lung cancer.

Note. From "New Therapeutic Strategies for Lung Cancer: Biology and Molecular Biology Come of Age," by P.A. Bunn, A. Soriano, G. Johnson, and L. Heasley, 2000, *Chest, 117,* p. 165S. Copyright 2000 by the American College of Chest Physicians. Reprinted with permission.

In a phase III study, patients with advanced NSCLC were given carboplatin and paclitaxel (Herbst et al., 2003). Patients were randomized to receive gefitinib or placebo in addition to chemotherapy. More than 2,000 patients were enrolled. Results found no survival benefit for the patients given gefitinib. Tissue samples were collected when possible; at this writing, investigators are analyzing them to determine if a correlation exists between EGFR expression and survival.

In another study, pretreatment characteristics associated with response were evaluated in 140 patients treated in one of three gefitinib programs at a single institution (Shah et al., 2003). Results of multivariate analysis revealed that "presence of any bronchioloalveolar feature pathologically" and being a "never smoker" were the only independent predictors of response to gefitinib. The results of this trial, if confirmed, can direct future research into the mechanism of action of gefitinib and better design future trials with gefitinib or similar agents.

As a result of clinical trials performed in the United States and abroad, gefitinib was approved for use in Japan and in the United States, as noted above. In the United States, it is approved for third-line treatment in patients with advanced NSCLC. Gefitinib has added a new alternative to cytotoxic treatment for patients with NSCLC and has benefited many. Significant pulmonary toxicity has been observed in some patients in Japan. This toxicity consists of diffuse alveolar damage and has resulted in respiratory failure and death in some (Okamoto et al., 2003).

Erlotinib is another EGFR inhibitor that has shown promising results; this agent still is in clinical trials. Studies have demonstrated that it has activity and side effects similar to that seen with gefitinib. Preliminary results of a phase II trial of erlotinib in patients with BAC were reported at ASCO's annual meeting in May 2003 (Miller et al., 2003). This trial was initiated as a result of anecdotal reports of dramatic results in patients with BAC, which generally is considered chemotherapy resistant. Preliminary results demonstrated a 27% major objective response rate. The side effect profile is similar to that seen with gefitinib. Clinical trials with this agent are ongoing.

The trials reported here represent a small amount of the research that is being conducted with new therapies for NSCLC. To date, the agents summarized here are the best studied in NSCLC. Trials are examining the effects of vascular endothelial growth factor receptor tyrosine kinase inhibitors (e.g., SU6668), monoclonal antibodies directed at growth factor receptors (e.g., IMC-225, trastuzumab), and anti-angiogenesis agents (e.g., BAY12-9566) (Herbst & Giaccone, 2002).

Outcomes

As noted earlier, NSCLC kills more men and women in the United States than any other cancer. The five-year survival for patients with stage IB–IV ranges from 38% to 9%, respectively (Mountain, 1997). Stages IB through IV represent a wide range of patients, including those considered to be resectable, with locally advanced disease and advanced NSCLC. Despite these dismal statistics, some progress has been made in the treatment of all stages of disease. The knowledge gained in recent years about cancer genetics and molecular biology is changing the treatment of cancer, including NSCLC.

Several notable avenues of research exist for diagnosis and treatment of patients with resectable disease. The first involves the use and refinement of FDG-PET in staging and prediction of outcomes in surgically resectable patients, use of PET in restaging patients after induction therapy, and the correlation of FDG uptake and prognosis in NSCLC (MacManus, 2003). Although early results of this research are exciting, more data must be collected to determine the value of FDG-PET in these areas. The role of induction chemotherapy in patients with earlier-stage disease has shown promise in initial studies (Pisters et al., 2000). Trials continue both in the United States and Europe.

The continued study of molecular markers and their role in prognosis, staging, and early detection of disease is exciting. Multiple studies are under way (Lau et al., 2000). One study is examining sputum washings to detect the presence of K-*ras* mutations. This may become a marker of early disease, and results are promising (Rieger, 2001). Gene therapy offers another promising approach to treatment of NSCLC (Joyce & Houlihan, 2001). In particular, *p53* gene mutations are present in about 80% of patients with NSCLC. Preclinical studies have shown promising results (Toloza, Roth, & Swisher, 2000).

In patients with advanced disease, new treatments and new combinations continue to be studied. Research continues into the use of combined modality treatment. These focus on the optimum dose and sequencing of both chemotherapy and radiation therapy. The exploration of the role of targeted therapies continues. Investigators are examining the effects of these agents in multimodality therapy as well as their effect in long-term control of tumors.

The new millennium holds great promise for the management of NSCLC. Many clinicians hope for the time when NSCLC is considered to be a chronic disease. With the results of the research currently being conducted, this may not be unreasonable.

References

Alberts, W.M. (2003). Lung cancer guidelines: Introduction. American College of Chest Physicians Guideline. *Chest, 123*(1 Suppl.), 1S–2S.

Armstrong, J., & McGibney, C. (2000). The impact of three dimensional radiation on the treatment of non-small cell lung cancer. *Radiotherapy Oncology, 56,* 157–167.

Barkley, J.E., & Green, M.R. (1996). Bronchioloalveolar carcinoma. *Journal of Clinical Oncology, 14,* 2377–2386.

Beckles, M.A., Spiro, S.G., Colice, G.L., & Rudd, R.M. (2003). Initial evaluation of the patient with lung cancer. *Chest, 123*(Suppl. 1), 97S–104S.

Beckles, M.A., Spiro, S.G., Colice, G.L., Rudd, R.M., & the American College of Chest Physicians. (2003). The physiologic evaluation of patients with lung cancer being considered for resectional surgery. *Chest, 123*(Suppl. 1), 105S–114S.

Belani, C.P. (1993). Multimodality management of regionally advanced non-small cell lung cancer. *Seminars in Oncology, 20,* 302–314.

Bengtson, E.M., & Rigas, J.R. (1999). A brief historical review of the development of chemotherapy for the treatment of advanced non-small cell lung cancer: Why we should look beyond platinum. *Seminars in Oncology, 26,* 1–6.

Block, A.J. (Ed.). (2003). Diagnosis and management of lung cancer: ACCP evidence-based guidelines. *Chest, 123*(Suppl. 1), 1S–337S.

Bonomi, P., Kim, K., Fairclough, D., Cella, D., Kugler, J., Rowinsky, E., et al. (2000). Comparison of survival and quality of life in advanced non-small cell lung cancer patients treated with two dose levels of paclitaxel combined with cisplatin versus etoposide with cisplatin: Results of an Eastern Cooperative Oncology Group trial. *Journal of Clinical Oncology, 18,* 623–631.

British Thoracic Society (BTS). (2001). BTS guidelines: Guidelines on the selection of patients with lung cancer for surgery. *Thorax, 56,* 89–108.

Buccheri, G.F., Ferrigno, D., Curcio, A., Vola, F., & Rosso, A. (1989). Continuation of chemotherapy vs. supportive care alone in patients with inoperable non small lung cancer and stable disease after two or three cycles of MACC. *Cancer, 63,* 428–432.

Bunn, P.A., Soriano, A., Johnson, G., & Heasley, L. (2000). New therapeutic strategies for lung cancer. Biology and molecular biology come of age. *Chest, 117*(4 Suppl. 1), 163S–167S.

Bush, D.A., Slater, J.D., Bonnet, R., Cheek, G.A., Dunbar, R.D., Moyers, M., et al. (1999). Proton-beam radiotherapy for early-stage lung cancer. *Chest, 116,* 1313–1319.

Carney, D.N. (2002). Lung cancer: Time to move on from chemotherapy. *New England Journal of Medicine, 346,* 126–127.

Cella, D.F., Bonomi, A.E., Lloyd, S.R., Tulsky, D.S., Kaplan, E., & Bonomi, P. (1995). Reliability and validity of the Functional Assessment of Cancer Therapy—Lung (FACT—L) quality of life instrument. *Lung Cancer, 12,* 199–220.

Clinical practice guidelines for the treatment of unresectable non-small cell lung cancer. (1997). *Journal of Clinical Oncology, 15,* 2996–3018.

Cullen, M., Billingham, J., Woodraffe, C., Chetiyawardana, A.D., Gower, N.H., Joshi, R., et al. (1999). Mitomycin, ifosfamide, and cisplatin in unresectable non-small cell lung cancer: Effects on survival and quality of life. *Journal of Clinical Oncology, 17,* 3188–3194.

Curran, W.J. (2000). Radiotherapy for locally advanced lung cancer: An overview. In H.I. Pass, J.B. Mitchell, D.B. Johnson, A.T. Turrisi, & J.D. Minna (Eds.), *Lung cancer: Principles and practice* (2nd ed., pp. 823–828). Philadelphia: Lippincott Williams & Wilkins.

D'Amico, T.A., Aloia, T.A., Moore, M.B.H., Conlon, D.H., Herndon, J.E., Kinch, M.S., et al. (2001). Predicting the sites of metastases from lung cancer using molecular biologic markers. *Annals of Thoracic Surgery, 72,* 1144–1148.

Detterbeck, F.C., Jones, D.R., Kernstine, K.H., Naunheim, K.S., & American College of Chest Physicians. (2003). Lung cancer: Special treatment issues. *Chest, 123*(Suppl. 1), 244S–258S.

Eagle, K.A., Brundage, B.H., Chaitman, B.R., Ewy, G.A., Fleisher, L.A., Hertzer, N.R., et al. (1996). Guidelines for perioperative cardiovascular evaluation for noncardiac surgery: Report of the American College of Cardiology/American Heart Association task force on practice guidelines. *Journal of the American College of Cardiology, 27,* 910–948.

Ebright, M.I., Zakowski, M.F., Martin, J., Venkatraman, E.S., Miller, V.A., Bains, M.S., et al. (2002). Clinical pattern and pathologic stage but not histologic features predict outcome for bronchioloalveolar carcinoma. *Annals of Thoracic Surgery, 74,* 1640–1647.

Fell, S.C., & Kirby, T.J. (2002). Segmental resection. In F.G. Pearson, J.D. Cooper, J. Deslauriers, R.J. Ginsberg, C.A. Hiebert, G.A. Patterson, et al. (Eds.), *Thoracic surgery* (pp. 991–1004). New York: Churchill Livingstone.

Finkelstein, D.M., Ettinger, D.S., & Ruckdeschel, J.C. (1986). Long-term survivors in metastatic non-small cell lung cancer: An Eastern Cooperative Oncology Group Study. *Journal of Clinical Oncology, 4,* 702–709.

Fossella, F.V., DeVore, R., Kerr, R.N., Crawford, J., Natale, R.R., Dunphy, F., et al. (2000). Randomized phase III trial of docetaxel versus vinorelbine or ifosfamide in patients with advanced non-small cell lung cancer previously treated with platinum containing chemotherapy regimens. *Journal of Clinical Oncology, 18,* 2354–2362.

Fukuoka, M., Yano, S., Giaccone, G., Tamura, T., Nakagawa, K., Douillard, J.Y., et al. (2002). Final results from a phase II trial of ZD1839 (Iressa) for patients with advanced non-small cell lung cancer (IDEAL I) [Abstract]. *Proceedings of the American Society of Clinical Oncology, 21,* 298.

Gail, M.H., Eagan, R.T., Feld, R., Ginsberg, R., Goodell, B., Hill, L., et al. (1984). Prognostic factors in patients with resected stage I non-small cell lung cancer: A report from the lung cancer study group. *Cancer, 54,* 1802–1813.

Ginsberg, R.J. (2002). Preoperative assessment of the thoracic surgical patient: A surgeon's viewpoint. In F.G. Pearson, J.D. Cooper, J. Deslauriers, R.J. Ginsberg, C.A. Hiebert, G.A., Patterson, et al. (Eds.), *Thoracic surgery* (pp. 43–50). New York: Churchill Livingstone.

Ginsberg, R.J., & Port, J.L. (2000). Surgical therapy of stage I and non-T3N0 stage II non-small cell lung cancer. In H.I. Pass, J.B. Mitchell, D.B. Johnson, A.T. Turrisi, & J.D. Minna (Eds.), *Lung cancer: Principles and practice* (2nd ed., pp. 682–693). Philadelphia: Lippincott Williams & Wilkins.

Ginsberg, R.J., Vokes, E.E., & Rosenzweig, K. (2001). Non-small cell lung cancer. In V. DeVita, S. Hellman, & S. Rosenberg (Eds.), *Cancer: Principles and practice of oncology* (6th ed., pp. 925–983). Philadelphia: Lippincott Williams & Wilkins.

Greenberg, E.J., Chu, F.C.H., Dwyer, A.J., Ziminski, E.M., Dimich, A.B., & Laughlin, J.S. (1972). Effects of radiotherapy on bone lesions as measured by 47-Ca and 85-Sr local kinetics. *Journal of Nuclear Medicine, 13,* 747–751.

Haapoja, I.S. (2000). Paraneoplastic syndromes. In C.H. Yarbro, M.H. Frogge, M. Goodman, & S.L. Groenwald (Eds.), *Cancer nursing: Principles and practice* (5th ed., pp. 792–812). Sudbury, MA: Jones and Bartlett.

Haas, M.L. (2003). Separating out the differences between lung cancers. In M.L. Haas (Ed.), *Contemporary issues in lung cancer: A nursing perspective* (pp. 3–10). Sudbury, MA: Jones and Bartlett.

Haigentz, M., & Keller, S.M. (2002). Concepts in the intraoperative staging of lymph nodes in non-small cell lung cancer and the role of mediastinal lymph node dissection. *Lung Cancer Principles and Practice Updates, 2*(4), 1–12.

Handy, J.R., Asaph, J.W., Skokan, L., Reed, C.E., Koh, S., Brooks, G., et al. (2002). What happens to patients undergoing lung cancer surgery? Outcomes and quality of life before and after surgery. *Chest, 122,* 21–30.

Harpole, D.H., Herndon, J.W., Young, W.G., Wolfe, W.G., & Sabiston, D.C. (1995). Stage I non-small cell lung cancer: A multivariate analysis of treatment methods and patterns of recurrence. *Cancer, 76,* 787–796.

Hazuka, M.B., & Turissi, A.T. (1993). The evolving role of radiation therapy in the treatment of locally advanced lung cancer. *Seminars in Oncology, 20,* 173–184.

Herbst, R.S., & Giaccone, G. (2002). Novel molecular strategies in lung cancer: EGFR inhibition and anti-angiogenesis. *Lung Cancer Principles and Practice Updates, 2*(2), 1–19.

Herbst, R.S., Giaccone, G., Schiller, J., Miller, V., Natale, R., Rennie, P., et al. (2003). Subset analyses of INTACT results for gefitinib (ZD1839) when combined with platinum-based chemotherapy (CT) for advanced non-small cell lung cancer (NSCLC) [Abstract]. *Proceedings of the American Society of Clinical Oncology, 22,* 2523.

Hollen, P.J., Gralla, R.J., Kris, M.G., Cox, C., Belani, C.P., Grunberg, S.M., et al. (1994). Measurement of quality of life in patients with lung cancer in multicenter trials of new therapies. Psychometric assessment of the lung cancer symptom scale. *Cancer, 73,* 2087–2098.

Ingle, R.J. (2000). Lung cancers. In C.H. Yarbro, M.H., Frogge, M. Goodman, & S.L. Groenwald (Eds.), *Cancer nursing: Principles and practice* (5th ed., pp. 1298–1328). Sudbury, MA: Jones and Bartlett.

Jett, J.R., Scott, W.J., Rivera, M.P., & Sause, W.T. (2003). Guidelines on treatment of stage IIIB non-small cell lung cancer. *Chest, 123*(Suppl. 1), 221S–225S.

Johnson, B.E. (1995). Biologic and molecular prognostic factors-impact on treatment of patients with non-small cell lung cancer. *Chest, 107*(Suppl. 6), 287S–290S.

Johnson, D.H. (2000). Evolution of cisplatin-based chemotherapy in non-small cell lung cancer: A historical perspective and the Eastern Cooperative Oncology Group Experience. *Chest, 117*(4 Suppl. 1), 133S–137S.

Johnson, D.H., & Turrisi, A.T. (2000). Combined modality treatment for locally advanced unresectable non-small cell lung cancer. In H.I. Pass, J.B. Mitchell, D.B. Johnson, A.T. Turrisi, & J.D. Minna (Eds.), *Lung cancer: Principles and practice* (2nd ed., pp. 910–920). Philadelphia: Lippincott Williams & Wilkins.

Joyce, M., & Houlihan, N. (2001). Current strategies in the diagnosis and treatment of lung cancer. In S.M. Hubbard, M. Goodman, & M.T. Knobf (Eds.), *Oncology nursing updates, 8*(2), 1–15.

Karnofsky, D.A., & Burchenal, J.H. (1949). The clinical evaluation of chemotherapeutic agents in cancer. In C. MacLeod (Ed.), *Evaluation of chemotherapeutic agents* (pp. 191–205). New York: Columbia University Press.

Keller, S.M., Adak, S., Wagner, H., & Johnson, D.H. (2000). Mediastinal lymph node dissection improves survival in patients with stages II and IIIA non small cell lung cancer. *Annals of Thoracic Surgery, 70,* 358–365.

Kelly, K. (2000). Future directions for new cytotoxic agents in the treatment of advanced stage non-small cell lung cancer. In American Society of Clinical Oncology (Ed.), *American Society of Clinical Oncology 2000 educational book. Thirty-sixth annual meeting* (pp. 357–367). Alexandria, VA: Author.

Kris, M.G., Natale, R.B., Herbst, R.S., Lunch, T.J., Prager, D., Belani, C.P., et al. (2002). A phase II trial of ZD1839 (Iressa) in advanced non-small cell lung cancer (NSCLC) patients who had failed platinum and docetaxel based regimens (IDEAL II) [Abstract]. *Proceedings of the American Society of Clinical Oncology, 12,* 292.

Lau, C.L., D'Amico, T.A., & Harpole, D.H. (2000). Clinical and molecular prognostic factors and models for non-small cell lung cancer. In H.I. Pass, J.B. Mitchell, D.B. Johnson, A.T. Turrisi, & J.D. Minna (Eds.), *Lung cancer: Principles and practice* (2nd ed., pp. 602–611). Philadelphia: Lippincott Williams & Wilkins.

Lau, C.L., Moore, M.B.H., Brooks, K.R., D'Amico, T.A., & Harpole D.H. (2002). Molecular staging of lung and esophageal cancer. *Surgical Clinics of North America, 82,* 497–523.

Liptay, M.J., Masters, G.A., Winchester, D.J., Edelman, B.L., Garrido, B.J., Hirschtritt, T.R., et al. (2000). Intraoperative radioisotope sentinel lymph node mapping in non-small cell lung cancer. *Annals of Thoracic Surgery, 70,* 384–389.

Little, A.G., DeHoyos, A., Kirgan, D.M., Arcomano, T.R., & Murray, K.D. (1999). Intraoperative lymphatic mapping for non-small cell lung cancer: The sentinel node technique. *Thoracic and Cardiovascular Surgery, 117,* 220–234.

MacManus, M.P. (2003). The role of positron emission tomography in the prognosis and in restaging of non-small cell lung cancer. In American Society of Clinical Oncology (Ed.), *American Society of Clinical Oncology 2003 educational book* (pp. 790–796). Alexandria, VA: Author.

Maher, K.E. (2000). Radiation therapy: Toxicities and management. In C.H. Yarbro, M.H., Frogge, M. Goodman, & S.L. Groenwald (Eds.), *Cancer nursing: Principles and practice* (5th ed., pp. 1298–1328). Sudbury, MA: Jones and Bartlett.

Martel, M., TenHaken, R., & Hazuda, M. (1999). Estimation of tumor control probability model parameters from 3-D dose distributions of non small cell lung cancer patients. *Lung Cancer, 24,* 31–37.

Martinez, F.J., Iannettoni, M., & Paine, R. (2000). Medical evaluation and management of the lung cancer patient prior to surgery, radiation, or chemotherapy. In H.I. Pass, J.B. Mitchell, D.B. Johnson, A.T. Turrisi, & J.D. Minna (Eds.), *Lung cancer: Principles and practice* (2nd ed., pp. 602–611), Philadelphia: Lippincott Williams & Wilkins.

Martini, N. (1993). Operable lung cancer. *CA: A Journal for Clinicians, 43,* 201–214.

Martini, N., & Ginsberg, R.J. (2002). Lobectomy. In F.G. Pearson, J.D. Cooper, J. Deslauriers, R.J. Ginsberg, C.A. Hiebert, G.A. Patterson, et al. (Eds.), *Thoracic surgery* (pp. 981–990). New York: Churchill Livingstone.

Martini, N., Kris, M.G., Flehinger, B.J., Gralla, R.J., Bains, M.S., Burt, M.E., et al. (1993). Preoperative chemotherapy for stage IIIA (N2) lung cancer: The Memorial Sloan-Kettering experience with 136 patients. *Annals of Thoracic Surgery, 55,* 1365–1374.

Miller, V.A., Patel, J., Shah, N., Kris, M.G., Tyson, L., Pizzo, B., et al. (2003). The epidermal growth factor receptor tyrosine kinase inhibitor Erlotinib (OSI-774) shows promising activity in patients with bronchioloalveolar cell carcinoma (BAC): Preliminary results of a phase II trial [Abstract]. *Proceedings of the American Society of Clinical Oncology, 22,* 2491.

Moore-Higgs, G.J. (2003). New advances in radiotherapy for lung cancer. In M. Haas (Ed.), *Contemporary issues in lung cancer: A nursing perspective* (pp. 83–91). Sudbury, MA: Jones and Bartlett.

Mountain, C.F. (1997). Revisions in the international system for staging lung cancer. *Chest, 111,* 1710–1717.

Mountain, C.F., Libshitz, H.I., & Hermes, K.E. (1999). *Lung cancer. A handbook for staging, imaging, and lymph node classification.* Houston: The Clifton F. Mountain Foundation, Charles P. Young Company.

Naruke, T., Goya, T., Tsuchiya, R., & Suemasu, K. (1988). Prognosis and survival in resected lung carcinoma based on the new international staging system. *Thoracic and Cardiovascular Surgery, 96,* 440–447.

Nesbitt, J.C., Putnam, J.B., Walsh, G.L., Roth, J.A., & Mountain, C.F. (1995). Survival in early-stage non-small cell lung cancer. *Annals of Thoracic Surgery, 60,* 466–472.

Non-Small Cell Lung Cancer Collaborative Group. (1995). Chemotherapy in non small cell lung cancer: A meta-analysis using updated data on individual patients from 52 randomized clinical trials. *British Medical Journal, 311,* 899–909.

Okamoto, I., Fujii, K., Matsumoto, M., Terasaki, Y., Kihara, N., Kohrogi, H., et al. (2003). Diffuse alveolar damage after ZD1839 in a patient with non-small cell lung cancer. *Lung Cancer, 40,* 339–342.

Padilla, J., Calvo, V., Penalver, J.C., Zarza, A.G., Pastor, J., Blasco, E., et al. (2002). Survival and risk model for stage IB non-small cell lung cancer. *Lung Cancer, 36,* 43–48.

Pearson, F.G. (1994). Current status of surgical resection for lung cancer. *Chest, 106*(Suppl. 6), 337S–339S.

Pisters, K.M.W., Ginsberg, R.J., Giroux, D.J., Putnam, J.B., Kris, M.G., Johnson, D.H., et al. (2000). Induction chemotherapy before surgery for early-stage lung cancer: A novel approach. *Journal of Thoracic and Cardiovascular Surgery, 119,* 429–439.

PORT Meta-Analysis Trialists Group. (1998). Postoperative radiotherapy in non small cell lung cancer: Systematic review and meta-analysis of individual patient data from nine randomized controlled trials. *Lancet, 352*(9124), 257–263.

Quinn, K.L. (2003). Managing patients through thoracic surgery. In M. Haas (Ed.), *Contemporary issues in lung cancer: A nursing perspective* (pp. 33–48). Sudbury, MA: Jones and Bartlett.

Rieger, P.T. (2001). The future of cancer therapy. In P.T. Rieger (Ed.), *Biotherapy: A comprehensive review* (pp. 669–699). Sudbury, MA: Jones and Bartlett.

Robinson, L.A., Wagner, H., & Ruckdeschel, J.C. (2003). Treatment of stage IIIA non-small cell lung cancer. *Chest, 123*(Suppl. 1), 202S–220S.

Rosell, R., Li, S., Skacel, Z., Mate, J.L., Maestre, J., Canela, M., et al. (1993). Prognostic impact of mutated *k-ras* gene in surgically resected non-small cell lung cancer patients. *Oncogene, 8,* 2407–2412.

Ross, J. (2003). Biology of lung cancer. In M.L. Haas (Ed.), *Contemporary issues in lung cancer: A nursing perspective* (pp. 11–23). Sudbury, MA: Jones and Bartlett.

Rusch, V.W., Albain, K.S., Crowley, J.J., Rice, T.W., Lonchyna, V., McKenna, R., Jr., et al. (1993). Surgical resection of stage IIIA and IIIB non small cell lung cancer after concurrent induction chemoradiotherapy. *Journal of Thoracic and Cardiovascular Surgery, 105,* 97–104.

Salgia, R., & Skarin, A.T. (1998). Molecular abnormalities in lung cancer. *Journal of Clinical Oncology, 16,* 1207–1217.

Sause, W., Kolesar, P., Taylor, S., Johnson, D., Livingston, R., Komaki, R., et al. (2000). Final results on phase III trial in regionally advanced unresectable non-small cell lung cancer. *Chest, 117,* 358–364.

Schiller, J.H., Harrington, D., Belani, C.P., Langer, C., Sandler, A., Krook, J., et al. (2002). Comparison of four chemotherapy regimens for advanced non-small-cell lung cancer. *New England Journal of Medicine, 346,* 92–98.

Scott, W.J., Howington, J., Movsas, B., & American College of Chest Physicians. (2003). Treatment of stage II non-small cell lung cancer. *Chest, 123*(1 Suppl.), 188S–201S.

Shah, N.T., Miller, V.A., Kris, M.G., Patel, J., Venkatraman, E., Benporat, L., et al. (2003). Bronchioloalveolar histology and smoking history predict response to gefitinib [Abstract]. *Proceedings of the American Society of Clinical Oncology, 22,* 2524.

Shaw, G.L., Gazdar, A.F., Phelps, R., Linnoila, R.I., Ihde, D.C., Johnson, B.E., et al. (1993). Individualized chemotherapy for patients with non-small cell lung cancer specimens: Cancer determined by prospective identification of neuroendocrine markers and *in vitro* drug sensitivity testing. *Cancer Research, 53,* 5181–5187.

Shepherd, F.A., Dancey, J., Ramlau, R., Mattson, K., Grall, R., O'Rourke, M., et al. (2000). Prospective randomized trial of docetaxel versus best supportive care in patients with non-small cell lung cancer previously treated with platinum-based chemotherapy. *Journal of Clinical Oncology, 18,* 2095–2103.

Silvestri, G.A., Handy, J., Lackland, D., Corley, E., & Reed, C.E. (1998). Specialists achieve better outcomes than generalists for lung cancer surgery. *Chest, 114,* 675–680.

Smith, I.E., O'Brien, M.E.R., Talbot, D.C., Nicolson, M.C., Mansi, J.L., Hickish, T.F., et al. (2001). Duration of chemotherapy in advanced non-small cell lung cancer: A randomized trial of three vs six courses of mitomycin, vinblastine, and cisplatin. *Journal of Clinical Oncology, 19,* 1336–1334.

Smythe, W.R. & American College of Chest Physicians. (2003). Treatment of stage I non-small cell lung carcinoma. *Chest, 123*(Suppl. 1), 181S–187S.

Socinski, M.A., Morris, D.E., Masters, G.A., & Lilenbaum, R. (2003). Chemotherapeutic management of stage IV non-small cell lung cancer. *Chest, 123*(Suppl. 1), 226S–243S.

Socinski, M.A., Schell, M.J., Peterman, A., Bakri, K., Yates, S., Gitten, R., et al. (2002). A phase III trial comparing a defined duration of therapy vs continuous therapy followed by second-line therapy in advanced stage IIIB-IV non-small cell lung cancer. *Journal of Clinical Oncology, 20,* 1335–1343.

Speiser, B.L., & Kresl, J.J. (2000). Endobronchial and interstitial brachytherapy. In H.L. Pass, J.B. Mitchell, D.H. Johnson, & A.T. Turissi (Eds.), *Lung cancer: Principles and practice* (2nd ed., pp. 775–789). Philadelphia: Lippincott Williams & Wilkins.

Thomas, M. (2003). Advances in chemotherapy. In M. Haas (Ed.), *Contemporary issues in lung cancer: A nursing perspective* (pp. 49–82). Sudbury, MA: Jones and Bartlett.

Toloza, E.M., Roth, J.A., & Swisher, S.G. (2000). Molecular events in bronchogenic carcinoma and their implications for therapy. *Seminars in Surgical Oncology, 18,* 143–151.

Travis, W.D., Colby, T.V., Corrin, B., Shimosato, Y., & Brambilla, E. (1999). *Histological typing of lung and pleural tumors* (3rd ed.). Berlin: Springer Verlag.

Travis, W.D., Linder, J., & Mackay, B. (2000). Classification, histology, cytology, and electron microscopy. In H.L. Pass, J.B. Mitchell, D.H. Johnson, & A.T. Turissi (Eds.), *Lung cancer: Principles and practice* (2nd ed., pp. 453–495). Philadelphia: Lippincott William & Wilkins.

Tsuchiya, R. (2002). Bronchoplastic techniques. In F.G. Pearson, J.D. Cooper, J. Deslauriers, R.J. Ginsberg, C.A. Hiebert, G.A. Patterson, et al. (Eds.), *Thoracic surgery* (pp. 1005–1013). New York: Churchill Livingstone.

Veale, D., Kerr, N., Gibson, G.J., Kelly, P.J., & Harris, A.L. (1993). The relationship of quantitative epidermal growth factor receptor expression in non-small cell lung cancer to long term survival. *British Journal of Cancer, 63,* 130–133.

Wall, L.M. (2000). Changes in hope and power in lung cancer patients who exercise. *Nursing Science Quarterly, 13,* 234–242.

Waters, P.F. (2002). Surgical techniques pneumonectomy. In F.G. Pearson, J.D. Cooper, J. Deslauriers, R.J. Ginsberg, C.A. Hiebert, G.A. Patterson, et al. (Eds.), *Thoracic surgery* (pp. 974–981). New York: Churchill Livingstone.

Weisenburger, T.H. (2002). Radiotherapy for non-small cell lung cancer. In F.G. Pearson, J.D. Cooper, J. Deslauriers, R.J. Ginsberg, C.A. Hiebert, G.A. Patterson, et al. (Eds.), *Thoracic surgery* (pp. 874–883). New York: Churchill Livingstone.

Wu, Y.L., Huang, Z.F., Wang, S.Y., Yang, X.N., & Ou, W. (2002). A randomized trial of systematic nodal dissection in resectable non-small cell lung cancer. *Lung Cancer, 36,* 1–6.

Yarbro, C.H., Frogge, M.H., & Goodman, M. (Eds.). (2004). *Cancer symptom management* (3rd ed.). Sudbury, MA: Jones and Bartlett.

Yim, A.P.C. (2002). Video-assisted pulmonary resections. In F.G. Pearson, J.D. Cooper, J. Deslauriers, R.J. Ginsberg, C.A. Hiebert, G.A. Patterson, et al. (Eds.), *Thoracic surgery* (pp. 1073–1084). New York: Churchill Livingstone.

Zimmerman, P.V., Bint, M.H., Hawson, G.A.T., & Parsons, P.G. (1987). Ploidy as a prognostic determinant in surgically treated lung cancer. *Lancet, 2*(8558), 530.

CHAPTER 9

Symptom Management of Lung Cancer

Nancy G. Houlihan, RN, MA, AOCN®, Dana Inzeo, RN, MA, AOCN®,
Margaret Joyce, MSN, RN, AOCN®, and Leslie B. Tyson, MS, ANP-C, OCN®

Introduction

Managing the symptoms of the patient with cancer is key to an overall positive treatment outcome. Supportive interventions for specific side effects of therapy help to ensure safety, survival, and maintenance of a satisfactory quality of life (QOL). Since the late 1980s, much research has gone into the development of supportive measures for the management of disease and treatment-related symptoms. Oncology nurses have partnered with their colleagues in the search for evidence to better manage the care of patients. The result is a growing body of standards and guidelines for the supportive care of people undergoing treatment for cancer.

Symptom management is particularly poignant for those with lung cancer. The majority of patients have some symptoms at the time of diagnosis (Kvale, Simoff, & Prakash, 2003). Although treatment may relieve disease-related symptoms, treatment-related side effects result. As patients move through the continuum of the disease from aggressive therapies to palliative care, the focus of the interventions may change, but the significance of controlling symptoms remains constant. The most commonly occurring symptoms are cough, hemoptysis, dyspnea, fatigue, and pain (Hollen, Gralla, Kris, Eberly, & Potanovich, 1993). This chapter will review these most common symptoms and the related interventions. As most of the treatment side effects from chemotherapy are not specific to lung cancer, we have limited this section to thoracic radiation-induced symptoms.

Cough

Cough is one of the most frequent and distressing symptoms in patients with lung cancer. Technically, cough is a protective mechanism that allows people to clear secretions and inhaled particles from the airways; "pathologic cough" is the result of a disease process (McDermott, 2000). Chronic cough is defined as a cough that lasts longer than three weeks

(McDermott). In patients who are current or previous smokers, cough that occurs for the first time and lasts for months or cough that changes in character may suggest bronchogenic carcinoma (Irwin et al., 1998). Cough is estimated to occur in up to 65% of patients as the initial manifestation of lung cancer (Kvale et al., 2003). Approximately 70%–90% of patients with lung carcinoma will develop cough at some time during the course of their illness (Irwin et al.). Complications of cough include musculoskeletal pain, rib fractures, hemoptysis, fatigue, and insomnia.

The cough reflex consists of three phases. The first phase occurs with deep inspiration. This is followed by closure of the glottis with a rapid increase in pleural pressure, marking the second phase of the reflex. The final phase involves the opening of the glottis with a rapid release of the pleural pressure (McDermott, 2000). The cough reflex is initiated by stimulation of neural mucosal receptors located within the nasopharynx, larynx, trachea, and bronchial tree (McDermott). The neural mucosal receptors are stimulated by mechanical or chemical irritants, resulting in transmission of impulses via cranial nerves IX and X to the cough center in the medulla. Once the cough center is stimulated, cough occurs from the forceful contraction of the diaphragm and other expiratory muscles in the chest (McDermott).

Cough from lung cancer is more likely to occur in patients with tumors of the central airways, such as squamous cell carcinoma and small cell lung cancer. Tumors in the central airways can cause obstruction, either from intraluminal growth of tumor or extraluminal compression of the airways, and this almost always leads to dyspnea and cough (Kvale et al., 2003). Adenocarcinoma usually presents as a peripheral lesion and is, therefore, less often associated with cough; however, cough can be caused by tumor involvement of any part of the respiratory tract. Other causes of cough in patients with lung cancer include recent upper respiratory tract infection, pleural or pericardial effusion, radiation pneumonitis, vocal cord paralysis, and aspiration. Other causes of cough that are not related to cancer include asthma, postnasal drip, gastroesophageal reflux disease (GERD), chronic obstructive pulmonary disease (COPD), congestive heart failure (CHF), and medications, such as angiotensin converting enzyme (ACE) inhibitors. Cough may be dry or associated with production of sputum.

To treat cough adequately, the cause must be determined. A thorough history and physical exam will help to determine the cause. The cough history should include onset, duration, and precipitating factors; presence or absence of sputum production and the color and odor (if any) of sputum; and current medications. The history also should include the presence or absence of any other illnesses or conditions that can cause cough (e.g., asthma, COPD, GERD), occupational or environmental exposure to irritants, and smoking history. Physical exam focuses primarily on the upper and lower respiratory tract. The oropharynx may reveal the presence of mucus, erythema, or a "cobblestone" appearance of the mucosa, which suggests postnasal drip (McDermott, 2000). Examination of the chest and lungs may reveal signs of pleural or pericardial effusion, pneumonia, or airway obstruction. When auscultating the lungs, listen for wheezing or other adventitious sounds and the presence or absence of breath sounds. The presence of stridor on inspiration suggests airway obstruction. Percussion of the chest may reveal areas of dullness, which can be seen with pneumonia or pleural effusion. Jugular venous distension, wet crackles at lung bases, and an S3 gallop suggest CHF. Observation of the respiratory rate, presence or absence of peripheral edema, and vital signs, including temperature, also are important. Diagnostic tests include evaluation of sputum, if present; radiologic tests, such as computed tomography (CT) or chest x-ray; pulmonary function testing; and bronchoscopy.

As noted earlier, treatment of cough consists of treating the underlying cause. Treatment of postnasal drip includes antihistamines, intranasal steroids, and inhalers, such as Atrovent® (3M Pharmaceuticals, St. Paul, MN). Cough from postnasal drip should subside within days to weeks with the above treatment. Cough from GERD may respond to change in lifestyle and addition of H_2 antagonists. Bronchodilators and corticosteroids may be helpful in management of cough from COPD. If infection is suspected, a course of antibiotics is indicated. Cough from ACE inhibitors usually occurs within the first few weeks of treatment and resolves with discontinuation of the drug.

If cough is caused by central airway obstruction from tumor, bronchoscopic therapies using a rigid bronchoscope may provide relief. The rigid bronchoscope can be used to examine the airways, place a stent to open an obstructed airway, and facilitate laser resection of obstructing tumor (Kvale et al., 2003). In patients with lung cancer, these procedures usually are considered palliative and may not entirely relieve cough. Cough from pleural or pericardial effusion may be helped by removal of fluid.

Pharmacotherapy and promotion of comfort is the mainstay of treatment for patients with cough from advanced bronchogenic carcinoma. In patients in whom cough is the presenting symptom from disease in the airway, treatment with chemotherapy may lead to reduction in tumor and, therefore, reduction in cough. In these patients, return of cough often signals progression of disease. Pharmacologic management includes the use of nonopioid cough suppressants, bronchodilators, corticosteroids, and opioids. The most commonly used nonopioid antitussive agent is dextromethorphan; it is available over the counter and comes in pill or liquid form. It often is available in combination with guaifenesin (e.g., Humibid DM® [Adams Laboratories, Ft. Worth, TX], Robitussin® [Wyeth Consumer Healthcare, Madison, NJ]), which is used as both an expectorant and antitussive. These agents are often of little value in patients with cough from advanced cancer. Benzonatate (Tessalon Perles® [Forest Pharmaceuticals, St. Louis, MO]) has been shown to be helpful for some (Doona & Walsh, 1998). Benzonatate is a peripherally acting drug that is available by prescription. The recommended dose is 100–200 mg, three times a day. In patients in whom bronchospasm plays a role in cough, bronchodilator therapy using inhaled ipratropium (Atrovent) has been shown to be helpful. To date, no studies have documented the role of corticosteroids in the management of cough from cancer; however, if cough is related to effects of radiation therapy (e.g., radiation pneumonitis), corticosteroids may be helpful (Kvale et al., 2003).

Opioids are currently the best available treatment for intractable cough from lung cancer. The recent American College of Chest Physicians guidelines recommend the use of opioids in the management of cough (Kvale et al., 2003). The most commonly used opioid is codeine; it is a centrally acting agent. Codeine is available in both tablet and liquid form. Low doses (10–20 mg, every 4–6 hours) are often sufficient for cough suppression (McDermott, 2000). Hydrocodone is also available in tablet or liquid form and is a good alternative to codeine or in patients who cannot tolerate codeine. The lowest effective dose of opioids should be used, and caution is recommended with use of increasing doses, as respiratory depression and hypoventilation can occur.

Other measures, such as deep breathing exercises and effective coughing, may relieve symptoms and can be taught (Ingle, 2000). Patients who smoke cigarettes should be encouraged to stop. Air humidifiers may be helpful in the management of cough in a dry environment. Warm, humidified air decreases the viscosity of secretions, which also can be helpful for cough.

Hemoptysis

Hemoptysis is the expectoration of blood and results from bleeding in the lower respiratory tract. The blood may or may not be mixed with sputum. Hemoptysis is the initial presenting symptom in an estimated 7%–35% of patients with lung cancer. It is estimated to occur in 20% of patients with lung cancer at some point during the course of the illness, and approximately 3% will die of massive hemoptysis (Beckles, Spiro, Colice, & Rudd, 2003; Kvale et al., 2003). The severity of hemoptysis is determined by the amount of blood that is coughed up. Patients who expectorate 100–600 ml of blood in 24 hours are considered to have massive hemoptysis (Kvale et al.). Hemoptysis is one of the most frightening and distressing symptoms associated with lung cancer.

The blood supply to the lungs comes from a dual supply. The pulmonary circulation system contains both arteries and veins, and it serves the function of oxygenation and elimination of carbon dioxide from the body (Guimarães, 2002). The pulmonary artery and its branches supply 95% of the blood and are a low-pressure system (Beers & Berkow, 1999). The bronchial system is a high-pressure system supplying 5% of the blood (mostly to the airways and supporting structures) and originating from the aorta (Beers & Berkow). The normal anatomy of the lung predisposes itself to the symptom of hemoptysis (Henke, 2000). This includes the close anatomic relationship of blood vessels and airways and the presence of the alveolar-capillary membrane (where the exchange of gasses between alveoli and capillaries takes place). Hemoptysis can occur from bleeding at any level in the system but most often occurs from the bronchial system (Henke).

Hemoptysis has multiple noncancerous causes, including infection (e.g., pneumonia, abscess, aspergillosis, tuberculosis), CHF, pulmonary embolism, chronic bronchitis, and pulmonary edema. In patients with lung cancer, hemoptysis can occur as a result of tumor erosion of a blood vessel. A recent retrospective analysis at a tertiary referral hospital documented the diagnosis and severity of hemoptysis in 208 patients (Hirshberg, Biran, Glazer, & Kramer, 1997). Of the 208 patients evaluated, lung cancer was the cause in 39. Bronchiectasis was the most frequent diagnosis, occurring in 41 patients. Bronchitis and pneumonia occurred in 37 and 33 patients, respectively. The most common primary lung cancer associated with hemoptysis in this review was small cell lung cancer. The majority of patients had moderate hemoptysis caused from bronchitis and lung cancer. Moderate hemoptysis in this study was defined as less than 500 ml of blood expectorated in 24 hours.

Hemoptysis usually is easily distinguished from hematemesis. However, distinguishing hemoptysis from epistaxis (i.e., bleeding from the gums or nasopharynx) can be more difficult, necessitating a careful history (Guimarães, 2002). The history should include the amount and color of the blood; the duration of the bleeding; the presence of clots; the relationship of bleeding to rest or activity; the presence of chest pain, cough, or dyspnea; prior history of heart and lung diseases; and history of cigarette smoking. Additionally, a careful medication history should be ascertained, as aspirin, non-steroidal anti-inflammatory drugs, and anticoagulant medicines all can cause bleeding. Diagnostic tests include labora-

tory exams, chest x-ray, CT scan, and bronchoscopy. Laboratory tests should include a complete blood count to determine if anemia is present and check platelet count. Coagulation tests include prothrombin time and partial thromboplastin time. Chest x-ray may reveal pulmonary infiltrates, a cavitary lesion, or atelectasis. A normal chest x-ray does not rule out pulmonary pathology as a source of bleeding (Guimarães). A CT scan or perfusion scanning also may reveal a source of bleeding, such as a pulmonary embolus or air bronchograms. Air bronchograms suggest obstruction, bronchiectasis, and chronic bronchitis, all potential causes of hemoptysis.

The most useful exam in patients who have hemoptysis is bronchoscopy. Bronchoscopy can reveal the source of bleeding and provide the physician with a means of intervention at the time of the procedure. The rigid bronchoscope is preferred, as the lumen is wide enough for suctioning of blood and debris, ventilation of the nonbleeding lung, and use of endoscopic procedures to control bleeding (Guimarães, 2002).

Treatment of hemoptysis depends on the cause of bleeding and the amount of blood that is coughed up. For most patients, hemoptysis stops spontaneously. In those with recurrent hemoptysis or those who expectorate larger amounts of blood, bronchoscopy usually is needed to identify and treat the source of bleeding. Multiple methods of "local control" to stop bleeding from endobronchial lesions are available, and all require an endoscopic procedure. In patients in whom bronchoscopy reveals visible bleeding but no identifiable lesion, endoscopic measures, such as instillation of epinephrine solution, iced saline solution, and balloons, may be used (Kvale et al., 2003). Balloon tamponade has been shown to be effective in management of massive hemoptysis (Guimarães, 2002).

Electrocautery involves the use of electrical current to produce coagulation and vaporization of bleeding in endobronchial lesions (Prakash, 1999). Disadvantages of electrocautery include endobronchial fire, hemorrhage, and inadvertent shock to the operator or patient (Prakash). Argon plasma coagulation (APC) is a newer modality and a type of noncontact electrocautery (Morice, Ece, Ece, & Keus, 2001). A recently published study utilizing APC for control of hemoptysis and neoplastic airway obstruction showed that immediate, complete control of hemoptysis was accomplished in all patients with no recurrence of hemoptysis for a mean follow-up time of 97 +/– 91.9 days (Morice et al.). Nd:YAG laser is another older type of noncontact electrocautery; photocoagulation has been shown to be helpful in controlling bleeding in approximately 60% of patients (Hetzel & Smith, 1991). Each procedure has its advantages and disadvantages; the newer APC is associated with less risk of endobronchial fire and no risk of retinal injury, compared with Nd:YAG laser (Dumon, Shapshay, & Bourcerau, 1984; Geffin, Shapshay, & Bellack, 1980; Guimarães, 2002).

Photodynamic therapy (PDT) is another newer modality used in the palliative management of hemoptysis (Birn &

Kosco, 2004). PDT also requires endoscopy; it uses lasers to activate light-sensitive pharmaceuticals to treat the lesion. PDT requires IV administration of Photofrin® (Sanofi Pharmaceuticals Inc., New York, NY), a photosensitive antineoplastic agent, 40–50 hours before the endoscopic procedure. A nonthermal laser light is used to activate the pharmaceutical agent. Approximately 24–72 hours later, another bronchoscopy is required to remove necrotic debris and perform another treatment if needed. The primary adverse effect of PDT is photosensitivity. Patients need to protect themselves from the sun or bright lights for 4–6 weeks after therapy with PDT. Outdoor activities should occur after sundown, as sunscreens do not provide adequate protection (Birn & Kosco). If an endobronchial lesion is visible and is determined not to be resectable or amenable to one of the aforementioned treatments, a course of external beam radiation therapy is recommended (Kvale et al., 2003).

Conservative management is preferred in patients with advanced cancer and small amounts of hemoptysis (30–50 ml/day) (Henke, 2000; Ingle, 2000). Because infection is one cause of hemoptysis, a course of oral antibiotics should be started. Additionally, cough suppression with an opioid (codeine) given around the clock will help to minimize irritation. For many patients, hemoptysis can be managed successfully with the above regimen on an outpatient basis.

Although massive hemoptysis is rare, death from massive hemoptysis in patients with bronchogenic carcinoma is estimated at 59%–100% (Corey & Hla, 1987). Surgical management usually is not an option because the majority of patients have advanced disease. Intervention, if undertaken, usually begins with endotracheal intubation to maintain an adequate airway and measures to prevent asphyxiation. Some of the previously described endoscopic procedures have been used with success. Bronchial artery embolization via endoscopy also can be used (Guimarães, 2002). Other emergency and supportive care measures are used, as well. Hospitalization is recommended; the patient should lie with the bleeding lung dependent and in the Trendelenberg position to prevent aspiration of blood into the opposite lung (Guimarães). Blood transfusions, oxygen supplementation, and antitussive agents also may be used as needed. Overall, the prognosis is poor in patients with bronchogenic carcinoma and massive hemoptysis and, as noted, the majority do not survive.

Dyspnea

Prevalence

Dyspnea is a complex and distressing symptom and a difficult clinical problem to manage. It is aligned closely with a primal fear of death by suffocation, and, hence, it evokes a response that begs intervention from patients, caregivers, and health professionals. Ripamonti and Fusco (2002) re-

ported that the prevalence of dyspnea in an advanced cancer population increases from 15%–55.5% at referral to palliative care service to 18%–79% during the last week of life. As expected, dyspnea is more common among patients with lung cancer than the cancer population in general. The prevalence of dyspnea in patients diagnosed with lung cancer ranges from 55%–87% (Dudgeon, Kristjanson, Sloan, Lertzman, & Clement, 2001; Muers & Round, 1993; Smith et al., 2001; Tanaka, Akechi, Okuyama, Nishiwaki, & Uchitomi, 2001).

In a survey of 120 outpatients with stages I–IV lung cancer that evaluated QOL, dyspnea, and the relationship between the variables, 87% of study participants experienced dyspnea. Patients with high dyspnea scores had lower QOL ($p = 0.04$) (Smith et al., 2001). Dudgeon et al. (2001) evaluated 923 patients with cancer in the outpatient setting to assess the intensity of their dyspnea. They found that 46% of the patients had some shortness of breath. Only 4% of this study's participants had a diagnosis of lung cancer, and, for that subgroup, 84% reported dyspnea. Muers and Round (1993) evaluated the presence and severity of 12 symptoms including dyspnea in a study of 289 patients with non-small cell lung cancer. Subjects were assessed at presentation and every two months for one year or until death. Cough and breathlessness were the two most prevalent symptoms. Breathlessness of any grade was present in 216 patients (75%). Severe breathlessness was present in 8%, moderate breathlessness in 33%, and mild breathlessness in 34% of the same 216 subjects. Lastly, in a study of 157 outpatients with advanced lung cancer, Tanaka et al. (2001) found that 55% of subjects reported "clinical dyspnea," defined as dyspnea interfering with at least one of the following seven categories: work, walking, general activities, sleep (which comprise the physical domain) and mood, relationships, and enjoyment (which comprise the psychological domain). Dyspnea interfered with not only the physical domain (52%) but also with the psychological domain (23%). Although this review is not exhaustive, it indicates that dyspnea is a prevalent symptom in patients with lung cancer; it interferes with QOL and has an impact on functional and emotional status.

Definition

The term *dyspnea* generally is applied to the sensations that individuals with unpleasant or uncomfortable respiration experience. The American Thoracic Society (ATS) (1999), in a comprehensive consensus statement, defined dyspnea as a subjective experience of breathing discomfort that consists of qualitatively distinct sensations that vary in intensity. The symptom derives from interactions among multiple physiologic, psychological, social, and environmental factors and may induce secondary physiologic and behavioral responses. This definition stresses the subjective and multifactorial nature of the dyspnea experience.

Pathophysiology of Dyspnea

A unifying theory is that dyspnea results from a disassociation or a mismatch between central respiratory motor activity and incoming afferent information from receptors in the airways, lungs, and chest wall structures. In other words, a mismatch occurs between the motor command and the mechanical response, which produces a sensation of respiratory discomfort (ATS, 1999).

ATS (1999) classified physiologic causes of dyspnea and alternative targets for treatment as
- Heightened ventilatory demand, as demonstrated when the intensity of dyspnea increases with exertion or exercise.
- Increased impedance or resistance to ventilation as noted when the respiratory effort expended is out of proportion to the resulting level of ventilation. Asthma and COPD can narrow airways increasing resistance to ventilation.
- Abnormalities of the respiratory muscles such as weakness or mechanical inefficiency. The pressure-generating capacity of the muscles is decreased, creating a mismatch between the central respiratory drive and achieved ventilation. Malnutrition from cancer cachexia reduces both respiratory muscle strength and maximal voluntary ventilation.
- Abnormal central perception of dyspnea caused from increased respiratory drive, as seen with blood gas abnormalities of hypoxia or hypercapnia.

Like pain, dyspnea has an affective component. The stimulus intensity of "just noticeable difference" for shortness of breath may be the same among patients with similar lung pathology; however, the affective component can vary greatly and actually modulate the intensity of the symptom (Carrieri-Kohlman, Gormley, Douglas, Paul, & Stulbarg, 1996). Hence, the threshold perception of dyspnea varies widely with individuals and is related only moderately to the degree of pulmonary dysfunction. Frequently, a discrepancy is found between severity of disease and intensity of breathing discomfort (ATS, 1999). Cognitive variables that have been shown to modify dyspnea include anxiety, depression (Dudley, Martin, & Holmes, 1964; Gift, 1991; Smith et al., 2001), personality (Chetta et al., 1998), and the meaning of the symptom for the person (Cioffi, 1991).

Etiology of Dyspnea

Dyspnea in lung cancer frequently has multiple etiologies. Possible causes of dyspnea in the general cancer population are listed in Figure 9-1. In addition to the effect of the primary lung tumor, a combination of other factors commonly contributes to dyspnea, depending on stage of disease. These include pleural effusion, anemia, cachexia, and underlying COPD. Many factors can converge to cause and contribute to the symptom of dyspnea.

Figure 9-1. Causes of Dyspnea in Patients With Cancer

Dyspnea caused directly by cancer
- Pulmonary parenchymal involvement (primary or metastatic)
- Lymphangitic carcinomatosis
- Intrinsic or extrinsic airway obstruction by tumor
- Pleural tumor
- Pleural effusion
- Pericardial effusion
- Ascites
- Hepatomegaly
- Phrenic nerve paralysis
- Multiple tumor microemboli
- Pulmonary leukostasis
- Superior vena cava syndrome

Dyspnea caused indirectly by cancer
- Cachexia
- Electrolyte abnormalities
- Anemia
- Pneumonia
- Pulmonary aspiration
- Pulmonary emboli
- Neurologic paraneoplastic syndromes

Dyspnea from cancer treatment
- Surgery
- Radiation pneumonitis or fibrosis
- Chemotherapy-induced pulmonary toxicity
- Chemotherapy-induced cardiomyopathy
- Radiation-induced pericardial disease

Dyspnea unrelated to cancer
- Chronic obstructive pulmonary disease
- Asthma
- Congestive heart failure
- Interstitial lung disease
- Pneumothorax
- Anxiety
- Chest wall deformity
- Obesity
- Neuromuscular disorders
- Pulmonary vascular disease

Note. From "Dyspnea in Cancer Patients: Prevalence and Associated Factors," by D.J. Dudgeon, L. Kristjanson, J.A. Sloan, M. Lertzmanm, and K. Clement, 2001, *Journal of Pain and Symptom Management, 21*, p. 100. Copyright 2001 by Elsevier. Reprinted with permission.

Assessment

Assessment of dyspnea is a nursing challenge, not only because of its multiple causes but also because of its subjective nature. One of the main problems is the variable intensity of dyspnea according to activity level and time of the day (Bruera & Ripamonti, 1998). Any assessment of dyspnea should attempt to differentiate the intensity or quality of the sensation and the emotional or behavioral response to the discomfort.

Several standardized assessment tools such as the Oxygen Cost Diagram, the Baseline Dyspnea Index, and the Borg scale exist to measure dyspnea (ATS, 1999). A simple visual analog scale, which consists of a 100-mm line with anchors at each end to indicate the extremes of "not breathless at all" to "very breathless," can be used. Scoring is accomplished by measuring the distance from the bottom or left of the scale if horizontally oriented to the level indicated by the patient.

The most common method to assess dyspnea in the clinical setting is self-report of the level of activity at which the patient has difficulty breathing. Common activities associated with dyspnea are climbing stairs or walking up hill, walking fast on level ground, and shortness of breath with dressing or talking. Shortness of breath at rest or with no activity is most dire. One potential limitation of this assessment is that because the intensity of dyspnea depends on the rate of work performance, patients may reduce the rate of work performance and, thereby, minimize the reported intensity of the symptom. For example, a person may report the ability to climb a flight of stairs without reporting the frequent rest stops to reduce symptoms.

An evaluation of dyspnea includes a complete history of the symptom, its temporal onset (acute or chronic), descriptors, precipitating and relieving events or activities and associated symptoms, and response to medication or behavioral changes (Ripamonti & Fusco, 2002). A dyspnea-focused physical examination includes complete vital signs (blood pressure, pulse, respiratory rate, and temperature) and observation of respiratory mechanics, such as pursed lip breathing or the use of accessory muscles. Notice the presence of pallor (relative absence of oxyhemoglobin with its characteristic red color) or cyanosis at the fingertips, lips, and oral mucosa. Clubbing of the fingers and toes can be seen in patients with chronic hypoxia. Cardiac assessment includes auscultation of heart sounds, palpation of the central pulses, and observation of jugular venous distention. Lung auscultation is performed to evaluate for absent breath sounds or the presence of rales, rhonchi, wheezes, or a rub. Lung field percussion is performed to locate areas of dullness. Respiratory excursion and fremitus are assessed. Mental status signs of hypoxia include restlessness, anxiety, disorientation, and confusion (Shepherd & Geraci, 1999).

Pertinent basic diagnostic testing includes pulse oximetry at rest and with activity, complete blood count, and chemistry panel. A chest radiograph may be indicated to evaluate for infiltrates, effusions, and pneumothorax as well as heart size and position. Pulmonary function tests that measure lung volumes and gas diffusion may be helpful to diagnose a reversible airway obstruction or hypoxemia, which can be improved with therapy. A ventilation-perfusion scan can be obtained if pulmonary embolus is suspected. The choice of appropriate diagnostic tests should be guided by the stage of disease, usefulness of the resultant information for therapeutic intervention, and the patient's wishes.

Considering the complex multidimensional nature of dyspnea, differentiating an acute and possibly reversible cause of dyspnea is important. Although dyspnea is usually a progressive complication of the lung cancer trajectory, some patients present with a sudden onset or acute exacerbation of shortness of breath. This could be considered a medical emergency depending on the presenting context and broad differential diagnosis possibilities.

Treatment of Dyspnea

The therapeutic goals in treating dyspnea are to promote patient comfort, increase exercise tolerance, and promote physical and social well-being (Carrieri & Janson-Bjerklie, 1986). Modest alterations in a number of physiologic and psychological variables, as a result of a particular treatment, can culminate in a clinically meaningful reduction in symptoms (ATS, 1999).

The optimal treatment of dyspnea is to treat reversible causes with specific therapies and to use nonspecific or symptomatic therapy to treat irreversible causes. The following therapy options are organized according to categorical causes of dyspnea: lung tumor, cancer therapy, indirect consequence of cancer diagnosis, and nonspecific palliative measures.

Dyspnea Caused by Tumor

If the lung tumor itself is causing shortness of breath, appropriate treatment with surgery, radiation, or chemotherapy will reduce symptoms. Even a minor response to oncologic therapy can improve dyspnea. Airway obstruction can be relieved with tracheobronchial stenting or laser ablation, or it can be palliated with either external beam radiotherapy or brachytherapy (Dudgeon, 2002).

Malignant pleural effusions can compromise respiration in some circumstances. Thoracentesis aimed at removing pleural fluid is beneficial in relieving dyspnea if the lung reexpands. In most instances, the pleural fluid reaccumulates shortly after thoracentesis. If relief is obtained with initial removal of fluid, pleural drainage with a chest tube and instillation of a sclerosing agent, such as talc, can be an effective method to prevent reaccumulation of pleural fluid and associated shortness of breath (see Table 9-1).

Dyspnea Caused by Therapy

Certain chemotherapy agents or chest radiation can cause either acute or chronic pneumonitis. Corticosteroids, usually prednisone starting at 60–100 mg daily and tapered over days to weeks, are the mainstay of treatment. Occasionally, supportive oxygen and bronchodilators are required (Dudgeon, 2002). Certain chemotherapeutic agents, such as doxorubicin, can cause cardiomyopathy with risk of CHF and shortness of breath. Conventional therapy for CHF and possibly cardiology consultation are indicated.

Table 9-1. Symptom Management of Lung Cancer

Symptom	Cause	Signs and Symptoms	Management
Cough	Airway obstruction by tumor Gastroesophageal reflux disease Postnasal drip Smoking	Frequent and associated with distress Productive or nonproductive	Pharmacologic: Cough suppressants (opioids and nonopioids), corticosteroids, and bronchodilators Air humidifiers, fans Breathing exercises with effective cough instruction Smoking cessation
Hemoptysis	Tumor invasion of vasculature Inflammation from pneumonia, bronchitis, or bronchiectasis Bleeding diathesis Congestive heart failure	Coughed up blood in sputum • Mild: 30–50 ml per day • Moderate: 500 ml in 24 hours • Massive: more than 500 ml in 24 hours	Pharmacologic: Cough suppressants, codeine, antibiotics Bronchoscopy with laser, instillation of epinephrine solution, iced saline, balloon Intubation and palliative care
Dyspnea	Airway obstruction Pleural effusion Anemia Cachexia Underlying chronic obstructive pulmonary disease	Tachypnea Tachycardia O_2 saturation level low Pursed lip breathing Use of accessory muscles Decreased or absent breath sounds, rales, rhonchi, wheeze, or rub Excursion or fremitus Pallor Cyanosis Clubbing of fingers or toes Activity intolerance Mental status changes	Treat the cause (cancer therapy). • Administer oxygen. • Administer medications such as corticosteroids, bronchodilators, antibiotics, or opioids. • Transfuse with blood products or treat anemia with epoetin alfa. • Drain effusions. • Assess activity tolerance and plan activities. • Teach coping strategies. • Assess and treat anxiety.
Fatigue	Disease: Dyspnea, pain, emotional distress, sleep disturbance, paraneoplastic syndromes Pain medications Treatment (radiation and chemotherapy) Anemia Cachexia and anorexia	Patient complaint Activity intolerance Anxiety, depression Cognitive dysfunction	Pharmacologic: Epoetin alfa, iron supplements, psychostimulants, antidepressants, corticosteroids Behavioral: Activity planning, psychosocial referral, restorative interventions, sleep interventions, dietary restrictions
Pain	Tumor location and nerve involvement (Pancoast tumor or brachial plexus, pleural effusion, or chest wall invasion) Metastatic involvement (back pain related to spinal cord compression, bone pain, headache, or abdominal pain) Treatment-related: Surgery or procedures (incisional), peripheral neuropathies from chemotherapy	Patient complaint Activity intolerance Anxiety, depression	Treat the cause (cancer therapy). • Assess at each visit for location, quality, intensity, relieving and aggravating factors, satisfaction with control. • Administer medications such as opioids, nonsteroidal anti-inflammatory drugs, corticosteroids, diphosphonates, adjuvants. • Manage side effects of medications. • Consider appropriate alternative interventions such as nerve block, massage, acupuncture, or distraction. • Educate patient and caretaker about use of interventions.

(Continued on next page)

Table 9-1. Symptom Management of Lung Cancer (Continued)

Symptom	Cause	Signs and Symptoms	Management
Esophagitis	Radiation to lungs	Dysphagia Odynophagia Reflux Epigastric pain	Pharmacologic: Oral analgesics before eating ("magic mouthwash," Lortab® [Whitby Pharmaceutical, Richmond, VA] Rothwell's solution), opioids, antifungals Dietary: Soft, bland, high-calorie diet; thick, soft foods and fluids; avoid alcohol and tobacco Behavioral: Use straw to drink, eat slowly, chew completely, cut foods into small pieces, take antacids before eating, maintain hydration.
Pneumonitis	Radiation to lungs	Dyspnea Cough Fever Night sweats Low O_2 saturation	Pharmacologic: Corticosteroids, antibiotics, bronchodilators, sedatives, oxygen

Dyspnea as an Indirect Consequence of Cancer

Many complications of chronic illness can occur that cause or contribute to dyspnea. Some common situations encountered in lung cancer are pneumonia and anemia. Pneumonia can be treated with adequate antibiotic therapy and lead to relief of dyspnea. If appropriate to the patient's condition, anemia can be resolved with red cell transfusions or erythropoietin therapy. Short- and long-term benefits can be realized with improved function and comfort. Malnutrition, mineral and electrolyte deficiencies, and overall deconditioning also can contribute to dyspnea. Again, depending on the patient's status, attempts to correct these circumstances may improve dyspnea control.

Nonspecific Treatments of Dyspnea

Symptomatic management of dyspnea is based on three main elements: oxygen therapy, pharmacologic therapy, and general support measures and education. Usually a combination of these interventions is employed.

Oxygen Therapy

Patients who are hypoxemic on room air are quite likely to benefit from oxygen therapy (Bruera, deStoutz, Velasco-Leiva, Schoeller, & Hanson, 1993). Most authorities currently recommend oxygen for patients with hypoxic dyspnea, even in the face of increasing hypercapnia, to achieve and maintain an oxygen saturation greater than 88% (Dudgeon, 2002). However, the usefulness of oxygen for management of patients with cancer who have nonhypoxic dyspnea is questioned in the literature (Bruera & Ripamonti, 1998; Dudgeon). Oxygen may acutely reduce exertional dyspnea; however, an individual response to oxygen cannot be predicted with precision. Evidence indicates that oxygen does have beneficial symptomatic effects in COPD and probably CHF, but patients with

dyspnea from cancer most frequently have restrictive pulmonary failure and might not respond in the same way (Bruera & Ripamonti).

Airflow over the face and nasal mucosa during oxygen administration may itself ameliorate dyspnea through poorly understood mechanisms involving modulation of afferent information by input from cutaneous nerves. In a similar way, the movement of cool air with a fan has been observed clinically to reduce dyspnea. Stimulation of mechanoreceptors on the face or a decrease in temperature of the facial skin, both mediated through the trigeminal nerve, may alter afferent feedback to the brain and modify the perception of dyspnea (ATS, 1999).

Pharmacologic Therapy

Opioids have been explored as a means to relieve dyspnea presumably because of a known respiratory depressive effect or by altering perceptual sensitivity. Opioids may alleviate dyspnea by blunting perceptual responses so that for a given stimulus, the intensity of respiratory sensation is reduced (ATS, 1999). Strong evidence from a recent meta-analysis supports the use of oral and parenteral opioids to treat dyspnea. Jennings, Davies, Higgins, Gibbs, and Broadley (2002) analyzed 18 double-blind, placebo-controlled trials of opioids for treatment of dyspnea secondary to any cause. Nine studies involved the use of oral or parenteral opioids, and nine involved nebulized opioids. This systematic review showed a statistically significant positive effect of oral and parenteral opioids on the sensation of breathlessness ($p = 0.0008$).

The intermittent use of opioids (most frequently morphine) is recommended in a population of patients who already are receiving opioids chronically. The optimal dose has not been determined. Allard, Lamontagne, Bernard, and Tremblay (1999) evaluated 25% and 50% of a four-hourly opioid dose and found them equivalent in relieving dyspnea. Dyspnea reduction was relatively greater in patients with initially low and moderate dyspnea intensity. Allard et al. concluded that 25% of the four-hourly dose of an opioid may be sufficient to reduce dyspnea. The use of sustained-released morphine and slow-release morphine has not shown benefit compared to placebo in reducing breathlessness (Dudgeon, 2002; Ripamonti & Fusco, 2002).

Although the use of nebulized opioids to reduce dyspnea may be tempting, because of local action on pulmonary receptors, a meta-analysis failed to show a positive effect of nebulized opioids on the sensation of breathlessness (Jennings et al., 2002). A synthesis of evidence about the use of nebulized opioids to treat dyspnea concluded that although scientific evidence is lacking to support the use, lower level evidence notes a positive effect in individual clinical settings in patients such as those receiving systemic opioids or experiencing dyspnea at rest (Joyce, McSweeney, Carrieri-Kohlman, & Hawkins, 2004).

Anxiolytics have the potential to relieve dyspnea by depressing hypoxic or hypercapnic respiratory responses as well as by altering the emotional response (ATS, 1999). However, clinical trials to determine the effectiveness of anxiolytics for the treatment of breathlessness have had conflicting results. In some patients, a trial of a benzodiazepine may be reasonable, particularly in those with morbid anxiety or respiratory panic attacks (ATS), but evidence does not support the regular use of benzodiazepines in the management of dyspnea (Bruera & Ripamonti, 1998).

Because 90% of patients who develop lung cancer have a smoking history, a proportion of them may have untreated obstructive airway disease. These patients may benefit from simple bronchodilator therapy. Inhaled beta-2-adrenergic agonists (albuterol), inhaled anticholinergics, and sustained-release theophylline all have been shown to improve dyspnea in patients with stable COPD.

General Supportive Measures

The effects of cognitive, emotional, and behavioral factors on the conscious awareness of the demand to breathe can modulate the perception of dyspnea. Interventions that may assist patients to cope with their dyspnea are breathing retraining, positioning, exercise training, and education about medication use (Carrieri & Janson-Bjerklie, 1986). Pulmonary rehabilitation uses a combination of techniques to decrease energy expenditure and maximize ventilation. The benefit of pursed lip and diaphragmatic breathing retraining may be explained by the decrease in respiratory rate and the increase in tidal volume associated with their use. Positioning, such as leaning forward while sitting, may provide postural relief because of increased efficiency of the diaphragm. Patients themselves devise strategies to minimize energy expenditures. Relaxation training and similar techniques to reduce anxiety have been advocated and are clinically useful. Nurses are in

a unique position to educate patients about dyspnea coping strategies. A patient's beliefs in the effectiveness of coping strategies can affect the perception of dyspnea.

Conclusion

Dyspnea is a complex symptom that requires thorough assessment and attention. Effectively managing dyspnea is a clinical challenge and usually requires a combined approach of various interventions. Evidence is scant about the efficacy of many interventions primarily because of the difficulty of conducting research trials in the patient with cancer who is experiencing dyspnea. Nonetheless, dyspnea is prevalent in lung cancer and can prompt many healthcare encounters.

Fatigue

Cancer-related fatigue has been defined by the Fatigue Practice Guidelines Panel as "an unusual, persistent, subjective sense of tiredness related to cancer or cancer treatment that interferes with usual functioning" (Mock, 2001, p. 1700). Others have conceptualized fatigue as general muscle weakness, decreased motivation, and lack of mental alertness or energy level (Cella, 1997). However, the true definition of fatigue is whatever the patient states it is and should be considered a self-perceived state (Nail, 2002).

According to the National Comprehensive Cancer Network's (NCCN's) "Clinical Practice Guidelines in Oncology: Cancer-Related Fatigue" (2003), 75% of all patients with a metastatic cancer experience cancer-related fatigue. Fatigue occurs in 70%–100% of patients with cancer receiving treatment with chemotherapy, radiation, or both (Curt et al., 2000; Mock, 2001). Patients with cancer experience fatigue that affects them on multiple levels: cognitive, physical, emotional, psychosocial, and spiritual (Holley, 2000). Fatigue commonly is correlated with anxiety, depression, pain, and emotional stress (Richardson, 1995). Up to 50% of patients with cancer reported disturbing affective symptomatology, lack of motivation, anxiety, and sadness (Glaus, Crow, & Hammond, 1996). Approximately 25% of patients had significant cognitive disturbances or an inability to concentrate (Morrow, Andrews, Hickock, Roscoe, & Matteson, 2002). Fatigue interferes with attention, concentration, and the patient's ability to understand and retain disease- or treatment-related information. Compliance with treatment and willingness to participate in clinical trials also are compromised (Morrow et al.).

Illness-related fatigue differs from the fatigue that a healthy person experiences in that it tends to be more persistent, is of greater intensity, and is not relieved by rest. It also interferes with one's ability to carry out normal daily activities (Curt et al., 2000; Mock, 2001). For a healthy person, fatigue is described as physical exhaustion and sleepiness without weakness or associated affective responses (Glaus et al., 1996).

Piper (1993) distinguished between acute fatigue, experienced by a healthy person, and the more chronic or cyclical fatigue, which resembles the experience of cancer treatment–related fatigue.

Distress is another aspect closely related to the phenomenon of cancer-related fatigue. Patients with cancer have rated fatigue as more distressing than both pain and nausea, and they described fatigue as having the most profound effect on QOL. One study showed that fatigue was reported to significantly impair emotional well-being, relationships with others, and the ability to work, enjoy life, and care for family (Vogelzang et al., 1997). The experience of fatigue has been shown to increase concerns with mortality and survival in about one-third of the patients with cancer surveyed. Fatigue continues to be a distressing symptom even in patients who have completed treatment and are in remission.

Curt et al. (2000) found that 66% of patients experienced fatigue at least a few days each month, and about one-third of patients experienced fatigue on a daily basis. Almost all the patients (88%–91%) felt that fatigue was the one symptom that prevented them from living a "normal" life and participating in social activities. Fatigue was the reason that about two-thirds of patients needed to change their employment status, including using disability benefits. Because fatigue is not recognized currently as a valid reason for disability, patients also are faced with economic concerns (Curt et al.). Unlike pain and nausea, no medications ensure relief from this symptom (NCCN, 2003).

Fatigue studies, specifically in patients with lung cancer, have produced similar data. One study showed that more than half (52%) of patients with advanced lung cancer reported a level of fatigue that interfered with the ability to perform at least one daily physical activity, such as walking or working (Tanaka, Akechi, Okuyama, Nishiwaki, & Uchitomi, 2002). This study also highlighted that even fatigue rated low in severity (1–3 on a numerical 1–10 scale) still interfered with patients' daily life activities. Sarna and Brecht (1997) found that fatigue was among the most distressing and prevalent serious life disruptions among women with advanced lung cancer. Patients with advanced lung cancer who were over 65 reported fatigue more frequently during the first year after diagnosis than patients with breast cancer (Given, Given, Azzouz, & Stommel, 2001). Overall, patients with lung cancer experience a compromised QOL from fatigue related to their disease and treatment.

Despite the prevalence, fatigue remains the most ignored and undermanaged symptom (Mock, 2001). This has been attributed to the fact that it is poorly understood by both healthcare providers and patients (Nail, 2002). A lack of knowledge about underlying mechanisms and appropriate interventions prevents physicians and nurses from discussing fatigue symptoms with patients. A study found that 8% of patients never discussed fatigue with their healthcare providers because they believed it was an expected side effect of their

illness that had no treatment or that it was transient and would not persist for long (Curt et al., 2000). Other barriers were age (patients over 65 were least likely to discuss fatigue) and a reported fear that discussing fatigue with the physician would jeopardize continuation of their current treatment.

Assessment of fatigue must reflect the multiple dimensions of this symptom or phenomena. Ideally, fatigue should be assessed at the initial visit, during each patient interaction, and as indicated for changes in clinical status. Subjective and objective symptoms even can be assessed in very sick patients with advanced disease, such as patients with stage IV lung cancer (Stone et al., 1999). The cornerstone of any thorough assessment is history, physical examination, and comprehensive review of the fatigue. This includes reviewing patients' recent radiographic studies, laboratory values, current disease status, and type, duration, and response to treatment. Because fatigue is a highly subjective experience, patient self-report is essential. Clinicians also should ask family or support system members about any notable changes in patient behavior (NCCN, 2003). During self-report, healthcare providers must ask patients to characterize fatigue using terms such as "decreased energy," "muscular weakness," "dysphoric mood," "impaired cognitive functioning," or some combination of these. The onset and duration of the fatigue also is important in helping to differentiate between an acute and chronic fatigue syndrome.

Use of a fatigue measuring tool is helpful in quantifying the level of fatigue and as a benchmark for gauging success of the interventions. A simple unidimensional scale can be used, such as a verbal rating of mild, moderate, or severe or a numerical 1–10 scale commonly used for pain. The National Cancer Institute's Common Toxicity Criteria rating scale uses a 0–4 scale. These scales typically measure intensity or distress. Multidimensional fatigue scales focus on different aspects of fatigue. Examples of these are the Profile of Mood States (Cella et al., 1987), the Piper Fatigue Self-Report Scale (Piper et al., 1998), the Functional Assessment of Cancer Therapy–Lung Cancer (FACT–L) (Cella et al., 1995), and the Lung Cancer Symptom Scale (LCSS) (Hollen et al., 1993). Use of these scales can be time-consuming and, therefore, less practical in clinical practice settings. The routine use of three simple questions has been shown to be useful in assessing the severity and impact of fatigue on the patient over time. The healthcare provider begins by asking the patient if he or she is experiencing any fatigue. If the patient replies yes, the provider asks the patient how severe the fatigue has been on average over the past week using a 1–10 scale and how much the fatigue has been interfering with ability to function, again on a 1–10 scale (Curt et al., 2000; Lesage & Portenoy, 2002).

The most common treatable causes for fatigue in the patient with lung cancer are dyspnea, pain, emotional distress, cachexia and anorexia, sleep disturbance, medication interactions, and exercise intolerance (Mock, 2001; NCCN, 2003; Stone et al.,1999). Cancer treatments, including chemotherapy, radiation, and pain medications, are other potential causes of fatigue. Common comorbidities in patients with lung cancer, such as asthma, emphysema, hypertension, CHF, and diabetes mellitus, also may contribute, as do specific physiologic properties of lung cancer, including anemia, cachexia, paraneoplastic syndromes, stress, and mood disorders (Gutstein, 2001).

Emotional distress commonly presents as depression or anxiety. Piper (1993) and Winningham et al. (1994) have hypothesized that the fatigue experience in patients with lung cancer could be a combination of symptoms, treatment, and stress. The severity of emotional distress and physical distress are directly proportional (Kou & Fung-Chi, 2002). Therefore, the concurrent relationship between these two psychological states could result in a fatigue syndrome that is difficult to treat.

Contributing Factors and Management

As stated previously, the goal of assessment is to uncover the underlying etiology so that specific treatments can be designed. The following section will describe contributing factors and management.

Dyspnea has been identified as the symptom most closely associated with cancer-related fatigue. Dyspnea is one of the most common and distressing symptoms reported in advanced lung cancer, with 80% of patients experiencing some degree of shortness of breath (Cooley, 2000). Difficulty breathing combined with the emotional stress of coughing, shortness of breath, and the site of bloody sputum strongly contribute to the fatigue syndrome (Kuo & Fung-Chi, 2002). Shortness of breath or dyspnea also causes exercise intolerance.

Dyspnea and fatigue produce similar feelings and limitations in patients and are difficult to differentiate. Interventions are similar and somewhat interchangeable. At present, the most commonly used interventions for dyspnea are supplemental oxygen and medications, such as opioids, bronchodilators, steroids, and diuretics (Luce & Luce, 2001). Some research has been conducted on the use of behavioral interventions, which have been shown to have a positive effect on relief of dyspnea. These include breathing exercises and emotional support to decrease anxiety (Inzeo & Tyson, 2003).

Pain syndromes specific to lung cancer vary according to the location of the lung tumor and sites of metastatic disease, with patients often experiencing pain in the chest wall, vertebrae, and brachial plexus (Silvestri, 2000). The experience of acute or chronic pain contributes to fatigue in that patients with pain experience insomnia, depression, and exercise intolerance, and treatments prescribed to relieve pain and distress, especially narcotic analgesics and antianxiety drugs, are sedating. Effective methods found to control pain related to lung cancer are use of oral, transdermal, rectal, or parenteral opioids, as well as nonopioid analgesics (Paice & Fine, 2001).

Long-acting preparations can reduce sedating effects, thereby reducing fatigue. Devine and Westlake (1995) conducted a meta-analysis that supports the use of muscle relaxation or guided imagery for the relief of both pain and anxiety. Studies currently are being conducted on the use of acupuncture in the relief and control of pain and dyspnea (Filshie, Penn, Ashley, & Davis, 1996). However, data are too preliminary to support this intervention.

Fatigue is often a presenting symptom of lung cancer, before treatment even begins. It has been reported to significantly increase during treatment with chemotherapy and radiation and persist for years after treatment ends (Richardson, Ream, & Wilson-Barnett, 1998). Patterns of fatigue depend on the timing and treatment schedule for the chemotherapy regimen (e.g., every 21 days, weekly, continuous infusion). As the time period between treatments increases, fatigue duration is shorter. In general, fatigue seems to peak 4–5 days after treatment, rise again around the nadir period, and decrease just prior to the next scheduled treatment. One study showed that fatigue associated with etoposide and cisplatin, drugs commonly used for lung cancer, was so severe that patients on this regimen experienced anticipatory fatigue prior to receiving the treatment (Richardson et al.).

Radiation is another important treatment modality for lung cancer. Although the etiology is unclear, a strong association has been found between radiation and fatigue (Hickok, Morrow, McDonald, & Bellg, 1996). Incidence is site-specific, as most patients with lung cancer experience fatigue with radiation to the chest (93%) and pelvis (65%) (King, Nail, Kreamer, Strohl, & Johnson, 1985). Fatigue is reported to start three weeks after the initiation of treatment and last for up to three months post-treatment in about one-third of these patients. Pain or depression can exacerbate radiation-related fatigue. Because radiation treatments have a limited duration, fatigue does improve once treatment is completed.

One of the initial presenting symptoms in lung cancer is unexplained or unintentional weight loss (Brown, 2002). In addition to those patients who present with weight loss, 46%–61% of patients with lung cancer continue to lose weight during treatment and approximately 15% experience cachexia (Chute et al., 1985; DeWys et al., 1980). Cachexia is a syndrome characterized by anorexia, weakness, fatigue, weight loss, muscle wasting, impaired immune response, decreased motor ability, and mood disorder (Costa & Donaldson, 1980; Lindsey, 1986; Morrison, 1989) Effective interventions for cancer-related cachexia and anorexia can reduce feelings of fatigue. These include interventions such as nutritional education about increasing food intake and pharmacologic progestational agents, such as Megace® (Bristol-Myers Squibb, New York, NY), corticosteroids, hydrazine, and cytohapatine (Gagnon & Bruera, 1998; Goldberg & Loprinzi, 1999; Maltoni et al., 2001).

Approximately 50%–60% of patients with lung cancer experience disease- or treatment-related anemia (Crawford et al., 2002; Glaspy, 2001). Chemotherapy-induced anemia occurs as the result of the direct myelosuppressive effect of particular agents and as a secondary decrease in the production of erythropoietin related to renal impairment. Platinum-based chemotherapeutic agents (e.g., cisplatin, carboplatin), which are commonly used in lung cancer, have a significant effect on the renal system with decreased erythropoietin production. Retrospective chart reviews have shown that patients with lung cancer receiving platinum-based chemotherapy require blood transfusions 30%–40% more than patients treated for other cancers that do not receive a platinum-based therapy (American Society of Clinical Oncology [ASCO], 1997; Wood & Hrushesky, 1995). Many of the single-agent chemotherapies used in lung cancer, including docetaxel, paclitaxel, gemcitabine, vinorelbine, and topotecan, also have been proven to produce mild to moderate anemia (Groopman & Itri, 1999). In addition, patients with lung cancer have about a 33%–47% chance of developing severe anemia if they have been treated with radiation therapy, multiple regimens of chemotherapy, or chemotherapy and radiation concomitantly (Crino et al., 1997).

Randomized, controlled studies on the effects of anemia on patients with cancer undergoing treatment have supported that mild to moderate anemia was a frequent and significant contributor to fatigue. Epoetin alfa (Epogen® [Amgen, Thousands Oaks, CA], Procrit® [Ortho Biotech, Bridgewater, NJ]) has been shown to effectively improve mild to moderate anemia and have a significant impact on overall QOL, despite disease response to chemotherapy. QOL studies confirmed that treatment of mild to moderate anemia with epoetin alfa had a meaningful impact on cancer-related fatigue, energy, activity level, and overall QOL (Crawford et al., 2002; Demetri, Kris, Wade, Degos, & Cella, 1998; Gabrilove et al., 2001; Glaspy, 2001; Glaus et al., 1996). Epoetin alfa has been approved in the United States for the treatment of anemia in patients with solid tumors receiving chemotherapy (Abels, 1992).

Epoetin alfa is able to improve anemia in approximately 60%–80% of patients with lung cancer receiving a platinum-based chemotherapy regimen and in close to 40% of patients receiving nonplatinum-based chemotherapy. Current guidelines for hemoglobin levels higher than 11 g/dl are 10,000 units via subcutaneous injection three times per week or 40,000 units via subcutaneous injection weekly (Gabrilove & Jakubowski, 1990). Iron supplements, such as daily doses of ferrous sulfate, should be prescribed in conjunction with epoetin alfa. For patients who are refractory, escalating the dose to 60,000 units weekly can increase hemoglobin recovery by 20% (Glaspy, 2001). Weekly dosing should continue until hemoglobin rises above 12 g/dl, at which time injections can be discontinued and patients should be observed. If anemia recurs, epoetin alfa can be reinitiated at the previous dose (Glaspy). Darbepoetin alfa (Aranesp® [Amgen]) was approved in 2002 as a longer-acting form of epoetin alfa requiring less-frequent dosing. Despite the success of epoetin alfa, about 20%–40% of patients still require blood transfusion (Del Mastro, Gennari, & Donati, 1999).

Depression is another problem that occurs frequently in patients with lung cancer. Several research studies show that 25%–70% of patients with advanced lung cancer experience depression (Aass, Fossa, Dahl, & Moe, 1997; Zigmond & Snaith, 1983). The severity of depression is related directly to the severity of symptoms or functional limitations. Depression and symptom distress have been correlated closely with fatigue and compromised QOL (Newall, Sanson-Fischer, Girgis, & Ackland, 1999). However, a study by Visser and Smets (1998) did not support a cause-and-effect relationship between depression and fatigue. Rather, the study found that the two symptoms have a concurrent relationship, with both symptoms negatively affecting overall QOL. Effectively treating depression with antidepressants and counseling can improve sleep, cognition, tolerance of treatment, fatigue, and overall QOL (Hopwood & Stephens, 2000).

Fatigue can have an adverse effect on cognitive function in patients with cancer. Careful assessment of mental status changes in patients with lung cancer is required to distinguish fatigue from disease-related changes such as central nervous system (CNS) metastases, paraneoplastic syndromes, electrolyte imbalances, or drug interactions.

The NCCN practice guidelines (2003) offer some general guidelines for fatigue management. Educating patients about fatigue can prepare them for the effect that treatment will have on their ability to perform usual activities. Patients must be informed that fatigue is an expected response from the cancer and treatment and is not a sign of treatment efficacy or disease progression. Counseling on useful strategies for coping with fatigue should include energy conservation and distraction. Although maintaining a normal level of activity is important physically and emotionally, patients should be encouraged to prioritize activities, pace themselves according to their energy level, delegate more activities to others, and postpone any unnecessary activities or plan to do them when they experience peak energy levels. Distracting activities, such as bird-watching, have been shown to improve fatigue and cognition, although the mechanism of action is unknown (Cimprich, 1992).

Other nonpharmacologic management strategies, including activity enhancement and psychosocial interventions, may be helpful. Activity enhancement or exercise can counteract the toxic effects of treatment, which, combined with inactivity, can result in a decreased activity tolerance and fatigue. Prolonged bed rest or periods of inactivity result in loss of muscle mass, plasma volume, and cardiac output, which, in turn, cause even normal levels of activity to be difficult. Several studies have shown that exercise can prevent development or reduce intensity of fatigue in patients with cancer during and after treatment (Dimeo, 2001). One study reported a reduction in fatigue and improvement of psychological distress in patients who followed an exercise program while in the hospital receiving high-dose chemotherapy regimens (Dimeo, Steiglitz, Novelli-Fischer, & Keue, 1999). Although the usefulness of exercise in reducing cancer-related fatigue is well documented, patients with lung cancer may be unable to perform any level of exercise. These patients may benefit from a consult with a physical therapist for an appropriate exercise regimen or rehabilitation program. Before any exercise program is initiated, careful consideration must be given to the presence of bone metastasis, neutropenia, thrombocytopenia, anemia, anticoagulant therapy, fever, pain, or other complications from treatment (NCCN, 2003). For those with lung cancer, evaluation of oxygen saturation levels before, during, and after exercise also is recommended to prevent excessive dyspnea.

Because of the strong correlation between emotional distress and fatigue, patients with lung cancer must be offered counseling on stress management, anxiety, and depression. Patients may benefit from referral for psychiatric intervention, support groups, or evaluation for mood-elevating medication. Restorative therapy can be helpful for attentional fatigue, or a decreased ability to concentrate. Restorative interventions, such as bird-watching or sitting outdoors, have been shown to improve concentration and problem-solving abilities in patients with cancer-related fatigue (Cimprich, 1992, 1993). Sleep interventions also have proven to be helpful. Patients with sleep disturbances require direction on strategies to improve sleep quality. These include maintaining a consistent bedtime, limiting daytime napping, avoiding caffeine, and limiting stimulating activities prior to bedtime (Berger & Farr, 1999).

Several pharmacologic agents that serve as psychostimulants are prescribed for fatigue. Methylphenidate and dextroamphetamine serve as CNS stimulants to enhance alertness, attention, and vigilance. Glucocorticoid steroids are prescribed for patients with lung cancer–related fatigue to enhance mood, increase appetite, and increase energy level. Antidepressants can be integral to the treatment of patients with cancer-related fatigue and depression. Bupropion can serve to decrease fatigue, improve mood, and assist with smoking cessation efforts in patients with lung cancer (Burks, 2001).

Many patients with cancer-related fatigue turn to herbal remedies for relief from fatigue. Gingko biloba is a popular herbal remedy shown to have a modest activity against tumor necrosis factor (TNF) (Kurzrock, 2001). Future research on this herbal regimen may prove to be very useful in the development of effective interventions for cancer-related fatigue.

Further research into the basic mechanisms of fatigue should lead to development of more effective management strategies. Studies currently are under way to uncover the role of cytokines (TNF, interleukin [IL]-6, IL-1) in cancer-related fatigue. Increased knowledge in this area could lead to the evaluation of cytokine inhibitors, such as selective cyclo-oxygenase (COX)-2 inhibitors, as modulators of fatigue (Kurzrock, 2001). Monoclonal antibodies, such as infliximab, can be used to neutralize cytokines and reduce fatigue (Kurzrock). Furthermore, improved fatigue assessment tools may influence more specific and effective treatments (Gutstein, 2001).

Pain

Many patients with lung cancer experience pain (Irvine, Vincent, Graydon, Bubela, & Thompson, 1994). A prospective study of patients with lung or colon cancer showed that more than 33% had more than one area of moderate pain over a four-week period. Approximately 90% of the patients had pain more than 25% of the time, and 50% reported that pain interfered with their daily life activities, sleep, mood, and overall enjoyment of life (Portenoy et al., 1992).

Pain associated with lung cancer has a variable presentation and is related to location of tumor and underlying etiology. Radicular chest wall pain is seen in patients with chest wall or mediastinal tumor involvement. Pleuritic pain is often a presenting symptom of pleural invasion with effusion. Mediastinal lymphadenopathy, or tumors located near the mediastinum, can cause pain related to pressure on neighboring nerves, such as the phrenic and vagus nerves. Nonspecific and vague noncardiac chest pain commonly occurs as a result of tumor compression of surrounding structures.

Pancoast lung tumors, or tumors of the superior sulcus of the lung apex, usually are associated with severe pain. These tumors directly invade and destroy the first rib and involve the brachial plexus and stellate ganglion in the surrounding area. Pancoast syndrome is characterized by shoulder or scapular pain and radicular pain that may include muscle wasting in the ulnar nerve region (i.e., elbow, hand, or medial forearm); Horner's syndrome, characterized by ptosis, miosis, hemianhydrosis, and enophthalmus; and rib erosion. The most common initial presentation (90%) of this lung tumor is shoulder pain, bone pain from rib erosion, and associated neuropathic pain (Busick, Fretz, Galvin, & Peterson, 1999; Ginsberg, Vokes, & Rosenzweig, 2001). Management of this type of tumor-related pain will be discussed later.

Metastatic disease causes pain in the site of metastases. The most common sites of metastasis are contralateral lung, bone, brain, adrenal gland, pericardium, and liver. Lung, bone, and liver metastases are the most frequently reported sites (Ginsberg, et al., 2001). Skeletal metastases occur in up to 30% of patients and generally present as localized pain. Liver metastases occur in 10%–20% of patients; symptoms can include a nonspecific presentation of abdominal discomfort and bloating or a more severe pain from hepatomegaly and ascites (Fretz & Peterson, 1999).

Lung cancer is often fatal, with 86% of patients with lung cancer dying from the disease. As death approaches, pain tends to increase; about half of patients with lung cancer experience pain in the last few days of life (McCarthy, Phillips, Zhong, Drews, & Lynn, 2000; Weiss, Emanuel, Fairclough, & Emanuel, 2001). More than half of terminally ill patients report pain associated with the primary tumor, regional metastasis, or distant metastatic sites. Palliation of pain is essential for ensuring comfort at the end of life (Kvale et al., 2003; Weiss et al.). Approximately 60%–90% of patients with advanced disease and 30% of patients with active metastatic disease experience some degree of pain. An alarming 50%–80% of patients who are not in hospice care report inadequate pain control (Von Roenn, Cleeland, Gonin, Hatfield, & Pandya, 1993).

Inadequate treatment of cancer pain may result in fatigue, depression, anxiety, and overall compromised QOL. Furthermore, decreased activity, anorexia, and sleep deprivation caused by pain further weaken already debilitated patients. Despite increased knowledge about the use of narcotic and non-narcotic analgesics and alternate pain management techniques, physicians continue to underassess and underprescribe pain medication. Barriers to prescribing maximum doses of pain medication include poor pain assessment by healthcare providers and concerns over side effects (Van Roenn et al., 1993). Physicians without specialized oncology training tend to have a conservative view of cancer pain treatment and place a lower priority on pain management (Cleeland, Cleeland, Dar, & Rinehardt, 1986).

Compounding the problem, patients often under-report pain and avoid the use of narcotics because of a fear of addiction. Patients often place a low priority on pain management because of their general lack of understanding about analgesic drug therapy and the physiology of cancer (Yeager, McGuire, & Sheidler, 2000).

The first step in effective pain management is a basic understanding and assessment of cancer-related pain. A thorough history and physical are needed to classify the pain as somatic, visceral, or neuropathic in nature (Staats, 2002). Somatic pain, the type of pain experienced with bone metastases, usually is localized, is caused by inflammation, and originates from peripheral and sensory efferent nerves. Visceral pain is more generalized, described as a deep ache, cramping, squeezing, or pressure-like pain. Visceral pain usually is caused by pressure on an organ by a tumor, such as a lung tumor stretching the thoracic viscera (Foley, 2001; Staats). Neuropathic pain results from pressure, injury, inflammation, or damage to either peripheral or central nerves (Staats). This kind of pain can develop as a result of tumor compression or infiltration of peripheral or spinal cord nerves caused by surgery, irradiation, or chemotherapy (Foley). Patients with lung cancer often present with both somatic and visceral pain; neuropathic pain occurs in about 15%–20% of this population (Weiss et al., 2001). Identifying the classification of the pain is essential for prescribing the most appropriate combination of pain management strategies.

Patients with neuropathic pain generally report a burning sensation that radiates with a vice-like quality and that may be associated with sensory perception loss. Because of the location of many lung tumors, patients can experience pain from pressure on the brachial plexus or lumbosacral plexopathies. Pancoast tumors, as previously mentioned, are the main cause of brachial plexopathies in patients with lung cancer (Busick et al., 1999). Metastatic lung cancer to the lumbosacral spine causing compression will present as a lumbrosacral plexopathy. In addition, patients with lung cancer report neuropathic pain at lung surgery incision sites and previous chest tube drainage sites.

Tumor-related paraneoplastic syndromes and certain chemotherapies can cause peripheral neuropathy. Frequently used chemotherapeutic agents for lung cancer, such as the vinca-alkaloids, platinums, and taxanes, can cause peripheral nerve injury or damage, which can be painful. The most frequently cited agents are vincristine, cisplatin, and paclitaxel (Lipton et al., 1989; Martin & Hagen, 1997). Chemotherapy-related neuropathies usually present distally and bilaterally and are characterized by sensory complaints of numbness and paresthesias.

Pain assessment also must incorporate measurement of pain intensity. The most frequently used scale to quantify pain and measure the success of pain treatment intervention is the 0–10 numeric scale, used in conjunction with questions about location, quality, duration, aggravating and relieving factors, present pain medications, and impact of pain on QOL. Three other scales frequently are used that serve not only to quantify the intensity of the pain but also to measure the multiple dimensions of the pain syndrome. The Brief Pain Inventory addresses the relevant aspects of pain (i.e., history, intensity, location, and quality) and the impact it has on one's ability to carry out activities of daily living (Daut, Cleeland, & Flanery, 1983). The McGill Pain Questionnaire is a complete, yet complex, scale that provides a methodologic approach to assess the sensory, affective, and evaluative components of pain (Graham, Bond, Gertrovitch, & Cook, 1980). The use of this scale in the patient with lung cancer presents challenges in terms of complexity and level of cognitive difficulty. The Memorial Pain Assessment Card consists of three visual analog scales that measure pain intensity, pain relief, and mood. This tool tends to provide a broader, more global assessment of pain (Fishman et al., 1986). Although not all scales are appropriate or feasible for routine assessment of the patient with lung cancer–related pain, the most appropriate scale should be integrated into the assessment to better define the impact of the pain symptomatology.

One of the most effective strategies for pain management is to assess pain at every patient encounter. A trusting relationship between patient and practitioner is critical for open, honest communication. Patients must feel that their complaints of pain are real and not just the result of inadequate coping (Arathuzik, 1991; Wolff, 1985). When patients present with a report of pain, a careful history of the pain must follow. This includes identification of the location, quality, aggravating and relieving factors, timing, onset, associated symptoms, impact on daily life and psychological well-being, and response to analgesics for the pain in the past.

A medical and neurologic examination allows healthcare providers to examine sites of pain and identify potential associated physical or neurologic signs. This examination includes review of all laboratory and radiologic tests for other potential causes. Once pain is treated, assessment should focus on the success of the intervention and changes in the pain status and psychological well-being. Patients and caregivers must be educated about pain and how it impacts all aspects of living. Healthcare providers must dispel myths of addiction and demonstrate how pain management is integral to the success and continuation of the treatment plan

The management of cancer-related pain is a complex process that is most successful when viewed as a holistic treatment approach. First, treatment must be focused on eradicating the underlying etiology. In patients with lung cancer, this involves treatment of the cancer with chemotherapy, radiation, or surgery. The next step is to use pharmacologic agents to change perceptions of pain (relieve the sensation of pain). Finally, psychological and emotional components of the pain syndrome must be addressed (Yeager et al., 2000).

Because advanced-stage lung cancer is an incurable disease, treatment eventually reaches the palliative phase. Studies have suggested that even in cases in which chemotherapy will not improve survival time, chemotherapy does have an effect on pain relief (Kvale et al., 2003). However, much of the evidence is anecdotal, and much more research is needed in this area.

Radiotherapy is an important treatment modality for pain relief in the patient with lung cancer. Most commonly, it is used to treat painful bone metastases, epidural cord compressions, Pancoast tumors, headaches from brain metastasis, and specific sites of disease causing severe pain (Jenis, Dunn, & An, 1999; Strohl, 2000; Tong, Gillick, & Hendrickson, 1982). The Radiation Therapy Oncology Group showed that 90% of patients with bone lesions experienced some relief of their pain, and 54% reported complete relief from pain (Tong et al.). Radiation to tumors that are compressing nerve roots, such as Pancoast tumors or epidural lesions, also provides relief from the associated neuropathies. Patients with lung cancer who present with sudden onset of back pain radiating to the arms or legs, accompanied by weakness, sensory disturbance, or sphincter dysfunction, must be evaluated for spinal cord compression. Spinal cord compression is treated with corticosteroids and radiation therapy to the lesion (Jenis et al.). Surgical intervention is indicated for intractable pain, spinal instability, or neurologic deterioration from vertebral collapse or failure of conservative treatment (Jenis et al.).

The primary approach to pain relief is pharmacologic management. Analgesic medications are divided into three main categories: nonopioid analgesics, opioids, and adjuvant analgesic drugs (Foley, 2001). According to the World Health Organization (WHO) Cancer Pain Relief Program (1986), nonopioid drugs should be considered as first-line treatment for mild to moderate pain. In cancer-related pain, nonsteroidal anti-inflammatory drugs (NSAIDs) and acetaminophen are useful in the management of mild to moderate somatic pain from metastatic bone lesions; pain from mechanical compression of muscles, tendons, pleura, or peritoneum; and nonobstructive visceral pain (Strohl, 2000; Ventafridda, Fochi, DeConno, & Sganzerla, 1980). If the pain worsens despite use of these medications, opioids can be added for a synergistic effect. Use of NSAIDs plus opioids can reduce the required dose of opioids, resulting in fewer side effects (WHO).

If NSAIDs do not relieve the pain, narcotic analgesia usually is required. Oral narcotic medications commonly are used because of convenience, effectiveness, and cost. Codeine sulfate, propoxyphen, and oxycodone usually are tried first because they have a greater analgesic effect than nonopioids and can be effective in controlling most pain. However, these medications have a low therapeutic dosing ceiling, which limits their use. Morphine and morphine derivatives are used for moderate to severe pain. The combination of a controlled-release preparation, such as MS Contin® (Purdue Pharma, L.P., Stamford, CT) or OxyContin® (Purdue Pharma, L.P.), plus an immediate-release preparation, such as morphine sulfate immediate release or oxycodone, are used to provide baseline pain control, along with "as needed" coverage for breakthrough pain. This regimen provides maximum 24-hour pain control with less frequent dosing and less severe adverse effects such as constipation or sedation.

Additional routes of administration include transdermal, rectal, IV, and intramuscular. Transdermal administration (patch) is an effective way to deliver a short-acting opioid on a continuous basis. This time-released route of administration bypasses the gastrointestinal system, which is useful for patients with dysphagia, obstruction, or refractory nausea and vomiting, and only requires changing every three days. The drug that is most frequently used in transdermal patches is fentanyl. Rectal administration of narcotics is useful in homebound patients who are either unresponsive or unable to swallow. Morphine, hydrocodone, and oxymorphone can be administered rectally as suppositories (Beaver & Feise, 1977). IV narcotics generally are used in the inpatient setting or via patient-controlled analgesia pumps in the home for patients with refractory or difficult pain control needs. This route of administration allows for rapid titration of doses for patients in acute pain crises. Intramuscular injections of narcotic analgesics are avoided in patients with lung cancer because this route of administration is painful and inconvenient, and the rate of absorption tends to be too variable (Kvale et al., 2003).

The primary side effects of narcotics are sedation, respiratory depression, nausea, vomiting, and constipation

(Palomano, McGuire, & Sheidler, 2000). Treatment for narcotic-induced sedation is discussed in the section on adjuvant therapy. Severe respiratory depression can be reversed quickly with naloxone (Narcan®, Endo Pharmaceuticals, Chadds Ford, PA) (Palomano et al.). However, naloxone should be used judiciously in patients with advanced lung cancer where respiratory depression is desired to reduce air hunger. Reversing respiratory depression may lead to dyspnea and pain, causing further discomfort. Opioid-induced nausea and vomiting can be managed with antiemetics (Palomano et al.). Constipation tends to be the most distressing for patients with lung cancer. Constipation should be anticipated in patients beginning narcotic pain regimens and should be treated prophylactically. Every patient should be assessed for bowel function at every encounter and educated about increasing fluid and fiber intake, bowel regimens consisting of ducosate sodium and a senna product, and reporting constipation to healthcare providers. Severe constipation may necessitate use of cathartic agents (Palomano et al.).

Adjuvant analgesics are not categorized as pain relievers; rather, they enhance the action of analgesics for maximum pain control. Classifications of these drugs include antidepressants, anticonvulsants, psychostimulants, corticosteroids, antihistamines, and bisphosphonates (Palomano et al., 2000). Tricyclic antidepressants have been found to be the most useful in the management of pain. In cancer-related pain, they are used in the treatment of neuropathic pain from peripheral neuropathy (Portenoy et al., 1992). Amitriptyline is used most commonly. Furthermore, treatment of underlying depression is effective in improving overall pain control and QOL. Anticonvulsants, such as phenytoin or carbamazepine, are the primary treatment for trigeminal and post-treatment neuropathies. Psychostimulants primarily are used to counteract the sedating side effects of narcotic medications by elevating mood and increasing alertness, ability to concentrate, and motor activity. Amphetamines and methylphenidate are used most commonly because they are powerful CNS stimulators (Portenoy et al.).

Corticosteroids are useful in decreasing sedation, relieving inflammation, and reducing cerebral or spinal cord edema in the context of brain metastases or lesions compressing the spinal cord. Hydroxyzine is the most commonly studied antihistamine for its analgesic effect in cancer-related pain. Although its mechanism of action is unclear, evidence supports use of this drug to decrease anxiety and nausea related to opioid use (Paice & Fine, 2001). Bisphosphonates act by inhibiting the bone-resorption effects of osteoclasts. These drugs, such as pamidronate and zoledronic acid, are given monthly to patients with metastatic lung cancer to the bone to strengthen the diseased bone, prevent idiopathic fracture, and promote pain relief. These drugs also are useful in treating hypercalcemia in patients with bone disease (Paice & Fine; Palomano et al., 2000).

Despite the use of the previously mentioned medications, a subgroup of patients still do not achieve adequate response. These patients seem to experience an unsatisfactory balance between the dose of pain medications and the adverse effects. In these patients, more individualized and alternate strategies should be employed. According to Portenoy (1999), four primary strategies are applied to the management of pain in patients with cancer who do not respond appropriately to initial opioid therapy. First, higher doses of narcotics can be prescribed if more aggressive management of side effects is employed. This is known as expanding the therapeutic window. This would involve more frequent use of psychostimulant drugs to treat the opioid-induced somnolence and mental clouding. The next strategy of opioid rotation involves switching to an equivalent dose of a different drug when the first drug seems to be ineffective. Invasive techniques, such as intraspinal opioid therapy, may need to be considered to allow for increased analgesic effects with lower doses of medication. Lastly, nonpharmacologic techniques may be helpful, including anesthesia (nerve block), neurostimulation (transcutaneous electrical nerve stimulation), surgery (cordotomy), rehabilitation (physical therapy), psychological support, and complementary medicines (Portenoy).

Although the primary treatment for cancer-related pain is analgesics, other treatment strategies can augment pain control in patients with lung cancer. Despite the lack of research in this area, complementary approaches, such as massage, acupuncture, and distraction with humor and music, are gaining interest as interventions for pain control (Beck, 1991). Further research and medical advancements in the treatment of lung cancer-related pain are critical. Research must focus on developing a better understanding of the mechanism of pain in the clinical setting and providing greater support and acceptance of innovative methods for the treatment of cancer-related pain.

Specific Treatment-Related Side Effects: Radiation

Pneumonitis

Radiation pneumonitis (RP) is a term used to describe a constellation of clinical, radiographic, and histologic findings reflecting lung injury from radiation. Symptomatic RP occurs in approximately 20% of patients and is classified as a continuum of clinical findings ranging from mild cough and exertional dyspnea to death from respiratory failure (Robnett et al., 2000).

Advances in the understanding of underlying molecular mechanisms have created a clear distinction between acute RP and late radiation lung fibrosis. Classical radiation pneumonitis (CRP), which ultimately leads to pulmonary fibrosis, primarily is caused by radiation-induced local cytokine production confined to the field of radiation (Morgan & Breit, 1995). The initial injury occurs during the first month and results in damage to the pneumocytes, endothelial cells, and interstitium, leading to release of surfactant and exudate into the alveoli and interstitial edema (Abratt & Morgan, 2002). The second phase, termed the intermediate or acute pneumonitis phase, lasts from one to several months. Inflammatory response, with capillary obstruction and an increase in leukocytes, plasma cells, macrophages, fibroblasts, and collagen fibers, continues. The alveolar septa become thickened, and the alveolar space becomes smaller. In the late phase, occurring at six months and longer, fibrosis develops with loss of capillaries, increase in the thickness of alveolar septa, and obliteration of the alveolar space (Abratt & Morgan).

Acute RP following fractionated irradiation, also known as sporadic pneumonitis, has been found to be a different syndrome than CRP. It is a bilateral lymphocytic alveolitis or hypersensitivity pneumonitis associated with unpredictable and sporadic onset, dyspnea out of proportion to the volume of lung irradiated, and symptom resolution without sequelae within six to eight weeks. It occurs in a minority of patients. In some patients, chest x-ray may show infiltrates within the radiated field, which may resolve over time or lead to an area of scarring and reduction in lung volume (Abratt & Morgan, 2002; Morgan & Breit, 1995). The exact etiology is unknown, but the generalized lymphocytic response is in keeping with an immunologically mediated response against damaged lung tissue (Abratt & Morgan).

Many studies have investigated risk factors for RP, allowing for high-risk groups to be identified and treatment tailored appropriately. The most consistently reported factors include low pretreatment performance status, comorbid lung disease, smoking history, and low pulmonary function tests. Studies of treatment-related factors, such as radiation dose, dose per fraction, field size, and concurrent chemotherapy, offer conflicting results but also seem to have contributing effects (Inoue et al., 2001; Robnett et al., 2000).

Cough is a common but temporary side effect that occurs during radiation. It is caused by irritation of the main bronchus and larger bronchioles from a decrease in mucus production (McDonald, Rubin, Phillips, & Marks, 1995). One to three months following completion of radiation, pneumonitis symptoms include dyspnea, productive cough, fever, and night sweats. Clinical characteristics may include pleural friction rub, pleural effusion, and radiographic evidence of infiltrate or consolidation that conforms to the radiation field (Knopp, 1997). Symptoms vary depending on the volume of the field and dose of radiation delivered. Doses greater than 25–30 Gy to a large volume of lung can produce earlier, more severe symptoms at three to six weeks and include acute respiratory distress with significant cough, dyspnea, fever, and tachycardia. An accelerated version of the syndrome may develop within a period of days after receiving concomitant chemotherapy (Knopp).

The acute, symptomatic phase of pneumonitis can be managed with supportive interventions. Corticosteroid therapy is the most common intervention with 30–60 mg prednisone given daily (approximately 1 mg/kg) for 2–3 weeks and a slow taper over 3–4 weeks or more (McDonald et al., 1995). Although use of steroids has been the standard for managing RP symptoms, studies have documented no significant difference in survival rate in patients receiving corticosteroid therapy (Inoue et al., 2001). Antibiotics may be necessary in the presence of secondary infection. Oxygen, bronchodilators, and sedatives to help to control anxiety, dyspnea, and cough also may be needed (Knopp, 1997).

The final, regenerative phase of RP may be characterized by lung fibrosis, a late effect of radiation, taking 6–24 months to evolve. Pulmonary fibrosis is a consequence of the repair process initiated by tissue injury and the resulting release of cytokines and chemotactic factors for fibroblasts, including transforming growth factor-beta, fibronectin, and platelet-derived growth factor (Abratt & Morgan, 2002). Interstitial and arteriolar fibrosis begins with swelling of the small vessel endothelial cells leading to partial obstruction and decreased blood flow (McDonald et al., 1995). It results in decreased lung compliance affecting total lung capacity and forced vital capacity and decreased perfusion to the radiated field. Progressive dyspnea and death frequently occur (Abratt & Morgan).

Fibrosis depends on many factors, but the volume of lung radiated above 20–30 Gy seems to have the most significance (Abratt & Morgan, 2002). The degree of impairment is related to radiation volume and dose, preexisting compromise, and additional effects of chemotherapy. Although steroids may reverse symptoms of pneumonitis within hours of initiation, they do not prevent or reverse the fibrotic phase. Fibrosis can occur without previous symptoms of pneumonitis, but once pneumonitis occurs, fibrosis is almost certain (Knopp, 1997).

Prevention is the primary goal in managing the pulmonary side effects of radiation. Treatment planning must include preassessment for underlying pulmonary impairment and careful attention to radiation volume and dose and chemotherapy treatments, particularly with concurrent schedules. Use of dose-volume histograms and calculation of dose distribution (lung mean dose or normalized total mean dose) to minimize the volume of lung irradiated, particularly for those at high risk, may reduce the risk of late side effects (Abratt & Morgan, 2002; Lebesque et al., 1997; McDonald et al., 1995).

Pharyngitis and Esophagitis

The epithelial cells of the pharynx and esophagus are highly radiosensitive and often in the field of the radiation treatment area. Radiation to the lungs and adjacent lymph nodes is associated with inflammation or ulceration of the mucosal lining of the pharynx and esophagus, which frequently leads to dose-limiting toxicity. Addition of concurrent chemotherapy regimens may compound the complications. Studies using endoscopic examination of the esophagus have revealed that clinical symptoms often do not reflect the extent of mucosal damage (Suzuki, Kobayashi, & Kitamura, 1997). Pharyngitis and, particularly, esophagitis can lead to serious complications and greatly affect QOL by causing pain and the inability to eat or drink. In addition, interruptions or delays in treatment schedules may be required, compromising the overall efficacy of treatment.

Symptoms occur approximately 2–3 weeks from the start of treatment and may occur sooner if concurrent chemotherapy is administered. Symptoms may resolve during radiation or last until after completion. Patients with pharyngitis complain of fullness in the throat with difficulty swallowing, with or without soreness. Patients with esophagitis tend to have more severe symptoms as a result of inflammation and denudation of the surface epithelium of the esophagus (Knopp, 1997). Dysphagia and edema occur with progressive therapy. Coarse foods and extreme food temperatures can further traumatize the mucosa, and patients complain of epigastric discomfort, esophageal reflux, and pain on swallowing certain or all foods. Disruption of the normal mucosal barrier can lead to invasive fungal infections from *Candida albicans,* part of the normal gastrointestinal flora. Esophageal candidiasis has been reported to be associated with half the cases of radiation pneumonitis (Suzuki et al., 1997). Chronic esophagitis may occur as a result of a herpetic or fungal infection. Esophageal stenosis, or necrosis leading to fistula, can occur several months after treatment, although it is rare and usually associated with prior surgery or tumor progression (Knopp).

Measures to relieve symptoms include gargling with saline before and after meals and taking liquid analgesics to control pain 30–60 minutes before meals. Combinations or "cocktails" of local anesthetics, antacids, and antihistamines, often referred to as "magic mouthwash," can provide effective relief. An example of contents is equal parts of dyclonine 0.5%, Maalox® (Novartis, Mississauga, ON), and diphenhydramine powder. Another mixture used is Kaopectate® (Pfizer, New York, NY), diphenhydramine elixir, and viscous lidocaine. Patients are instructed to swallow 10 cc every four to six hours as needed (Knopp, 1997; Suzuki et al., 1997). Lortab® elixir (Whitby Pharmaceutical, Richmond, VA) also has been found to reduce pain associated with radiation esophagitis. One teaspoon of Lortab contains 12.5 mg of hydrocodone barbiturate, 120 mg acetaminophen, and 7% alcohol. Patients are instructed to take one teaspoon one-half hour before meals as needed (Madeya, 1996). Another recommended mixture for pain control and to reduce candidiasis is Rothwell's solution, which contains 14.5 ml nystatin suspension, 24 ml tetracycline syrup, 120 mg hydrocortisone powder, and 650 mg diphenhydramine powder (Knopp). Fungal infections require treatment with oral or IV antifungals. Antacids can provide comfort and reduce additional ulceration from reflux (Suzuki et al.)

Dietary measures include a soft, bland diet with the addition of high-caloric snacks and supplements. Patients report that thick, soft food and fluids are more tolerable than water or juices. Recommendations include avoiding spicy or irritating foods, alcohol, and tobacco; sitting upright to eat and remaining sitting or standing after meals for at least 15 minutes; drinking liquids through a straw to ease swallowing; eating slowly, chewing completely, and cutting foods into small pieces; taking antacids before meals; and crushing allowable medications that are difficult to swallow. Rarely do patients require enteral feedings as is seen frequently with radiation therapy to the head and neck areas. Maintenance of fluid hydration is key, and patients should be encouraged to drink large volumes of fluids, especially when other nutritional intake is impossible. IV fluid hydration may be necessary during highest acuity.

Studies of dosimetric predictors of radiation esophagitis have identified variables to include in treatment planning. These parameters, which include mean dose to affected areas, may provide methods for prevention of esophagitis and pharyngitis (Hirota et al., 2001).

Summary

Nursing care of those with lung cancer covers all aspects of treatment across the continuum of the disease. A snapshot of lung cancer includes those undergoing induction therapy prior to surgical resection and hoping for cure; those with advanced disease at diagnosis undergoing chemotherapy with the goal of living longer; those for whom available therapy has been exhausted and are receiving palliation only; and finally, the survivors who are living each day, coping with sequelae of illness and treatment, hoping for a disease-free life. All patients require ongoing management of disease and treatment-related needs with an emphasis on improving or maintaining their QOL. Nursing interventions include direct care delivery; education about the illness and treatments to promote adaptation and safety related to self-care measures; support, counseling, and referral for psychosocial adjustment; management and palliation of symptoms; and coordination of end-of-life needs.

As with all chronic diseases, education of patients and caregivers about available resources for services and support is an important component of assisting development of effective coping strategies. Appendix 1 contains many lung cancer resources for patients and professionals.

References

Aass, N., Fossa, S.D., Dahl, A.A., & Moe, T.J. (1997). Prevalence of anxiety and depression in cancer patients seen at the Norwegian Radium Hospital. *European Journal of Cancer, 33,* 1597–1604.

Abels, R.I. (1992). Use of recombinant human erythropoietin in the treatment of anemia in patients who have caner. *Seminars in Oncology, 19*(3 Suppl. 8), 29–35.

Abratt, R.P., & Morgan, G.W. (2002). Lung toxicity following chest irradiation in patients with lung cancer. *Lung Cancer, 35*(2),103–109.

Allard, P., Lamontagne, C., Bernard, P., & Tremblay, C. (1999). How effective are supplementary doses of opioids for dyspnea in terminally ill cancer patients? A randomized continuous sequential clinical trial. *Journal of Pain and Symptom Management, 17,* 256–265.

American Society of Clinical Oncology. (1997). Clinical practice guidelines for the treatment of unresectable non-small cell lung cancer. *Journal of Clinical Oncology, 15,* 2996–3018.

American Thoracic Society. (1999). Dyspnea mechanisms, assessment and management: A consensus statement. *American Journal of Respiratory and Critical Care Medicine, 159,* 321–340.

Arathuzik, D. (1991). The appraisal of pain and coping in cancer patients. *Western Journal of Nursing Research, 13,* 714–731.

Beaver, W.T., & Feise, G.A. (1977). A comparison of the analgesic effects of oxymorphones by rectal suppository and intramuscular injection in patients with postoperative pain. *Journal of Clinical Pharmacology, 17,* 276–291.

Beck, S.L. (1991). The therapeutic use of music for cancer-related pain. *Oncology Nursing Forum, 18,* 1327–1337.

Beckles, M.A., Spiro, S.G., Colice, G.L., & Rudd, R.M. (2003). Initial evaluation of the patient with lung cancer. Symptoms, signs, laboratory tests, and paraneoplastic syndromes. *Chest, 123*(Suppl. 1), 97S–104S.

Beers, M.H., & Berkow, R. (Eds.). (1999). *The Merck manual, centennial edition.* Whitehouse Station, NJ: Merck Research Laboratories.

Berger, A.M., & Farr, L. (1999). The influence of daytime inactivity and nighttime restlessness on cancer-related fatigue. *Oncology Nursing Forum, 26,* 1663–1671.

Birn, C.S., & Kosco, P. (2004). Flexible scopes and photodynamic therapy [Continuing education program]. *Nursing Spectrum.* Retrieved January 14, 2004, from http://nsweb.nursingspectrum.com/ce/ce264.htm

Brown, J.K. (2002). A systematic review of the evidence on symptom management of cancer-related anorexia and cachexia. *Oncology Nursing Forum, 29,* 517–532.

Bruera, E., deStoutz, N., Velasco-Leiva, A., Schoeller, T., & Hanson, J. (1993). Effects of oxygen on dyspnoea in hypoxaemic terminal-cancer patients. *Lancet, 342*(8862), 13–14.

Bruera, E., & Ripamonti, C. (1998). Dyspnea in patients with advanced cancer. In A. Berger, R.K. Portenoy, & D.E. Weissman (Eds.), *Principles and practice of supportive oncology* (pp. 295–308). Philadelphia: Lippincott Williams & Wilkins.

Burks, T.F. (2001). New agents for the treatment of cancer-related fatigue. *Cancer 92*(6 Suppl.), 1714–1718.

Busick, N.P., Fretz, P.C., Galvin, J.R., & Peterson, M.W. (1999). Pancoast tumors. In J.R. Galvin & M.W. Peterson (Eds.), *Lung tumors: A multidisciplinary database.* Iowa City, IA: University of Iowa. Retrieved May 8, 2003, from http://www.vh.org/adult/provider/radiology/LungTumors/ParaneoplasticProcesses/Text/PancoastSyndrome.html

Carrieri, V.K., & Janson-Bjerklie, S. (1986). Dyspnea. In V.K. Carrieri, A. Lindsey, & C.M. West (Eds.), *Pathophysiologic phenomena in nursing human responses to illness* (pp. 191–218). Philadelphia: W.B. Saunders.

Carrieri-Kohlman, V., Gormley, J.M., Douglas, M.K., Paul, S.M., & Stulbarg, M.S. (1996). Differentiation between dyspnea and its affective components. *Western Journal of Nursing Research, 18,* 626–642.

Cella, D. (1997). The Functional Assessment of Cancer–Anemia (FACT-An scale): A new tool for the assessment of outcomes in cancer anemia and fatigue. *Seminars in Hematology, 34*(Suppl. 2), 13–19.

Cella, D., Bonomi, A., Lloyd, S., Tulsky, D., Bonomi, P., & Kaplan, E. (1995). Reliability and validity of the Functional Assessment of Cancer Therapy–Lung (FACT-L) quality of life instrument. *Lung Cancer, 12,* 199–220.

Cella, D.F., Jacobsen, P.B., Orav, E.J., Holland, J.C., Silberferb, P.M., & Rafla, S. (1987). A brief POMS measure of distress for cancer patients. *Journal of Chronic Diseases, 40,* 939–942.

Chetta, A., Gerra, G., Foresi, A., Zaimovic, A., DelDonno, M., Chittolini, B., et al. (1998). Personality profiles and breathlessness measurement in outpatients with different grading of asthma. *American Journal of Respiratory and Critical Care Medicine, 157,* 116–122.

Chute, C.G., Greenberg, E.R., Baron, J., Korson, R., Baker, J., & Yates, J. (1985). Presenting conditions of 1539 population based lung cancer patients by cell type and stage in New Hampshire and Vermont. *Cancer, 56,* 2107–2111.

Cimprich, B. (1992). Attentional fatigue following breast cancer surgery. *Research Nursing Health, 15,* 199–207.

Cimprich, B. (1993). Development of an intervention to restore attention in cancer patients. *Cancer Nursing, 16,* 83–92.

Cioffi, D. (1991). Beyond attentional strategies: A cognitive-perceptual model of somatic interpretation. *Psychological Bulletin, 109,* 25–41.

Cleeland, C.S., Cleeland, L.M., Dar, R., & Rinehardt, L.C. (1986). Factors influencing physician management of cancer pain. *Cancer, 58,* 796–800.

Cooley, M.E. (2000). Symptoms in adults with lung cancer: A systematic research review. *Journal of Pain and Symptom Management, 19,* 137–153.

Corey, R., & Hla, K.M. (1987). Major and massive hemoptysis: Reassessment of conservative management. *American Journal of Medical Science, 294,* 301–309.

Costa, G., & Donaldson, S. (1980). Nutritional effects of cancer and its therapy. *Nutrition and Cancer, 2,* 22–29.

Crawford, J., Cella, D., Cleeland, C.S., Cremieux, P.Y., Demetri, G.D., Sarokhan, B.J., et al. (2002). Relationship between changes in hemoglobin level and quality of life during chemotherapy in anemic patients receiving epoetin alfa therapy. *Cancer, 95,* 888–895.

Crino, L., Scagliotti, M., Marangolo, F., Figoli, F., Cleric, M., DeMarinis, V., et al. (1997). Cisplatin-gemcitabine combination in advanced non-small cell lung cancer: A phase II study. *Journal of Clinical Oncology, 15,* 297–303.

Curt, G., Breitbart, W., Cella, D., Groopman, J.E., Horning, S.J., Itri, L.M., et al. (2000). Impact of cancer-related fatigue on the lives of patients: New findings from the fatigue coalition. *Oncologist, 5,* 353–360.

Daut, R.L., Cleeland, C.S., & Flanery, R.C. (1983). The development of the Wisconsin Brief Pain Questionnaire to assess pain in cancer and other diseases. *Pain, 17,* 197–210.

Del Mastro, L., Gennari, A., & Donati, S. (1999). Chemotherapy of non-small cell lung cancer: Role of erythropoietin in the management of anemia. *Annals of Oncology, 10*(Suppl. 5), S91–S94.

Demetri, G.D., Kris, M., Wade, J., Degos, L., & Cella, D. (1998). Quality-of-life benefit in chemotherapy patients treated with epoetin alfa is independent of disease response or tumor type: Results from a prospective community oncology study. Procrit Study Group. *Journal of Clinical Oncology, 16,* 3412–3425.

Devine, E., & Westlake, S. (1995). The effects of psychoeducational care provided to adults with cancer: Meta-analysis of 116 studies. *Oncology Nursing Forum, 22,* 1369–1381.

DeWys, W.D., Begg, C.H., Douglass, H.O., Engstrom, P.R., Ezdinli, E.Z., Horton, J., et al. (1980). Prognostic effects of weight loss prior to chemotherapy in cancer patients. *American Journal of Medicine, 69,* 491–497.

Dimeo, F.C. (2001). Effects of exercise on cancer-related fatigue. *Cancer, 92*(Suppl. 6), 1689–1693.

Dimeo, F.C., Steiglitz, R.D., Novelli-Fischer, U., & Keue, J. (1999). Effects of physical activity on the fatigue and psychological status of cancer patients during chemotherapy. *Cancer, 85,* 2273–2277.

Doona, M., & Walsh, D. (1998). Benzonatate for opioids-resistant cough in advanced cancer. *Palliative Medicine, 12,* 55–58.

Dudgeon, D.J. (2002). Managing dyspnea and cough. *Hematology/Oncology Clinics of North America, 16,* 557–577.

Dudgeon, D.J., Kristjanson, L., Sloan, J.A., Lertzman, M., & Clement, K. (2001). Dyspnea in cancer patients: Prevalence and associated factors. *Journal of Pain and Symptom Management, 21*(2), 95–102.

Dudley, D.L., Martin, C.J., & Holmes T.H. (1964). Psychophysiologic studies of pulmonary ventilation. *Psychosomatic Medicine, 26,* 645–659.

Dumon, J.F., Shapshay, S., & Bourcerau, J. (1984). Principles for safety in application of neodymium-YAG laser in bronchology. *Chest, 86,* 163–168.

Filshie, J., Penn, K., Ashley, S., & Davis, C. (1996). Acupuncture for the relief of cancer-related breathlessness. *Palliative Medicine, 10,* 145–150.

Fishman, B., Pasternak, S., Wallerstein, S.L., Houde, R.W., Holland, J.C., & Foley, K.M. (1986). The Memorial Pain Assessment Card: A valid instrument for the assessment of cancer pain. *Cancer, 60,* 1151–1157.

Foley, K.M. (2001). Supportive care and quality of life: Management of cancer pain. In V.T. DeVita, S. Hellman, & S.A. Rosenberg (Eds.), *Cancer: Principles and practice of oncology* (6th ed., pp. 2977–3011). Philadelphia: Lippincott Williams & Wilkins.

Fretz, P.C., & Peterson, M.W. (1999). Clinical signs and symptoms. In J.R. Galvin & M.W. Peterson (Eds.), *Lung tumors: A multidisciplinary database.* Iowa City, IA: University of Iowa. Retrieved on May 8, 2003, from http://www.vh.org/adult/provider/radiology/LungTumors/ClinicalPresentation/Text/InitialEvaluation.html

Gabrilove, J.L., Cleeland, C.S., Livingston, R.B., Sarokham, B., Winer, E., & Einhorn, L. (2001). Clinical evaluation of once-weekly dosing of epoetin alfa in chemotherapy patients: Improvements in hemoglobin and quality of life are similar to three-times weekly dosing. *Journal of Clinical Oncology, 15,* 1218–1234.

Gabrilove, J.L., & Jakubowski, A. (1990). Hematopoietic growth factors: Biology and clinical application. *Journal of the National Cancer Institute, 10,* 73–77.

Gagnon, G., & Bruera, E. (1998). A review of the drug treatments of cachexia associated with cancer. *Drugs, 55,* 675–688.

Geffin, B., Shapshay, S.M., & Bellack, G.S. (1980). Flammability of endotracheal tubes during ND-YAG laser application in the airway. *Anesthesiology, 89,* 124–128.

Gift, A. (1991). Psychologic and physiologic aspects of acute dyspnea in asthmatics. *Nursing Research, 40,* 196–199.

Ginsberg, R.J., Vokes, E.E., & Rosenzweig, K. (2001). Non small cell lung cancer. In V.T. DeVita, S. Hellman, & S.A. Rosenberg (Eds.), *Cancer: Principles and practice of oncology* (6th ed., pp. 925–983). Philadelphia: Lippincott Williams & Wilkins.

Given, B., Given, C., Azzouz, F., & Stommel, M. (2001). Physical functioning of elderly patients prior to diagnosis and following initial treatment. *Nursing Research, 50,* 222–232.

Glaspy, J. (2001). Anemia and fatigue in cancer patients. *Cancer, 92*(Suppl. 6), 1719–1724.

Glaus, A., Crow, R., & Hammond, S.A. (1996). A qualitative study to explore the concept of fatigue/tiredness in cancer patients and in healthy individuals. *Supportive Care in Cancer, 4,* 82–96.

Goldberg, R.M., & Loprinzi, C.L. (1999). Cancer anorexia/cachexia. In C.F. von Guten (Ed.), *Palliative care and rehabilitation of cancer patients* (pp. 31–41). Boston: Kluwer Academic.

Graham, C., Bond, S.S., Gertrovitch, M.M., & Cook, M.R. (1980). Use of the McGill Pain Questionnaire in the management of cancer pain: Replicability and consistency. *Pain, 8,* 337–387.

Groopman, J.E., & Itri, L. (1999). Chemotherapy induced anemia in adults: Incidence and treatment. *Journal of the National Cancer Institute, 91,* 1616–1634.

Guimarães, C.A. (2002). Massive hemoptysis. In F.G. Pearson, J.D. Cooper, J. Deslauriers, R.J. Ginsberg, C.A. Hiebert, G.A. Patterson, et al. (Eds.), *Thoracic surgery* (2nd ed., pp. 717–736). New York: Churchill Livingstone.

Gutstein, H.B. (2001). The biological basis of fatigue. *Cancer, 92*(Suppl. 6), 1678–1683.

Henke, C.S. (2000). Hemoptysis. In D. Camp-Sorrell & R.A. Hawkins (Eds.), *Clinical manual for the oncology advanced practice nurse* (pp. 137–140). Pittsburgh, PA: Oncology Nursing Society.

Hetzel, M.R., & Smith, S.G. (1991). Endoscopic palliation of tracheobronchial malignancies. *Thorax, 46,* 325–333.

Hickock, J.T., Morrow, G.R., McDonald, S., & Bellg, A.J. (1996). Frequency and correlates of fatigue in lung cancer patients receiving radiation therapy: Implications for management. *Journal of Pain and Symptom Management, 11,* 370–377.

Hirota, S., Tsujino, K., Endo, M., Kotani, Y., Satouchi, M., Kado, T., et al. (2001). Dosimetric predictors of radiation esophagitis in patients treated for non-small cell lung cancer with carboplatin/paclitaxel/radiotherapy. *International Journal of Radiation Oncology, Biology, Physics, 51,* 291–295.

Hirshberg, B., Biran, I., Glazer, M., & Kramer, M. (1997). Hemoptysis: Etiology, evaluation, and outcome in a tertiary referral hospital. *Chest, 112,* 440–444.

Hollen, P., Gralla, R., Kris, M., Eberly, S., & Potanovich, L. (1993). Quality of life assessment in individuals with lung cancer: Testing the Lung Cancer Symptom Scale (LCSS). *European Journal of Cancer, 29A*(Suppl. 1), S51–S58.

Holley, S. (2000). Cancer-related fatigue: Suffering a different fatigue. *Cancer Practice, 8,* 87–95.

Hopwood, P., & Stephens, R.J. (2000). Depression in patients with lung cancer: Prevalence and risk factors derived from quality of life data. *Journal of Clinical Oncology, 18,* 893–903.

Ingle, R.J. (2000). Lung cancers. In C.H. Yarbro, M.H. Frogge, M. Goodman, & S.L. Groenwald (Eds.), *Cancer nursing: Principles and practice* (5th ed., pp. 1298–1328). Sudbury, MA: Jones and Bartlett.

Inoue, A., Kunitoh, H., Sekine, I., Sumi, M., Tokuuye, K., & Saijo, N. (2001). Radiation pneumonitis in lung cancer patients: a retrospective study of risk factors and the long-term prognosis. *International Journal of Radiation Oncology, Biology, Physics, 49,* 649–655.

Inzeo, D., & Tyson, L. (2003). Nursing assessment and management of dyspneic patients with lung cancer. *Clinical Journal of Oncology Nursing, 7,* 332–333.

Irvine, D., Vincent, L., Graydon, J., Bubela, N., & Thompson, L. (1994). The prevalence and correlates of fatigue in patients receiving treatment with chemotherapy and radiation. *Cancer Nursing, 17,* 367–378.

Irwin, R.S., Boulet, L.P., Cloutier, M.M., Fuller, R., Gold, P.M., Hoffstein, V., et al. (1998). Managing cough as a defense mechanism and as a symptom. A consensus panel report of the American College of Chest Physicians. *Chest, 114*(Suppl. 2), 133S–181S.

Jenis, L.G., Dunn, E.J., & An, H.S. (1999). Metastatic disease of the cervical spine: A review. *Clinical Orthopedics, 359,* 89–103.

Jennings, A.L., Davies, A.N., Higgins, J.P., Gibbs, J.S., & Broadley, K.E. (2002). A systematic review of the use of opioids in the management of dyspnea. *Thorax, 57,* 939–944.

Joyce, M., McSweeney, M., Carrieri-Kohlman, V.L., & Hawkins, J. (2004). Evidence synthesis: The use of nebulized opioids in the management of dyspnea. *Oncology Nursing Forum, 31,* 551–561.

King, K.B., Nail, L.M., Kreamer, K., Strohl, R.A., & Johnson, J.E. (1985). Patient's descriptions of experience of receiving radiation therapy. *Oncology Nursing Forum, 12,* 55–61.

Knopp, J.M. (1997). Lung cancer. In K.H. Dow, J.D. Bucholtz, R.R. Iwamoto, V.K. Fieler, & L.J. Hilderley (Eds.), *Nursing care in radiation oncology* (2nd ed., pp. 293–315). Philadelphia: W.B. Saunders.

Kuo, T., & Fung-Chi, M. (2002). Symptom distresses and coping strategies in patients with non-small cell lung cancer. *Cancer Nursing, 25,* 309–317.

Kurzrock, R. (2001). The role of cytokines in cancer-related fatigue. *Cancer, 92*(Suppl. 6), 1684–1688.

Kvale, P.A., Simoff, M., & Prakash, U.B.S. (2003). Palliative care. *Chest, 123*(Suppl. 1), 284S– 311S.

Lebesque, J.V., Kwa, S.L.S., Theuws, J.C.M., Bentel, G., Marks, L.B., Munley, M.T., et al. (1997). Radiation pneumonitis as a function of dose and volume; an analysis of pooled data of 442 patients. *International Journal of Radiation Oncology, Biology, Physics, 39,* 197–203.

Lesage, P., & Portenoy, R. (2002). Management of fatigue in the cancer patient. *Oncology, 16,* 373–389.

Lindsey, A.M. (1986). Cancer cachexia: Effects of the disease and its treatments. *Seminars in Oncology Nursing, 2,* 19–29.

Lipton, R.B., Apfel, S.C., Dutcher, J.P., Rosenberg, R., Kaplan, J., Berger, A., et al. (1989). Taxol produces a predominantly sensory neuropathy. *Neurology, 39,* 368–373.

Luce, J.M., & Luce, J.A. (2001). Management of dyspnea in patients with far advancing lung diagnosis. *JAMA, 285,* 1331–1337.

Madeya, M.L. (1996). Oral complications from cancer therapy: Part 2—Nursing implications for assessment and treatment. *Oncology Nursing Forum, 23,* 808–819.

Maltoni, M., Nanni, O., Scarpi, E., Rossi, D., Serra, P., & Amadon, D. (2001). High dose progestins for the treatment of cancer anorexia-cachexia syndrome: A systematic review of randomized clinical trials. *Annals of Oncology, 12,* 289–300.

Martin, L.A., & Hagen, N.A. (1997). Neuropathic pain in cancer patients: Mechanisms, syndromes, and clinical controversies. *Journal of Pain and Symptom Management, 14,* 99–117.

McCarthy, E.P., Phillips, R.S., Zhong, Z., Drews, R.E., & Lynn, J. (2000). Dying with cancer: Patients' function, symptoms, and care preferences as death approaches. *Journal of American Geriatric Society, 48*(Suppl. 5), S110–S121.

McDermott, M.K. (2000). Cough. In D. Camp-Sorrell & R.A. Hawkins (Eds.), *Clinical manual for the oncology advanced practice nurse* (pp. 127–130). Pittsburgh: Oncology Nursing Society.

McDonald, S., Rubin, P., Phillips, T., & Marks, L. (1995). Injury to the lung from cancer therapy: Clinical syndromes, measurable endpoints, and potential scoring systems. *International Journal of Radiation Oncology, Biology, Physics, 31,* 1187–1203.

Mock, V. (2001). Fatigue management: Evidence and guidelines for practice. *Cancer, 92*(Suppl. 6), 1699–1707.

Morgan, G.W., & Breit, S.N. (1995). Radiation and the lung: A re-evaluation of the mechanisms mediating pulmonary injury. *Inter-national Journal of Radiation Oncology, Biology, Physics, 31,* 361–369.

Morice, R.C., Ece, T., Ece, F., & Keus, L. (2001). Endobronchial argon plasma coagulation for treatment of hemoptysis and neoplastic airway obstruction. *Chest, 119,* 781–787.

Morrison, S.D. (1989). Cancer cachexia. *Cancer Growth Process, 3,* 176–213.

Morrow, G.R., Andrews, P.L.R., Hickock, J.T., Roscoe, J.A., & Matteson, S. (2002). Fatigue associated with cancer and its treatment. *Supportive Cancer in Care, 10,* 389–398.

Muers, M.F., & Round, C.E. (1993). Palliation of symptoms in non-small lung cancer: A study by the Yorkshire Regional Cancer Organization thoracic group. *Thorax, 48,* 339–343.

Nail, L.M. (2002). Fatigue in patients with cancer. *Oncology Nursing Forum, 29,* 537–544.

National Comprehensive Cancer Network. (2003). *Clinical practice guidelines in oncology: Cancer-related fatigue.* Retrieved June 3, 2003, from http://www.nccn.org/physician_gls/f_guidelines .html

Newall, S., Sanson-Fischer, R.W., Girgis, A., & Ackland, S. (1999). The physical and psycho-social experiences of patients attending an outpatient medical oncology department: A cross-sectional study. *European Journal of Cancer Care, 8,* 73–82.

Paice, J.A., & Fine, P.G. (2001). Pain in the end of life. In B.F. Ferrell & N. Coyle (Eds.), *Textbook of palliative nursing* (pp. 76–90). New York: Oxford University Press.

Palomano, R.C., McGuire, D.B., & Sheidler, V.R. (2000). Management of cancer pain. In S.L. Groenwald, M.H. Frogge, M. Goodman, & C.H. Yarbro. (Eds.), *Cancer nursing: Principles and practice* (5th ed., pp. 657–690). Sudbury, MA: Jones and Bartlett.

Piper, B. (1993). Fatigue. In V. Carrieri-Kohlman, A. Lindsey, & C. West (Eds.), *Pathophysiological phenomena in nursing: Human response to illness* (pp. 279–302). Philadelphia: W.B. Saunders.

Piper, B.F., Dibble, S.L., Dodb, M.J., Weiss, M.C., Slaughter, R.E., & Paul, S.M. (1998). The revised Piper Fatigue Scale: Psychometric evaluation in women with breast cancer. *Oncology Nursing Forum, 25,* 677–684.

Portenoy, R. (1999). Managing cancer pain poorly responsive to systemic opioids therapy. *Oncology, 3,* 25–29.

Portenoy, R., Miransky, J., Thaler, H.T., Hornung, J., Bianchi, C., Cibas-Kong, I., et al. (1992). Pain in ambulatory patients with lung or colon cancer: Prevalence, characteristics, and impact. *Cancer, 70,* 1616–1624.

Prakash, U.B.S. (1999). Advances in bronchoscopic procedures. *Chest, 116,* 1403–1408.

Richardson, A. (1995). Fatigue in cancer patients: A review of the literature. *European Journal of Cancer Care, 4,* 20–32.

Richardson, A., Ream, E., & Wilson-Barnett, J. (1998). Fatigue in patients receiving chemotherapy: Patterns of change. *Cancer Nursing, 21,* 17–30.

Ripamonti, C., & Fusco, F. (2002). Respiratory problems in supportive care. *Cancer, 10,* 204–216.

Robnett, T., Machtay, M., Vines, E., McKenna, M., Algazy, K., & McKenna, W.G. (2000). Factors predicting severe radiation pneumonitis in patients receiving definitive chemoradiation for lung cancer. *International Journal of Radiation Oncology, Biology, Physics, 48,* 89–94.

Sarna, L., & Brecht, M.L. (1997). Dimensions of symptom distress in women with advanced lung cancer: A factor analysis. *Heart and Lung, 26,* 23–30.

Shepherd, S., & Geraci, S. (1999). The differential diagnosis of dyspnea: A pathophysiologic approach. *Clinician Reviews, 9*(4), 52–72.

Silvestri, G.A. (2000). Palliation for the dying patient with lung cancer. *Respiratory Care, 45,* 1490–1496.

Smith, E.L., Hann, D.M., Ahles, T.A., Furstenberg, C.T., Mitchell, T.A., Meyer, L., et al. (2001). Dyspnea, anxiety, body consciousness and quality of life in patients with lung cancer. *Journal of Pain and Symptom Management, 21,* 323–329.

Staats, P.S. (2002). Pain management and beyond: Evolving concepts and treatments involving cyclooxygenase inhibition. *Journal of Pain and Symptom Management, 24,* 54–59.

Stone, P., Hardy, J., Broadley, K., Tookman, A.J., Kurowska, A., & Hern, R.A. (1999). Fatigue in advanced cancer: A prospective controlled cross sectional study. *British Journal of Cancer, 79,* 1479–1486.

Strohl, R. (2000). Bone metastasis. In D. Camp-Sorell & R. Hawkins (Eds.), *Clinical manual for the oncology advanced practice nurse* (pp. 611–614). Pittsburgh, PA: Oncology Nursing Society.

Suzuki, M., Kobayashi, J., & Kitamura, S. (1997). Radiation esophagitis in the treatment for lung cancer. *Lung Cancer, 18*(Suppl. 1), 206–211.

Tanaka, K., Akechi, T., Okuyama, T., Nishiwaki, Y., & Uchitomi, Y. (2001). Prevalence and screening of dyspnea interfering with daily life activities in ambulatory patients with advanced lung cancer. *Journal of Pain and Symptom Management, 23,* 484–489.

Tanaka, K., Akechi, T., Okuyama, T., Nishiwaki, Y., & Uchitomi, Y. (2002). Impact of dyspnea, pain, and fatigue on daily life activities in ambulatory patients with advanced lung cancer. *Journal of Pain and Symptom Management, 23,* 417–423.

Tong, D., Gillick, L., & Hendrickson, F.R. (1982). The palliative of symptomatic osseous metastases: Final results of the study by the Radiation Therapy Oncology Group. *Cancer, 50,* 893–899.

Ventafridda, V., Fochi, V., DeConno, D., & Sganzerla, E. (1980). Use of non-steroidal anti-inflammatory drugs in the treatment of pain in cancer. *British Journal of Clinical Pharmacology, 10*(Suppl. 2), 3435–3465.

Visser, M.R.M., & Smets, E.M.A. (1998). Fatigue, depression, and quality of life in cancer patients: How are they related? *Supportive Cancer in Care, 6,* 101–108.

Vogelzang, N.J., Breitbart, W., Cella, D., Curt, G.A., Groopman, J.E., Horning, S.J., et al. (1997). Patient, caregiver, and oncologist perceptions of cancer-related fatigue: Results of a tripart assessment survey. *Seminars in Hematology, 35*(3 Suppl. 2), 4–12.

Von Roenn, J.H., Cleeland, C.S., Gonin, R., Hatfield, A.K., & Pandya, K. (1993). Physician attitudes and practice in cancer pain management. *Annals of Internal Medicine, 119,* 121–126.

Weiss, S.C., Emanuel, L.L., Fairclough, D.L., & Emanuel, E.J. (2001). Understanding the experience of pain in terminally ill patients. *Lancet, 357*(9265), 1311–1315.

Winningham, M., Nail, L., Barton-Burke, M., Brophy, L., Cimprich, B., Jones, L., et al. (1994). Fatigue and the cancer experience: The state of knowledge. *Oncology Nursing Forum, 21,* 23–36.

Wolff, B.B. (1985). Ethnocultural factors influencing pain and illness behavior. *Clinical Journal of Pain, 1,* 23–30.

Wood, P.A., & Hrushesky, W.J.M. (1995). Cisplatin-associated anemia: An erythropoietin deficiency syndrome. *Journal of Clinical Investment, 95,* 1650–1659.

World Health Organization. (1986). *Cancer pain relief.* Geneva: Author.

Yeager, K.A., McGuire, D.B., & Sheidler, V.R. (2000). Assessment of cancer pain. In S.L. Groenwald, M.H. Frogge, M. Goodman, & C.H. Yarbro (Eds.), *Cancer nursing: Principles and practice* (5th ed., pp. 633–656). Sudbury, MA: Jones and Bartlett.

Zigmond, A.S., & Snaith, R.P. (1983). The hospital anxiety and depression scale. *Acta Psychiatrica Scandinavica, 67,* 361–370.

APPENDIX

Appendix 1. Resources Related to Lung Cancer

Cancer/Lung Cancer Information

Alliance for Lung Cancer Advocacy, Support and Education (ALCASE)
P.O. Box 849, Vancouver, WA 98666
Phone: 360-696-2436 or 800-289-2436
Web site: www.alcase.org
ALCASE is the only nonprofit organization dedicated solely to supporting and improving the quality of lives of people with lung cancer. ALCASE should be your first source for information and support following a lung cancer diagnosis.

American Cancer Society
National Home Office, 1599 Clifton Road, Atlanta, GA 30329
Phone: 800-ACS-2345
Web site: www.cancer.org
ACS is a nationwide, community-based organization that conducts cancer advocacy and research activities and provides patient education and support services. Information available in Spanish.

American Lung Association
1740 Broadway, New York, NY 10019
Phone: 212-315-8700
Web site: www.lungusa.org
The mission of ALA is to prevent lung disease and promote lung health, with special emphasis on asthma, tobacco control and environmental health. Information available in Spanish.

American Society of Clinical Oncology (ASCO)
1900 Duke Street, Suite 200, Alexandria, VA 22314
Phone: 703-299-0150
Web site: www.asco.org
ASCO is a professional organization for cancer specialists. New findings in cancer research are presented each year at its annual conference. Conference abstracts are posted on the ASCO Web site.

Lung Cancer Online
Web site: www.lungcanceronline.org
Comprehensive directory to lung cancer information and resources for patients and their families. Edited by Karen Parles.

Lungcancer.org
Web site: www.lungcancer.org
Lung cancer information for patients, healthcare professionals and the media. Sponsored by Cancercare® and the Oncology Nursing Society.

National Cancer Institute (NCI)
Public Inquiries Office, Building 31, Room 10A31, Bethesda, MD 20892-2580
Phone: 800-4-CANCER (NCI's Cancer Information Service)
Web site: www.cancer.gov
NCI offers extensive up-to-date online and print information on lung cancer and its treatment, including clinical trials. Information available in Spanish.

People Living with Cancer
Web site: www.plwc.org
Oncologist-approved information for people with cancer. Maintained by ASCO.

Steve Dunn's Cancerguide
Web site: www.cancerguide.org
Steve Dunn, a kidney cancer survivor, provides a patient's perspective and valuable advice on how to find the answers to your questions about cancer and, most importantly, how to know which questions to ask.

Print Publications
ALCASE publications include a lung cancer manual and newsletters for patients (*Spirit and Breath*) and physicians (*Quarterly Scan*).
Henschke, Claudia, et al. *Lung Cancer: Myths, Facts, Choices – and Hope*. New York: W.W. Norton, 2002.
In Touch Magazine: The Good Health Guide to Cancer Prevention and Treatment. Subscription available by phone at 877-246-8682 or online at www.intouch.com. Must join to have access.
Johnston, Lorraine. *Lung Cancer: Making Sense of Diagnosis, Treatment & Options*. Sebastopol, CA: O'Reilly & Associates, 2001.

Caregivers and Home Care

Family Caregiver Alliance
690 Market Street, Suite 600, San Francisco, CA 94104
Phone: 415-434-3388
Web site: www.caregiver.org
Caregiver resources include an online support group and an information clearinghouse. Information available in Spanish.

National Family Caregivers Association
10400 Connecticut Avenue, #500, Kensington, MD 20895-3944
Phone: 800-896-3650
Web site: www.nfcacares.org
Provides education, information, support and advocacy services for family caregivers.

CAREGIVERS (Association of Cancer Online Resources)
Web page: www.acor.org click on "mailing lists" then select "CAREGIVERS."
Online discussion group for caregivers of cancer patients.

Caring for the Caregiver (National Coalition for Cancer Survivorship)
Web site: www.canceradvocacy.org

Guide for Cancer Supporters: Step-by-Step Ways to Help a Relative or Friend Fight Cancer (R.A. Bloch Cancer Foundation)
Web site: www.blochcancer.org

(Continued on next page)

Appendix 1. Resources Related to Lung Cancer *(Continued)*

Caregivers and Home Care *(cont.)*

Print Publications

Houts, Peter S. and Julia A. Bucher, Eds. *Caregiving: A Step-by-Step Resource for Caring for the Person with Cancer at Home*. Atlanta, GA: American Cancer Society, 2000.

Children

Kids Konnected
27071 Cabot Road, Suite 102, Laguna Hills, CA 92653
Phone: 949-582-5443
Web site: www.kidskonnected.org
Provides extensive support resources and programs for children who have a parent with cancer.

What Do I Tell the Children? – A Guide for a Parent with Cancer (Cancer BACUP)
Web page: www.cancerbacup.org

Print Publications

Ackerman, Abigail and Adrienne Ackerman. *Our Mom Has Cancer*. Atlanta, GA: American Cancer Society, 2000.
Harpham, Wendy S. *When a Parent Has Cancer: A Guide to Caring for Your Children*. Companion book: *Becky and the Worry Cup*. New York: HarperCollins, 1997.

Clinical Trials Resources

There is no single resource for locating clinical trials for lung cancer. It makes sense to check all of the resources listed below repeatedly because new trials are continually added. There are also clinical trials services emerging that help to match patients to clinical trials. Some of these services can be useful for obtaining information and saving time, but it is important to read the company's privacy statement and know whether the company is being paid for recruiting patients before using them.

NCI Clinical Trials
Phone: 800-4-CANCER
Web site: www.cancer.gov/clinical_trials/
NCI offers comprehensive information on understanding and finding clinical trials, including access to the NCI/PDQ Clinical Trials Database.

NIH/NLM Clinical Trials
Web site: www.clinicaltrials.gov
Clinical trials database service developed by the National Institutes of Health's National Library of Medicine.

CenterWatch Clinical Trials Listing Service
Web site: www.centerwatch.com
Listing of clinical trials conducted by drug companies.

Clinical Trials Resources (Lung Cancer Online)
Web page: www.lungcanceronline.org/treatment-experimental/clinicaltrials.html

In addition to linking to the major clinical trials resources listed above, Lung Cancer Online provides links to NCI-designated cancer centers and hospitals with lung cancer programs that are likely to be conducting clinical trials in lung cancer. These sites can be contacted directly for information on available lung cancer trials. Links to some clinical trials services can also be found in Lung Cancer Online's clinical trials section.

NCI Clinical Trials and Insurance Coverage
Web page: www.cancer.gov/clinical_trials/ Type "insurance" in the search box.
Excellent in-depth guide to clinical trials insurance issues.

Print Publications

Finn, Robert. *Cancer Clinical Trials: Experimental Treatments & How They Can Help You*. Sebastopol, CA: O'Reilly & Associates, 1999.
Mulay, Marilyn. *Making the Decision: A Cancer Patient's Guide to Clinical Trials*. Sudbury, MA: Jones & Bartlett Publishers, 2002.

Complementary and Alternative Medicine (CAM)

American Academy of Medical Acupuncture
Web site: www.medicalacupuncture.org
Professional site with articles on acupuncture, a list of frequently asked questions and an acupuncturist locator.

Commonweal
P.O. Box 316, Bolinas, CA 94924
Phone: 415-868-0970
Web site: www.commonweal.org
Provides information on complementary approaches to cancer care, including the full-text of Michael Lerner's 1994 book, *Choices in Healing: Integrating the Best of Complementary Approaches to Cancer*, published by MIT Press (updated version available in print).

National Center for Complementary and Alternative Medicine (NCCAM)
Web site: www.nccam.nih.gov
Offers information on complementary and alternative medicine therapies, including NCI/PDQ expert-reviewed fact sheets on individual therapies and dietary supplements.

NCI Office of Cancer Complementary and Alternative Medicine (OCCAM)
Web site: www.cancer.gov/occam
Information clearinghouse supporting the NCI's CAM activities.

Print Publications

American Cancer Society's Guide to Complementary and Alternative Cancer Methods. Atlanta, GA: American Cancer Society, 2000.
Benson, Herbert. *The Relaxation Response*. New York: Avon Books, 1975.

(Continued on next page)

Appendix 1. Resources Related to Lung Cancer *(Continued)*

Complementary and Alternative Medicine *(cont.)*

Cassileth, Barrie R. *The Alternative Medicine Handbook: The Complete Reference Guide to Alternative and Complementary Therapies.* New York: W.W. Norton & Company, 1998.
Kaptchuk, Ted J. *The Web That Has No Weaver: Understanding Chinese Medicine.* Columbus, OH: McGraw-Hill, 2000.

Diet and Nutrition

American Institute for Cancer Research
1759 R Street, NW, Washington, DC 20009
Phone: 800-843-8114 or 202-328-7744 (in DC)
Web site: www.aicr.org
Supports research on diet and nutrition in the prevention and treatment of cancer. Provides information to cancer patients on nutrition and cancer, including a compilation of healthy recipes. Maintains a nutrition hotline for questions relating to nutrition and health.

Nutrition (American Cancer Society)
Web page: www.cancer.org (Enter "nutrition" in the search box.)
Nutrition resources include: ACS guidelines on nutrition, dietary supplement information, nutrition message boards and tips on low-fat cooking and choosing healthy ingredients.

Drugs/Medications

MEDLINEplus: Drug Information
Web page: www.medlineplus.gov (Click on the "drug information" button.)
A guide to over 9,000 prescription and over-the-counter medications provided by U.S. Pharmacopeia (USP).

Print Publications
Consumers Guide to Cancer Drugs. Atlanta, GA: American Cancer Society, 2000.

Employment, Insurance, Financial and Legal Resources

Americans with Disabilities Act (U.S. Department of Justice)
Web site: www.usdoj.gov

Cancer Legal Resource Center
919 S. Albany Street, Los Angeles, CA 90019
Phone: 213-736-1455
A joint program of Loyola Law School and the Western Law Center for Disability Rights. Provides information and educational outreach on cancer-related legal issues to people with cancer and others impacted by the disease.

Centers for Medicare & Medicaid Services (CMS) (formerly the Health Care Financing Administration [HCFA])
Web site: www.cms.hhs.gov

Oversees administration of:
• Medicare – federal health insurance program for people 65 years or older and some disabled people under 65 years.
Phone: 800-633-4227
Web site: www.medicare.gov
• Medicaid – federal and state health insurance program for certain low-income people. Contact your state Medicaid offices for further information.
• Health Insurance Portability and Accountability Act (HIPPA) – insurance reform that may lower your chance of losing existing coverage, ease your ability to switch health plans, and/or help you to buy coverage on your own if you lose your employer's plan and have no other coverage available.
Web page: www.cms.hhs.gov Enter "HIPPA" into the search box.

Family and Medical Leave Act (FMLA)
Web site: www.dol.gov
U.S. Department of Labor Web page providing information about the FMLA.

Health Insurance Association of America (HIAA)
1201 F Street, NW, Suite 500, Washington, DC 20004-1204
Phone: 202-824-1600
Web site: www.hiaa.org
Provides insurance guides for consumers. Topics include health insurance and managed care, disability income, long-term care and medical savings accounts.

Hill-Burton Program (Health Resources and Services Administration)
Phone: 301-443-5656, or 800-637-0742 (800-492-0359 in Maryland)
Web page: www.hrsa.gov:80/OSP/dfcr/obtain/obtain.htm
Facilities that receive Hill-Burton funds from the government are required by law to provide services to some people who cannot afford to pay. Information on Hill-Burton eligibility and facility locations is available via phone or Internet.

Patient Advocate Foundation
753 Thimble Shoals Boulevard, Suite B, Newport News, VA 23606
Phone: 800-532-5274
Web site: www.patientadvocate.org
Nonprofit organization helps patients to resolve insurance, debt and job discrimination matters relative to cancer. Patient resources include: *The National Financial Resources Guidebook for Patients: A State-by-State Directory, Your Guide to the Appeals Process* and the *Managed Care Answer Guide*, among others.

Social Security Administration (SSA)
Web site: www.ssa.gov
Oversees two programs that pay benefits to people with disabilities:
• *Social Security Disability Insurance* – pays benefits to you and certain members of your family if you have worked long enough and paid Social Security taxes.
• *Supplemental Security Income* – supplements Social Security payments based on need.

(Continued on next page)

129

Appendix 1. Resources Related to Lung Cancer *(Continued)*

Employment, Insurance, Financial and Legal Resources *(cont.)*

Veterans Health Administration
810 Vermont Avenue, NW, Washington, DC 20420
Phone: 202-273-5400 or 877-222-8387 (Health care benefits)
Web site: www.va.gov/vbs/health
Eligible veterans and their dependents may receive cancer treatment at a Veteran's Administration Medical Center.

Print Publications
Hoffman, Barbara. *Working It Out: Your Employment Rights as a Cancer Survivor.* Silver Spring, MD: National Coalition for Cancer Survivorship, undated. This booklet can be ordered from the NCCS at 877-622-7937.
Landry, David S. *Be Prepared: The Complete Financial, Legal and Practical Guide to Living with Cancer, HIV and other Life-Challenging Conditions.* New York: St. Martin's Press, 1998.

Financial Assistance Programs

Air Care Alliance
Phone: 888-260-9707
Web site: www.aircareall.org
Network of organizations willing to provide public benefit flights for health care.

Finding Ways to Pay for Care (National Coalition for Cancer Survivorship)
Web page: www.canceradvocacy.org (Select "Programs" and then "Cancer Survival Toolbox.")

NeedyMeds
Web site: www.needymeds.com
Information on patient assistance programs and other programs that help people obtain medications, supplies and equipment.

Hospice and End-of-Life Issues

Partnership for Caring
1620 Eye Street, NW, Suite 202, Washington, DC 20006
Phone: 202-296-8071 or 800-989-9455
Web site: www.partnershipforcaring.org
Comprehensive information and resources covering end-of-life issues, including advanced directives.

CANCER-HOSPICE (Association of Cancer Online Resources)
Web site: www.acor.org (Click on "Mailing Lists" and then select "CANCER-HOSPICE.")
Online discussion group for cancer patients dealing with hospice issues.

Growth House
Web site: www.growthhouse.org
Extensive, annotated directory to hospice and end-of-life resources. Organized by topic.

Home Care Guide for Advanced Cancer (American College of Physicians)
Web page: www.acponline.org/public/h_care/
Guide for family and friends caring for advanced cancer patients who are living at home.

Hospice Net
Web site: www.hospicenet.org
Provides comprehensive information to patients and families facing life-threatening illness. Extensive resources addressing end-of-life issues from both patient and caregiver perspectives.

Patient Advocacy Skills

Cancer Survival Toolbox (National Coalition for Cancer Survivorship)
Web page: www.canceradvocacy.org (Select "Programs" and then "Cancer Survival Toolbox.")
Topics include: communication skills, finding information, solving problems, making decisions, negotiating and standing up for your rights. (Also available as audiotapes at 877-866-5748.)

Information for the Asking: Questions to Help You Get the Information You Need from Your Healthcare Provider (ALCASE)
Web page: www.alcase.org

Print Publications
Anderson, Greg. *50 Essential Things to Do When the Doctor Says It's Cancer.* New York: Penguin Books, 1993.
Oster, Nancy et al. *Making Informed Medical Decisions: Where to Look and How to Use What You Find.* Sebastopol, CA: O'Reilly & Associates, Inc., 2000.
Willis, Joanie. *The Cancer Patient's Workbook.* New York: Dorling Kindersley Publishing, Inc., 2001.

Physician and Hospital Locators

American Society of Clinical Oncology (ASCO)
Web page: www.asco.org (Click on "About ASCO" then click the "Find an Oncologist" button.)

American College of Surgeons (ACS) Commission on Cancer
Web page: www.facs.org (Use the "Public Information" tab then choose "Protecting Your Health.")
Listing of ACS Commission on Cancer's Approved Hospital Cancer Programs.

American Medical Association (AMA) Physician Select
Web page: www.ama-assn.org
Provides professional information on licensed U.S. physicians.

Cardiothoracic Surgeons Network (CTSNet)
Web page: www.ctsnet.org (Click on the "members" button.)
Database of cardiothoracic surgeons who are members of the American Association of Thoracic Surgery (AATS), the Society

(Continued on next page)

Appendix 1. Resources Related to Lung Cancer *(Continued)*

Physician and Hospital Locators *(cont.)*

Cardiothoracic Surgeons Network *(cont.)*
of Thoracic Surgeons (STS) or the European Association for
Cardio-Thoracic Surgery.

Lung Cancer Online: Lung Cancer Programs
Web site: www.lungcanceronline.org
Directory of institutions with multidisciplinary lung cancer pro-
grams, including NCI-designated cancer centers.

Prevention and Risk Assessment
Prevention (American Cancer Society)
Web page: www.cancer.org (Enter "prevention" in the search
box.)
Comprehensive section on prevention covers topics such as environmental and occupational cancer risks, exercise, tobacco
and cancer, nutrition for risk reduction and prevention and detection programs.

Your Cancer Risk (Harvard Center for Cancer Prevention)
Web site: www.yourcancerrisk.harvard.edu
Online lung cancer risk assessment tool.

Research Resources and Reference

PubMed: MEDLINE (National Library of Medicine)
Web site: www.ncbi.nlm.nih.gov/PubMed/
Provides free online access to MEDLINE, a database of over 11
million citations to the medical literature.

Medscape
Web site: www.medscape.com (Enter "Lung Cancer Resource
Center" in the search box.)
Medscape is an excellent source for latest news in lung cancer
research, including access to summaries of cancer conferences.
Aimed at health care professionals. Registration required for free
access to Medscape.

Merriam Webster Medical Dictionary
Web site: www.intelihealth.com (Enter "Merriam Webster" in the
search box.)
Registration required for free access to Intelihealth.

Print Publications
Laughlin, Edward H. *Coming to Terms with Cancer: A Glossary
of Cancer-Related Terms.* Atlanta, GA: American Cancer Society, 2002.

Smoking Cessation

Freedom from Smoking (American Lung Association)
Web page: www.lungusa.org/ffs
Free online smoking cessation program designed to educate and
modify smoking behavior patterns. This interactive course can
be accessed 24 hours a day, 7 days a week.

Office of the Surgeon General: Tobacco Cessation
Web page: www.surgeongeneral.gov/tobacco/default.htm
See especially the "You Can Quit Smoking Consumer Guide."
Also available by calling 202-401-4357.

Quitnet
Web site: www.quitnet.org
Comprehensive Web site for smoking cessation needs. Offers
interactive personalized quitting tools, quitting guides, smoking
cessation program locators, 24-hour online support/discussion,
and links to smoking, tobacco and cessation-related information and resources.

Support Services

**Alliance for Lung Cancer Advocacy, Support and Educa-
tion (ALCASE)**
P.O. Box 849, Vancouver, WA 98666
Phone: 360-696-2436 or 800-289-2436
Web site: www.alcase.org
ALCASE offers a phone buddy program (individual patient-to-
patient support) and maintains a geographic listing of in-person
lung cancer support groups.

Association of Cancer Online Resources (ACOR)
Web site: www.acor.org (Click on "Mailing Lists.")
ACOR offers online support groups for cancer patients. Lung
cancer lists include: a general list (LUNG-ONC), and specific lists
for small cell lung cancer (LUNG-SSLC), non-small cell lung cancer (LUNG-NSCLC) and bronchioloalveolar (LUNG-BAC).

Cancer Care
275 Seventh Avenue, New York, NY 10001
Phone: 212-712-8080 or 800-813-4673
Web site: www.cancercare.org
Provides comprehensive support services and programs to
people with cancer.

Cancer Survivors Network
Web site: www.acscsn.org
ACSCSN is the American Cancer Society's online patient com-
munity.

R.A. Bloch National Cancer Foundation
4400 Main Street, Kansas City, MO 64111
Phone: 816-932-8453 or 800 433-0464
Web site: www.blochcancer.org
Provides Bloch-authorized cancer books free of charge, a
multidisciplinary referral service and patient-to-patient phone
support.

Vital Options International
15060 Ventura Boulevard, Suite 211, Sherman Oaks, CA 91403
Phone: 818-788-5225
Web site: www.vitaloptions.org
Produces "The Group Room," a weekly, syndicated radio call-in
show (with simultaneous Web cast) covering important and
timely topics in cancer.

(Continued on next page)

Appendix 1. Resources Related to Lung Cancer *(Continued)*

Support Services *(cont.)*

Wellness Community
35 East Seventh Street, Suite 412, Cincinnati, OH 45202
Phone: 513-421-7111 or 888-793-WELL
Web site: www.wellness-community.org
Provides educational programs and support groups for people with cancer and their families.

Talking About Cancer (American Cancer Society)
Web page: www.cancer.org (Enter "Talking About Cancer" in the search box.)
Discusses how to talk about your cancer with family, friends, your health care providers and your employer. Includes resources for locating in-person and online support groups.

Print Publications
Coping with Cancer. Cancer magazine available free of charge in oncology offices or by subscription at 615-791-3859 or www.copingmag.com
Holland, Jimmie C. and Sheldon Lewis. *The Human Side of Cancer.* New York: HarperCollins Publishers, 2000.
Schimmel, S.R., and B. Fox. *Cancer Talk: Voices of Hope and Endurance from "The Group Room," the World's Largest Cancer Support Group.* New York: Broadway Books, 1999.

Symptoms, Side Effects, and Complications

Fatigue
Cancer Fatigue.org
Web site: www.cancersymptoms.org (formerly www.cancerfatigue.org)
Information about cancer-related fatigue for patients and caregivers.

CANCER-FATIGUE (Association of Cancer Online Resources)
Web page: www.acor.org (Click on "Mailing Lists" and then select "CANCER-FATIGUE.")
Online discussion list covering cancer and treatment-related fatigue.

NCCN Cancer-Related Fatigue Treatment Guidelines for Patients
Web page: www.nccn.org/patient_gls/_english/_fatigue/index.htm

Print Publications
Harpham, Wendy S. "Resolving the Frustration of Fatigue." *CA: A Cancer Journal for Clinicians* 49 (1999): 178-189.
Outstanding article by a patient/physician discusses cancer-related fatigue and how to deal with it.

Nausea and Vomiting

NCCN Nausea and Vomiting Treatment Guidelines for Patients with Cancer
Web page: www.nccn.org/patient_gls/_english/_nausea_and_vomiting/index.htm

NCI/PDQ Nausea and Vomiting
Web page: www.cancer.gov (Enter "nausea" in the search box.)
Expert-reviewed information summary about cancer-related nausea and vomiting.

Nutritional Problems

NCI/PDQ Nutrition
Web page: www.cancer.gov (Enter "nutrition" in the search box.)
Expert-reviewed information summary about the causes and management of nutritional problems occurring in cancer patients.

Oral Complications

Oral Health, Cancer Care and You (National Institute of Dental and Craniofacial Research)
Web site: www.nohic.nidcr.nih.gov

NCI/PDQ Oral Complications of Chemotherapy and Head/Neck Radiation
Web page: www.cancer.gov (Enter "oral complications" in the search box.)

Pain

The National Pain Foundation (NPF)
P.O. Box 102605, Denver, CO 80250-2605
Web site: www.painconnection.org
NPF Web site offers online education and support communities for pain patients and their families, including cancer pain and palliative care resources.

CANCER-PAIN (Association of Cancer Online Resources)
Web page www.acor.org (Click on "Mailing Lists" and then select "CANCER-PAIN.")
Online discussion list about pain associated with cancer and its treatments.

NCCN Cancer Pain Treatment Guidelines for Patients
Web page: www.nccn.org/patient_gls/_english/_pain/index.htm

NCI/PDQ Pain
Web page: www.cancer.gov (Enter "pain" in the search box.)
Expert-reviewed information summary about cancer-related pain. Includes discussion of approaches to the management and treatment of cancer-associated pain.

Print Publications
Abrahm, Janet L. *A Physician's Guide to Pain and Symptom Management in Cancer Patients.* Baltimore, MD: The Johns Hopkins University Press, 2000.
Aimed at health care professionals, this practical and comprehensive textbook is also an excellent resource for patients.

(Continued on next page)

Appendix 1. Resources Related to Lung Cancer *(Continued)*

Peripheral Neuropathy

The Neuropathy Association
60 East 42nd Street, Suite 942, New York, NY 10165
Phone 212-692-0662
Web site: www.neuropathy.org

CANCER-NEUROPATHY (Association of Cancer Online Resources)
Web page: www.acor.org (Click on "Mailing Lists" and then select "CANCER-NEUROPATHY.")
Online discussion group for patients dealing with cancer induced neuropathy or its treatments.

Print Publications
Almadrones, L.A. and R. Arcot. "Patient Guide to Peripheral Neuropathy" *Oncology Nursing Forum* 26, no. 8 (1999): 1359-1362.

Pleural Effusion

Chemical Pleurodesis for Malignant Pleural Effusion (Cancer Supportive Care)
Web page: www.cancersupportivecare.com/pleural.html
Carolyn Clary-Macy, RN, provides a clear explanation of chemical pleurodesis for malignant pleural effusion. Aimed at patients.

Sexual Effects

CANCER-FERTILITY & CANCER-SEXUALITY (Association of Cancer Online Resources)
Web page: www.acor.org (Click on "Mailing Lists" and then select "CANCER-FERTILITY" and/or "CANCER SEXUALITY.")
Online discussion lists about fertility and sexuality issues associated with cancer.

NCI/PDQ Sexuality and Reproductive Issues
Web page: www.cancer.gov (Enter "sexuality" in the search box.)
Expert-reviewed information summary about factors that may affect fertility and sexual functioning in people who have cancer.

Tests and Procedures

Diagnostic Imaging (MEDLINEplus)
Web page: www.nlm.nih.gov/medlineplus/diagnosticimaging.html

Laboratory Tests (MEDLINEplus)
Web page: www.nlm.nih.gov/medlineplus/laboratorytests.html

Print Publications
Margolis, Simeon, Ed. *The Johns Hopkins Consumer Guide to Medical Tests: What You Can Expect, How You Should Prepare, What Your Results Mean.* Baltimore, MD: The Johns Hopkins University Press, 2001.

Treatment Information and Guidelines

NCCN Lung Cancer Treatment Guidelines for Patients
Web page: www.nccn.org/patient_gls/_english/_lung/index.htm

NCI/PDQ Non-small Cell Lung Cancer Treatment & Small Cell Lung Cancer Treatment
Web page: www.cancer.gov (Enter "Lung Cancer" in the search box and then select "Lung Cancer Home Page.")
Expert-reviewed summaries about the treatment of NSCLC and SCLC.

Chemotherapy and You (NIH/NCI)
Web page: www.cancer.gov (Enter "Chemotherapy and You" in the search box.)
Also available in print by calling 800-4-CANCER.

Radiation Therapy and You (NIH/NCI)
Web page: www.cancer.gov (Enter "Radiation Therapy and You" in the search box.)
Also available in print by calling 800-4-CANCER.

Your Surgery
Web site: www.yoursurgery.com (Select "Chest" and then "Thoracotomy.")
Detailed explanation of thoracotomy, including discussion of lobectomy and pneumonectomy.

Print Publications
McKay, Judith and Nancee Hirano. *The Chemotherapy and Radiation Therapy Survival Guide.* Oakland, CA: New Harbinger Publications, Inc., 1998.
Olson, Kaye. *Surgery and Recovery.* Traverse City, MI: Rhodes & Easton, 1998.

Survivorship Issues

LT-SURVIVORS (Association of Cancer Online Resources)
Web page: www.acor.org (Click on "Mailing Lists" and then select "LT-SURVIVORS.")
Forum for discussion of issues of concern to long-term cancer survivors.

Print Publications
Harpham, Wendy S. *After Cancer: A Guide to Your New Life.* New York: W.W. Norton & Company, 1994.

Women and Minorities

National Women's Health Information Center
8550 Arlington Boulevard, Suite 300, Fairfax, VA 22031
Phone: 800-994-9662
Web site: www.4women.gov

Office of Minority Health
P.O. Box 37337, Washington, DC 20013-7337
Phone: 800-444-6472
Web site: www.omhrc.gov

Note. From *100 Questions and Answers About Lung Cancer* (pp. 179–197), by K. Parles, 2002, Sudbury, MA: Jones and Bartlett. Copyright 2002 by Jones and Bartlett. Reprinted with permission. (Updated to reflect information as of the time of this publishing.)

Index

The letter *f* after a page number indicates that relevant content appears in a figure; the letter *t,* in a table.